Of Motherhood and Melancholia

# Of Motherhood and Melancholia
## *Notebook of a Psycho-ethnographer*

Lou-Marié Kruger

UNIVERSITY OF KwaZulu-Natal PRESS

Published in 2020 by University of KwaZulu-Natal Press
Private Bag X01
Scottsville, 3201
Pietermaritzburg
South Africa
Email: books@ukzn.ac.za
Website: www.ukznpress.co.za

ISBN: 978 1 86914 434 0
e-ISBN: 978 1 86914 435 7




Managing editor: Sally Hines
Editor: Alison Lockhart
Layout: Patricia Comrie
Proofreader: Catherine Munro
Cover design: Artworks
Cover artwork: *Girl with Blue Hands* by Tanya Poole

For Mia

It may be difficult for us to imagine how restricted a life so many of our fellow human beings lead, what little living they manage to do. There is, of course, the wonder of birth (impossible to recollect), some mother's milk (sometimes not), the affection of relatives (often thoroughly disrupted), perhaps some schooling (mostly not), a bit of play (amid pestilence and panic), and then things end (without a rumble). The world goes on as if nothing much has happened.

— Amartya Sen, 'Foreword' to Paul Farmer's *Pathologies of Power*

# Contents

# Prologue

*'It may be difficult for us to imagine . . .'* *

In the clinic, each day brings a harvest of tales of woe.

— Paul Farmer, 'Foreword'

How do we psychoanalysts make contact with the other whose experience is not just unformulated, but seems unspeakable? And how do our violated and frozen patients attempt to speak to us?

— Donna Orange, 'Speaking the Unspeakable'

'Feel my hands – they are always wet,' Wendy Winters says and holds up her hands to me. In the blue blazer of her school uniform (the dress is mustard yellow), she carries a red facecloth, specifically for drying her hands. She seems to know what information I need; I don't have to ask questions. She does not look me in the eye, her head is slightly lowered, her shoulders seem tense.

'I am on the till at Meatrite. My aunties have been working there for more than ten years. My mother's name is Anna Winters. My dad's name is Piet Soldaat. My mother was nineteen when she got pregnant with me, and twenty when she had me. My mother and father were together for two years and then my father started stealing things from our house for drinking money. Then he stole something from a car and went to jail. Then my grandfather said that he wasn't allowed to see me anymore.

---

* The quote in the subtitle of this chapter – 'It may be difficult for us to imagine . . .' – is from Sen, 2005: xi.

'Two years after that my mother married my stepdad. His name is Moos Winters. *Hy het my afgeskeep* [He neglected me]. My little sister and I were not treated the same by my stepdad. I cannot remember my real dad. The only good thing I remember about my stepdad is the prayer he taught me: "Gentle Jesus, meek and mild, look upon a little child. Amen."

'I was sent to school in pre-primary. When I got home from school the first day, my dad was there and I showed him my school dress. A few months later I went to the Pniel to live with my grandmother and grandfather. My grandmother spoiled me a lot. She always washed me. I remember in the mornings my grandmother washed me, and then she dressed me, while I was still sleeping on the chair.'

Wendy says that in Grade 1 she did not like her teacher. 'My stomach hurt,' she says. 'I had to read in front of the class. Every morning before school the uncles gave me sweets and medicine for my nerves. I then never really stayed with my mother, I cannot remember. My mother was like my older sister that left the house. My grandmother, I told everything. For me, my grandmother was my mother.

'The other one who lives in my grandmother's house is my mother's brother. He also drinks. But he doesn't drink like my stepfather. He doesn't bother anyone; he is just mellow. His name is David. My auntie also stays there with her child. My auntie is not married. My cousin and I share a room. My auntie has her own room. Then the other uncle who stays there is my grandfather's brother. He fell off a truck. He cannot speak right and he cannot walk right. My grandfather also was in an accident, a tractor accident. He has *spookpyne* [ghost pains] in the leg that was amputated after his accident. Then it's his knee, then his foot, then his toes. Always something hurting.'

In Grade 3, Wendy says, things took a turn for the worse. 'My best friend moved to Paarl. I had no one anymore. My mother decided then that I had to go up to the Kylemore to help her with the new baby. The second weekend I was there, my stepdad got drunk. I can't remember what he said, but I went to the bedroom to cry. He then told me I must not go on like that. He hurt me very much. After that he was drunk every weekend. Every weekend he hit my mother. I could not take it. I screamed when he hit her. Then he yelled at me, "*Jou ma se poes*" [Your mother's cunt]. The first time he hit me was when I was twelve years old. I was in Grade 7. He threw me against the floor. My mother got hysterical. That was enough. He was totally drunk. Then I told him, "Daddy has no respect for Mommy." Then he hit me in my face or slapped me. I cannot remember. I had to go to school the Monday. I said I fell in the bath.'

It did not help that her mother was also quite sickly. It is not clear what her illness was. Wendy says that her colon turned and then she went into a coma. 'She was in a coma. She was in Tygerberg Hospital for three days and then the colon turned back by itself. Then my mother and sister and little brother went to the Pniel to my grandmother and grandfather. I had to stay with my stepdad to cook for him. Since then it worked like that, from Grade 7 onwards. I helped my mother, then my dad hit me and then I would go to the Pniel for three months, back to my grandmother. Then my mom complained. Then I go back again to help her.'

School also had its own stresses. 'During primary school I was a very quiet child. I always tried, but the girls, they bullied me. They always made up stories. They gossiped about me.[1] I was not even there and then it is my fault. I was soft. In Grade 7 I thought enough is enough. Then I told that one girl she should meet me at the gate. I beat her up. Then the whole school turned for me. High school is okay. I once tried to get drunk. Three months ago, I hit my little brother. He hit me back. My aunt hit him. He wants to hit my aunt. And so it goes. Nobody wants to do something about the problem. My mother tries to fix everything, but she can't. My father doesn't help her. It isn't my responsibility.'

She repeats this sentence – 'It is not my responsibility' – and pauses for the first time. She looks me straight in the eye and holds out her hands again. 'Feel my hands,' she says.

Wendy Winters, a young woman of seventeen years old, told me this while I was working as a clinical psychologist at the primary health-care clinic serving the people of the Dwarsrivier Valley, or 'the valley', as it is informally called.[2] At the time, Wendy lived with her grandmother and grandfather in one of the towns in the valley, her mother and stepfather lived in another town. In valley terms, Wendy was doing relatively well. She was in Grade 12, achieving academically, aspiring to do a two-year diploma in marketing at a local college and she had a boyfriend whom she described as '*ordentlik*' (decent).[3] In a community where teenage pregnancy is rife, Wendy was a young woman who was determined not to be like her mother and aunts, and not to have a baby at a young age.[4]

Despite all her efforts and focus, she is severely anxious when I start seeing her. Her palms are always dripping wet, so wet that the red facecloth comes out frequently. She often has panic attacks and her underlying anxiety is visible in her small, stiff shoulders. Wendy's story contains many of the social problems present in the narratives of most women in the valley: poverty, violence, crime, substance abuse, occupational hazards, accidents, health problems, relationship problems. Many of them, like Wendy, are severely distressed, with the distress subjectively experienced as a wide range of emotions: anxiety, panic, fear, sadness, anger, rage, despondency, hopelessness, anomie and passivity. Wendy's distress manifests as a panic disorder and in sleeping problems, but eating problems and substance use are also rife. In low-income communities in South Africa and elsewhere, many women fulfil the criteria for anxiety or mood disorders and are diagnosed with these disorders by medical workers.[5]

Wendy's story, however, also reveals the factors that have been crucial in her resilience. She has been loved and cared for. She has had relationships within which she has felt, and still feels, special. Despite everything that has been difficult, she has learned some prayers and has some hopes. In Wendy's story we see a bizarre juxtaposition of agency and disempowerment: on the one hand, a sense of hope and entitlement and, on the other hand, what can be interpreted as a profound sense of dread – most poignantly inscribed on her body in her wet hands.

The majority of the inhabitants of Wendy's valley live in five settlements, urban nodes that are picturesquely integrated with orchards and vineyards.[6] Both the neighbouring towns, Stellenbosch and Franschhoek, are highly developed and are characterised by the wealth of the white inhabitants and the success of their tourist industries.[7] Many of the current inhabitants of the valley are so-called coloured farmworkers,[8] who have been forced off farms with the new labour laws that instituted a minimum wage for farm- and domestic workers, and are trying to get into the more formal labour market.[9] The women in the valley are now mostly domestic, factory and service workers, but many still do some seasonal work on farms.[10] The men in their lives (fathers, husbands, sons, partners) typically do manual work on farms and in factories. Unemployment figures are high. The communities of the valley may be seen as marginal in quite literal ways,[11] but in more symbolic ways they also occupy a borderland and seem to have always done so. In the 1840s, the first emancipated slaves were settled in the valley on land that was owned by and under the control of the church. The first inhabitants of this valley were therefore people struggling to make the transition between being slaves and being liberated.[12]

The physical landscape of the valley powerfully suggests the paradoxical existence of a post-apartheid South African context: the valley is both beautiful and terrifying. The communities of the valley are idealised in many ways – an idealisation that has everything to do with the beauty of the panoramas, the tranquillity of the landscape, the quaintness of the facades of the small houses and the brave little gardens. The streets of the towns seem friendly too: children play barefoot in the middle of roads, women chat to each other from washing line to washing line, men sit in doorways, watching or smoking. But the valley is deceptive in its tranquillity and beauty: the quaint towns are rife with social problems, infused with suffering. The suffering is directly related to the uneven ways in which processes of development and transformation are unfolding in contemporary South Africa. The valley can thus be regarded 'as a microcosm of the economic crisis of the wider South Africa'.[13] It displays some of the most brutal paradoxes of post-apartheid society, where transformation and the redistribution of wealth have simply meant that certain interests are privileged and resources are distributed for the benefit of some, at the expense of others.[14] Poverty in the valley, as in other places in the world, has been aggravated by structural forces associated with globalisation and transformation: individuals and communities are being pushed to the margins of society.[15] In the lives of men and women of the valley, what Robert Nixon has called the 'slow violence of poverty', is apparent:

> We are accustomed to conceiving violence as immediate and explosive, erupting into instant concentrated visibility. But we need to revisit our assumptions and consider the relative invisibility of slow violence. I mean a violence that is neither

spectacular nor instantaneous but instead incremental, whose calamitous repercussions are postponed for years or decades or centuries. I want, then, to complicate conventional perceptions of violence as a highly visible act that is newsworthy because it is focused around an event, bounded by time, and aimed at a specific body or bodies. Emphasizing the temporal dispersion of slow violence can change the way we perceive and respond to a variety of social crises, like domestic abuse or post-traumatic stress.[16]

In the valley, however, one also experiences a sense of anticipation. Changes in the country in general and in the valley specifically have created a moment of potential and tension; both the hope and dread that inevitably accompany development are palpable. It is clear that several development initiatives in the area have the potential to be beneficial for the local communities, but they can also entrench existing inequalities and further impoverish people. Individual agents may escape the entrapments of a vicious cycle of poverty and victimisation, or they may find that their agency is still limited or even more limited, despite – or because of – development and change.

Doing both clinical work and psychological research, I have been working with students in in the valley for almost two decades. My fellow researchers and I have interviewed people, we have conducted surveys, we have filled out questionnaires and we have observed. We do individual therapy, group therapy, couples therapy, psychoeducational evenings and parental guidance. We walk the streets, we stalk the clinic, we talk endlessly about our work. We write up our experiences in presentations, theses, dissertations, papers – some published, some not. It is difficult to articulate what we experience; it is even more difficult for us to capture the lived experience of poverty, particularly in academic journals and academic writing.[17]

In *Of Motherhood and Melancholia: Notebook of a Psycho-ethnographer* I write about almost two decades of clinical and research encounters I have had in the Dwarsrivier Valley.[18] In these pages, I aim to give an account of the complex realities and lived experiences of low-income mothers in post-apartheid South Africa.[19] I reflect on the emotional experience of poverty in one particular place, trying to show the impact of the 'slow violence of poverty' on the emotional lives of women.[20] I do so as a white, middle-class psychologist and my representation of the women is therefore always compromised: I am telling stories of encounters with low-income women from a very particular perspective.

Focusing specifically on maternal life in a semi-rural community, this book can be regarded as a South African case study, 'showing how particular events, unique occasions, an encounter here, a development there . . . woven together with a variety of facts and a battery of interpretations to produce a sense of how things go, have been going, and are likely to go'.[21] While this book can be seen as a case study of a place and a community, I also present the lives of individual people, individual case studies.[22] Paul Farmer, medical doctor and anthropologist, articulates the importance of showing the impact of larger processes on individual lives:

> Our job is to document, as meticulously and as honestly as we can, the complex workings of a vast machinery rooted in a political economy that only a romantic would term fragile. What is fragile is rather our enterprise of creating a more truthful accounting and fighting amnesia. We will wait for the 'glitch in the matrix' so that more can see clearly just what the cost is – not for us (for we who read the journals or engage in the social analyses are by definition shielded) – but for those who still set their backs to the impossible task of living on next to nothing while others wallow in surfeit.[23]

In his award-winning book *Pathologies of Power* Farmer emphasises the importance of biography:

> But the experience of suffering, it's often noted, is not effectively conveyed by statistics or graphs. In fact, the suffering of the world's poor intrudes only rarely into the consciousness of the affluent, even when our affluence may be shown to have direct relation to their suffering. This is true even when spectacular human rights violations are at issue, and it is even more true

when the topic at hand is the everyday violation of social and economic rights. Because the 'texture' of dire afflictions is better felt in the gritty details of biography.[24]

Economist Amartya Sen also emphasises the 'need to move beyond "the cold and often inarticulate statistics of low incomes" to look at the various ways in which agency – what [Sen] terms the "capabilities of each person" – is constrained'.[25] While Farmer states that individual case studies are crucial in revealing suffering because 'they tell us what happens to one or many people', he also argues that if we are to explain suffering, we must embed individual biography in the larger matrix of culture, history and political economy.[26] He insists on the need to 'study both individual experience and the larger social matrix in which it is embedded in order to see how various social processes and events come to be translated into personal distress and diseases'. He asks a pertinent question: by which mechanisms, precisely, do social forces – ranging from poverty to racism and gender – become embodied as individual experience?[27] He points out that simultaneous consideration of various social axes is imperative in efforts to discern a 'political economy of brutality'. Such social factors, he says, are differentially weighted in different settings and at different times.[28]

In this book, I am telling the story of a valley and its people, but I am also giving an account of an extended research and clinical encounter. In exploring the lived experience of motherhood, my starting point was not existing diagnostic categories or existing theories. It was the experiences of the mothers, as related to us by the women themselves, and our experiences as researchers and clinicians working with women in the field. This book is an attempt to describe low-income mothers' emotional distress, and their well-being, in their own terms and to show how they themselves understand their emotional lives and explain it to us as researchers and clinicians. The feature that seemed most prominent in their emotional worlds is how ordinary aspects of life, such as home, labour, love, work, food, pleasure, illness and death, become brutal. The book is subsequently organised around those themes.[29]

I started writing this book as a straightforward academic text, informed and shaped in very systematic ways by psychological theory and based on substantive empirical research and clinical data. However, in the process, the narratives of the women in the valley seemed to become more prominent and more important.[30] Their voices, juxtaposed with my own journal notes and the journal notes of students, seemed to better capture the lives of the women we encountered and the encounters themselves. The implicit argument here is that academic writing and language often serve to obscure the lives of the people being written about. This book is an indirect critique of how the poor and the 'slow violence of poverty' have been (mis)represented and systematically obscured in academic writing, albeit often inadvertently. Researchers and clinicians need to explore alternative ways of representation, write differently in an effort to disturb 'the normalized quiet of unseen power'.[31] Nixon writes that 'we also need to engage the representational, narrative and strategic challenges posed by the relative invisibility of slow violence':

> How can we convert into image and narrative the disasters that are slow moving and long in the making, disasters that are anonymous and star nobody, disasters that are attritional and of indifferent interest to the sensation-driven technologies of our image-worlds? How can we turn the long emergencies of slow violence into stories dramatic enough to rouse public sentiment and warrant political intervention, these emergencies whose repercussions have given rise to some of the more critical challenges of our time?[32]

This book is indirectly taking on the challenge posed by Nixon to devise arresting stories, images and symbols to make visible the lives of those permeated by slow violence, the ungrievable lives of the so-called disposables.[33] According to Nixon, 'in a world permeated by insidious unspectacular violence . . . writing can make the unapparent appear, rendering it tangible by humanizing drawn-out calamities inaccessible to the human senses'.[34] Writing itself seems to be crucial in making visible the lives of those on the margins.[35]

In my attempts to understand how individual biographies are embedded in larger matrices, I have found feminist relational psychoanalysis and discursive psychology particularly useful.[36] In my analysis I therefore pay close attention to detail and to social theory (typically associated with discursive psychology), but I also focus on individual biography and emotional subtexts (typically the terrain of psychoanalysis).[37] As Stephen Frosh, Ann Phoenix and Rob Pattman argue:

> Using psychoanalysis in qualitative studies involves conceptualizing individuals as embedded in social and cultural contexts with socially acceptable and powerful ways of being, but also as individually orientated to these contexts, uniquely invested in discourses in different ways influenced by conscious and unconscious wishes. Such an approach requires thinking about narratives as dynamic processes mediated by, but not reducible to, personal biographies, relational events, linguistic repertoires and subjective experiences.[38]

By using a case study approach, I implicitly argue that human beings are complex, multifaceted, situated, in process, under construction. I am able to consider multiple factors in looking at the community and the people: subjectivity, context, history, intersubjectivity, the material details of their lives, discourses, the unconscious, difference, theory and language.

My methodology also compels me to engage in the activity of continuous self-reflection or reflexivity.[39] This requires a continuous conversation about what I am doing, how I am doing it, what I am finding out and what I am doing with what I find out. It means that all aspects of research and clinical work are discussed, including traditionally hidden aspects.[40] The point is not to legitimise or prove what one already knows. It is to undertake to know how, and up to what limit, it is possible to know and think differently.

## The white writer

Obviously, it's a category I've been made aware of
from time to time.

It's been pointed out that my characters eat a lot of lightly braised asparagus
and get FedEx packages almost daily.[41]

Yet I *dislike* being thought of as a white writer.
. . .

But after a while, you start to feel like, to the world, white
is all you'll ever be.

And gradually, after all the struggling against,
after tasting your own fear of being

only what you are,
you accept –

Then, with fresh determination, you lean forward again.
You write whiter and whiter.
— Tony Hoagland, *Unincorporated Persons in the Late Honda Dynasty*

I try to write the book, I cannot finish it.

'Your outputs are too low,' my bosses grumble. 'You are no researcher,' they say, 'you are an expert in nothing. Your publication units are below the average of an associate professor.' Another colleague says patronisingly, 'You committed career suicide by focusing on clinical work and students and training. You are not a real academic, you know.'

*So, what am I then?* I think.

I clearly am someone who struggles to write.

Sometime in the struggle with writing this book, I write a letter to my friend, a novelist. We will call her N.

Dear N,

*Dankie tog* [Thanks so much], thank you for your wonderful, wonderful letter. As always.

By the way, '*Is fokken Ferdie van sy kop af*?' [Has fucking Ferdie lost his mind?] should be the title of your next novel. But first finish the one that you are busy with, the one that has no title yet. Or so you say.

Today N, I think I need to explain to you why I can't write a book.

You know that I write about this valley. My book starts with descriptions of the valley. Wanting to be a real researcher, I try to find others' descriptions of the valley. I want the earliest recorded descriptions of the valley. I find a quote of Lady Anne Barnard,[42] who passed through this valley in early 1800:

> The road from Stellenbosch leads thro' a pass formed between the above mountain and Simon's Berg, called Bange Kloof, or the tremendous passage. This last Parnassian Mountain with its high forked top has also its Helicon but no Apollo nor the Muses.[43]

I google the Helicon River.

> The people of Dion (Dium) say that at first this River flowed on land throughout its course. But, they go on to say, the women who killed Orpheus wished to wash off in it the blood-stains, and that the River sank underground, so as not to lend its waters to cleanse manslaughter.[44]

As a psychologist working in this valley, I can't believe my luck with this reference: women who get rid of bloodstains in an underground river. Psychoanalysis is alive and well and living in the valley. As I have told you, exactly because I am so very aware of violence against women, the most difficult topic that I write about is the rage of women: the murderous mothers, the violent females that we encounter in our work – vulnerable women certainly abandoned by gods and muses.

Then, of course, I think that this is far too corny. I can't use it.

Bange Kloof seems obvious. It means 'valley of fear'.

Then I see Lady Anne's beautiful words 'tremendous passage'

and I look up the word 'passage' in the *Oxford Dictionary*, which defines it as 'the act or process of moving through, under, over, or past something on the way from one place to another'. Then I decide my book is about passages – of pregnancy, of childbirth, of motherhood, of healing, of becoming a psychologist. And I write a drama queen paragraph about this, which is immediately deleted.

I only just stop myself from not also referring to the other definition of passage: 'a narrow way, typically having walls on either sides' (think of the valley, think of the birth passage!) or how the word is used in ornithology – to describe what 'migrating birds' do: the action of passing through a place en route to somewhere else.

I decide not to be seduced by Lady Anne's word 'tremendous'.

Then I look up the phrase 'rites of passage' and come across a reference to the book by Van Gennep and his idea of liminal (of threshold) rites, liminality, liminal personae, threshold people. And then I think threshold, margins, marginal maternities. And I think I cannot write further if I have not read more about marginality and liminality.

This continues with more searches for more definitions.

I wonder about Lady Anne and when she made the trip to the valley. I discover another diary of another early traveller to the valley, also under the impression of the deceptiveness of the valley:

> And, indeed, 'tis a Road full of dangers. 'Tis frequently infested with Lions, Tigers &c, is very steep, narrow and stony; and leads you on the Edges of precipices and Pits of Water.[45]

A Road full of dangers. Steep, narrow and stony . . . leads you on the Edges . . .

Then I realise Lady Anne probably has nothing to do with anything.

But I think I will double check and reread Antjie Krog's poetry collection, *Lady Anne.*

### *Lady Anne at the microwave oven*
oh my Afrikaner sisters in kombis and station wagons
with stylish sunglasses and hair tinted against the grey
bodies that jog and gym and yoga in flowery leotards
                        fiercely clinging to pliancy and Pill
as we flit past one another on the highways
stop in dusty clouds next to sportfields
attentively gesticulate the rhythm outside music studios
pray one another to tears during Bible study
I am wondering: what kind of breed are we?
in the merciless methodology of planning
I recognise the insanity of packing an oxwagon
the passion with which children are pushed to excel
and persevere smells of concentration camp and croup
and as we sit on sanderson linen and ooh and coo
and the men at the built-in bar drink desperately and talk
about tits
we know that we are the last
the last whose children are being tenderly blonded on
milk and honey
this is the end
behind us under us around us
structures that keep our kind in place
are crushing themselves to bits.[46]

This, my friend, is why I can't write.

I will write later about all the other things that haunt us as middle-class women: things like dogs and daughters and deadlines and other dictators.

Much love,
Lou-Marié

Writing this letter, I knew, however, that my problem with writing is not simply a problem of a wandering mind and too many free associations. It is the rather uninteresting paralysis of a white academic and writer involved in the paradoxical task of writing about the crumbling of structures 'that keep our kind in place'. It is the problem of 'white writing'.[47] Locked into the hierarchical position I occupy, writing seems to be an impossibility. In the words of South African author Marlene van Niekerk:

> You can no longer say even the most ordinary things with a clear conscience in this country. It's almost as if you can only quote. I had a garden in Africa. I wanted a garden in Africa. We used to have a garden in Africa. Roses, foxgloves, snowdrops, blue forget-me-nots. Richman poorman beggarman thief.[48]

I am yet another white woman trying to write South Africa. Lady Anne did not only write about the valley and its deceptive beauty, she also wrote about the town of Stellenbosch, the last town you pass before entering the valley:

> But the perfection of this place consists in its extreme coolness in the midst of the most sultry weather; it is built in long streets, perfectly regular, each street having on each side a row of large oaks, which shadow the tops of the houses, keeping them cool, and forming a shady avenue between, through which the sun cannot pierce. Whatever way one walks one finds an avenue, right or left, and each house has a good garden. Stellenbosch, therefore, though there may not be above a hundred families in it, covers a good deal of ground, and is so perfectly clean and well built that it appears to be inhabited only by people of small fortune. But I am told there are many very poor people in it, without the means of ever becoming richer.[49]

As a white academic and writer, I live on one of the long streets in the coolness of oak trees in sultry Stellenbosch, *'daai groen hel'* (that green hell), as a well-known Afrikaans writer refers to the town. I have a good garden and a perfectly clean and well-built house. I know, like other white women writers, that my privilege is built on crumbling structures, that in repeating the ditty 'richman poorman beggarman thief, richman poorman beggarman thief', richman is as close to thief as beggarman and, despite the fact that we know this, there are poor people who · certainly appear to be 'without the means of ever becoming richer'.

I know what is happening to me is what inevitably happens when a white South African meets a black or coloured South African in an encounter where power is not distributed equally – as researcher, as psychotherapist and as author. American poet Tony Hoagland is clear about what happens 'when a black man and a white man / turn their glances on each other':

> the air suddenly
> fills up with secret signs:
> Here is what we know:
> history is a car wreck from which
> our parents did not escape;
> our nation is a career criminal;
> we were raised to be liars and deniers.[50]

In the South African context, an encounter between a white person and a black or coloured person is even more loaded than in Hoagland's world: 'Because we have lived through apartheid, our bodies confer on us instant membership of different worlds – those who have benefited from unearned privilege and those who have not,' says South African psychologist Sally Swartz.[51] 'My skin immediately and irredeemably marks my privilege . . . I am a perpetrator.'[52] Skin colour and what it is associated with assumes central importance in any South African encounter.[53]

Nathan Trantraal, a prize-winning Afrikaans poet who identifies himself as a coloured South African, writes about white people's insistence on being white while oblivious of everyone who is not white in an essay titled 'Wat wiet 'n sak vanne tou af?' (What does a bag know about a string?):

VH1 Classics is on the TV. Mrs Kamfer vacuums the lounge where the TV is.

Mrs Kamfer stops the vacuum cleaner, stands still, gives a sudden laugh, a throwaway little laugh. And then she says, half to me and half to herself: 'A white man will do everything, except for stopping to be white. What does a bag know about his string?'

I don't know what a bag knows about his string, so I write it down so that I can ask her again some other time.

Mrs Kamfer, my wife Ronelda's mother, was a chronic white person roaster. Ronelda once told me that her mother was a maid with guerilla tendencies.

Ronelda's mother has now been dead for six years and I never asked her. Ronelda says her mother always had such sayings, it is the kind of thing that farm people do.

She also wondered what her mother meant and asked her mother what she meant with the string and the bag. White people exist in a bag, she says, like a shield, like a safe space, the rest of us who are not white, we are the strings or the straps and we carry the bag of whiteness around and the bag thinks he is the important one.[54]

Trantraal's story doesn't alleviate my sense of paralysis, but it implores me to confront the shield and the safe space of the bag of whiteness. I have to think about the problem of 'white writing'.[55] Homi K. Bhabha in 'The White Stuff' suggests that whiteness is naturalised by 'social power and epistemological privilege' and the only way to challenge this is to 'reveal within the very integuments of "whiteness", the agonistic elements that make it the unsettled, disturbed form of authority that it is'.[56] His metaphor (the integument of whiteness) is similar to Trantraal's, with an integument being 'something that covers or encloses; especially: an enveloping layer (such as a skin, membrane, or cuticle) of an organism or one of its parts'.[57]

In order to write about others, I have to reflect on myself: about that which keeps me safe and powerful, but paradoxically also makes me vulnerable; that which covers me and protects me, but also makes me impenetrable and dense. My view is always obscured, a biased understanding is guaranteed. I have to expose my biases, focus on my responsibility, give up on ideals of truth and completeness and usefulness.

I have to interrogate why I write, what my responsibility is, what my limitations are.

In short, I cannot escape some degree of self-reflection, painful as it may be for myself – and the reader.

## The psycho-ethnographer

> Great poets can tell their own stories without once saying 'I', and in doing so, lend their voice to all of humanity.
>
> — J.M. Coetzee in David Atwell, *J.M. Coetzee*

In A.S. Byatt's *The Biographer's Tale* (a novel about writing and research and all academic endeavours), the main character becomes a biographer in an attempt to escape the murky, shifty world of postmodern academia. But he soon laments about the imperative of self-reflection. He says:

> I seemed to understand that the imaginary narrative had sprung out of the scholarly one, and that the compulsion to invent was in some way related to my own sense that in constructing this narrative, I had to insert facts about myself, and not only dry facts, but my feelings, and now my interpretations. I have somehow been made to write my own story, to write in very different ways.[58]

This, Byatt's character says, is very difficult: 'If I were to write about myself, where would it start? Arbitrarily, let me decide, with my socks. Socks are a fact. Mine are not new, and all have matted patches under the metatarsal joint.'[59]

And so forth. Then he says: 'I detest autobiography. Slippery, unreliable, and worse, imprecise . . . Autobiography, as I write, is fashionable. The flavour of the moment . . . They are rather repulsive. I was brought up as a child to believe in self-effacement and as a student to believe in impersonality.'[60]

Like Byatt's tortured hero I, too, would prefer not to tell you about my socks.[61] I, too, want to resist having to write yet another middle-class, white woman writer's confession of coming to terms with lives so unlike her own.[62]

If I think about why I am working as an academic and clinician, why I am writing, I can quote the psychoanalyst and political philosopher Jane Flax: I am doing this work and this writing 'to be of use'.[63] Part of the paralysis of myself as writer has to do with the inevitable tension between the desire to know and the longing to help, the schism between epistemology and action/ethics/politics.[64]

This longing to be of use, in some form or another, is also present in the students who want to work with me. While this longing is by no means transparent, it can be tied to complicated human emotions such as shame, guilt, despair, envy, fear; a sense of profound – if bizarre – identification with the person who suffers and/or with intricate theoretical imperatives. But it does provide us with some standard against which to measure the value of our work.

The desire to be useful is idealistic, fraught for biographers (the writers of lives) in general.[65] Writing about the lives of the women I am working with inevitably constitutes a certain kind of betrayal, not least because my whiteness and my privilege obscure my view. However, not writing the stories would constitute a worse betrayal. 'Speaking is impossible,' writes Jacques Derrida when his friend Paul de Man dies, 'but so too would be silence or absence or a refusal to share one's sadness.'[66] The biographer Gail Hornstein, who wrote an authoritative biography of psychiatrist Frieda Fromm-Reichmann, articulates her own paralysis in the process of research:

> My problem is that I care so much about Frieda I have trouble writing about her, I am as concerned about hurting her as I am about telling what I know . . . I already know too many things about Frieda . . . To reveal them seems disloyal, not to do so seem worse . . . Part of the seductiveness of writing a life is that it fosters the fantasy of perfect understanding. You start by imagining your subject as misunderstood and unappreciated, someone in need of rescue. Then you convince yourself that you are the first to recognize her, to see fully who she was.[67]

This uncertainty hovers below the surface of all my writing. I know that if one insists on capturing the complexity of lives when writing, the writing will always constitute both tribute and betrayal, also of oneself.

Although a clinical psychologist by training, I now call myself a psycho-ethnographer. An ethnographer, because I am interested in the materiality of everyday life, the embodied experience of being poor and being a woman. Paul Farmer is my hero.[68] He says:

> The adverse outcomes associated with structural violence, death, injury, illness, subjugation, stigmatization, and even psychological terror – come to have their 'final common pathway' in the material. Structural violence is embodied as adverse events if what we study, as anthropologists, is the experience of people who live in poverty or are marginalized by racism, gender inequality, or a noxious mix of all of the above. The adverse events to be discussed here include epidemic disease, violations of human rights, and genocide.[69]

However, the relationship between anthropology and psychology always has been troubled.[70]

As a psychologist, I am interested in how what is on the outside becomes the inside: how the body, the house, the relationships, the street, the town, the valley, the country, the world is internalised and imprinted on the minds of individuals and groups. And vice versa.

In line with more postmodern readings of psychoanalytic theory, I struggle with the binary oppositions of individual and society and I am interested in the murky places where the individual internalises the social and where the individual constructs the social. I want to insist on being both social scientist/ethnographer and psychologist. Nancy Chodorow writes: 'By character, those who become social scientists tend intuitively to be paranoid externalizers who projectively see troubles and opportunities as coming from without; those who are analysts tend intuitively to be omnipotent (or depressive) narcissists who see the world as created from within.'[71] In her terms, I am sometimes paranoid and externalising, but mostly a melancholic, white, middle-class, female academic – hopelessly depressed in my (probably deluded) sense of omnipotence, the idea that I can have an impact on the world.

When I try to write I feel fragmented, muddled and incoherent.[72] I yearn for a coherent story that has a beginning, a middle and an end, a story that gets to the bottom of things,[73] a story that tells of a 'more profound, coherent and reasoned trajectory'.[74] Instead, the story that I end up trying to write is one of ambivalence and complexity – a rather melancholic one. 'Surprisingly, the prospect of reflecting upon my writing fills me with melancholy,' Flax writes. She says:

> Perhaps the unconscious effects of a still-powerful, though disavowed, enlightenment wish contribute to this mood. It would be pleasant to chart a straightforward and progressive course: from error to truth, from uncertainly to clarity, from confusion to complex simplicity, from relative poverty to the accumulation of theoretical access. Instead, I feel compelled to tell a more ambiguous story.[75]

Anthropologist Michael Jackson in *Life within Limits: Well-Being in a World of Want* says that through his 'scribbled notes', he was 'gathering glimpses into what it meant to be a stranger in a world where so much was unfamiliar and forbidding'.[76] He cites Jürgen Habermas's notion of 'purposeless journeys', the necessity of abandoning 'the search for the real or the essential; replacing it with an effort to give voice to the multitude of agents involved in the production of culture . . . any culture . . . resists final summation . . . could never be pinned down or fully known'. Perhaps the problem with white writing is not that we try to write, but that we think we can see and know it all; we assume we understand and assume that our limited diagnostic and explanatory systems, our statistics, can illuminate the lives of others.[77] Instead, perhaps we should be content with 'scribbled notes' of 'purposeless journeys'.

Michel Foucault reminds us of the whales beneath the surface:

> For my part, it has struck me that I might have seemed a bit like a whale that leaps up to the surface of the water disturbing it momentarily with a tiny jet of spray and lets it be believed, or pretends to believe, or wants to believe, or himself does in

fact indeed believe, that down in the depths where no one sees him anymore, where he is no longer witnessed or controlled by anyone, he follows a more profound, coherent and reasoned trajectory.[78]

Vincent James Stanzione talks about the 'pilgrimage of learning', a pilgrimage with 'no definitive point or termination', a pilgrimage 'that remains unfinished' and is only justified in 'knowing one's own humanness in the reflection of the only-too-human other'.[79]

Maybe if we can be more modest in our claims, more tentative in our conclusions, open up our work to the scrutiny of others in undefensive ways, our white writing can be part of a project where exclusions, misrecognitions and disavowals are seen as inevitable, not only personal, but also political. In engaging with critiques about our representations, we can interrogate ourselves about how our work as researchers and clinicians produces and reproduces larger societal discourses. We must stay vigilant with our readers and interlocutors about how our omissions fit in with larger structures of misrecognition – 'the growing amnesia about the poor amid the rising tides of economic liberalisation', the forces of globalisation and the politics of reform.[80]

I realise the only way that I know how to write about white writing is to try to put my work on the table, opening it up to a critical community willing to engage.

Maybe if we can get past our own fears of incompetence, of whiteness and of privilege, we might be able to focus on the human beings we encounter, the real relationships that are formed (flawed as they might be) and get past the paralysis.

If we perhaps understand how much we are in the bag, we will be more aware of the strings and of the role they fulfil and the strength they need to have, even if we can never get to see the strings with absolute clarity.

Jackson writes about ethnography:

Ethnography provides a method whereby the occluded, denigrated, or masked dimensions of our common humanity may be recovered, not through thought alone but through practical engagement with others in the world . . . this movement is not away from the empirical but toward it, and entails a radicalization of the empirical as encompassing what is illuminated as well as what lies in shadow, the fluid as well as the fixed, the transitive as well as the intransitive, the verbal as well as the nonverbal, the personal as well as the transpersonal, the worldly as well as the extra-worldly.[81]

In my writing there is a 'struggle with responsibility under conditions of disenchantment, disorder, and imperfection'.[82] It entails a recognition that the empiricist or modernist desire for order, certainty and total control of both the process and the results of research is impossible to fulfil – it is the giving up of innocence. These seemingly endless reflexive endeavours can highlight the melancholia and can feed the paralysis, but if the clinician and researcher persist, they can also be enabling.[83] In the words of Barbara Myerhoff:

> We can never return to our former easy terms with a world that carried on quite well without our administrations. We may find ourselves like Humpty-Dumpty, shattered wrecks unable to recapture a smooth, seamless innocence, or like the paralyzed centipede that never walked again once he was asked to consider the difficulty in manipulating all those legs. Once we take into account our role in our own productions, we may be led into new possibilities that compensate for this loss. We may achieve a greater originality and responsibility than before, a deeper understanding at once of ourselves and of our subjects.[84]

I also need to understand that what I am writing is neither the biographies of others nor an autobiography. This book is an attempt to write about an engagement, a series of encounters, thwarted and complex relationships. Jackson reflects on his bond with a region in north-eastern Sierra Leone and southern Guinea, where he does his fieldwork:

> But what about my paradoxical relationship with the Kurankoa, who have contributed so much to my own well-being, a significant part of the 'upstream region of myself' . . . I have to

admit that both my aesthetic and intellectual responses to my fieldwork experience have produced a little knowledge, to be sure, but more importantly perhaps, they bear witness to a struggle to cope with relationships that were never easy, a language that was never mastered, food that was never entirely palatable, customs that often seemed cruel and living conditions that were seldom comfortable. More like an arranged marriage than a love match, my bond with Kuranko was also a kind of bondage, a curious mix of obligation and affection. And yet, by seeing this relationship through, I have gained the satisfaction of survival – which is so much deeper than the satisfaction of success.[85]

If I think about this book and what it is for me, Hoagland comes to mind, 'But me, I have this strange conviction that I am going to be born.'[86]

# Home

*'. . . how restricted a life so many of our fellow human beings lead, what little living they manage to do'* *

Is there anything in the world sadder than a train standing in the rain?
— Pablo Neruda, *The Book of Questions*

I lost all airs. I really realised who I am because this is the type of place where the internal becomes external. Everything that is on the bottom comes up and people live within it. It is a very weird place. It makes you used to everything.
— Nathan Trantraal, in Murray la Vita, 'En ôs stuck innie mirrel'[1]

That is what going home means for me. It is to stand outside myself and watch my bourgeois life prodded and pushed and buffeted around by lives quite unlike my own. It is to surrender myself to a world so much bigger than I am and to the destiny of a nation I cannot control. In this surrender is an expansion, a flowering, of what it means to be alive.
— Jonny Steinberg, 'Why I'm Moving back to South Africa'

It is the beginning of the academic year. I am doing a home visit with a student. We are visiting the Smits, a family participating in an infant observation study.[2] My student has become uncomfortable – she says

---

* The quote in the subtitle of this chapter – '. . . how restricted a life so many of our fellow human beings lead, what little living they manage to do' – is from Sen, 2005: xi.

that there are men leering at her when she arrives every week to observe the baby. I agree to go with her to see the neighbourhood for myself.

I walk across the dusty back yard, aware of my designer jeans and Doc Martens. The air smells of soot and ash and my Issey Miyake perfume. I duck past the laundry on the washing lines – 'spiderwebs of intricate relationships seeking a form'?[3] I am stared at by two skinny dogs and three young men in the neighbouring yard. The men are standing at a fire, smoking. They are quiet. One of them stirs a pot on the fire. Loud music is blaring across the back yards: 'Keep the lights off. We have company.'[4]

The black sand that covers the yard is interposed with a cheerful flower bed, grassy verges and a rather sombre attempt at a vegetable garden. There is a dead television, some rubbish, the ashes of a burned-out fire in a tin can and a forlorn plastic chair between the second and third line of structures. An outside tap at the front right. I know from my student that there are 48 people living in this particular yard and that this is the only running water.

The main house in the Smits's yard is a brick structure painted a dirty shade of yellow. Their one-room house is set against the back wall of the pink house and made of wooden logs, with gaps where the logs join together. There are three other dwellings in the yard.

Eve Smit (nicknamed 'Koekie') is a short woman with spiky hair. Her two front teeth are missing. Jan Smit has soft brown eyes, rounded features and greying hair. He walks with a limp – he was born with one leg shorter than the other. Six-year-old Natasha (nicknamed 'Tietie') is big for her age, cheeky, with many tiny ponytails on the sides of her head. The baby, Milla, is plump and enchanting, with clever eyes.

Inside the house there is a dirt floor, covered partially with offcuts of carpet and linoleum. On the one side of a room divider is a double bed that takes up half the house. On the other side are two cupboards, one for clothes and one for food. The clothes cupboard is also a television stand and the food cupboard doubles up as a kitchen counter, with buckets and a two-plate stove on it. There also is a kitchen chair and several cardboard boxes. A twin-tub washing machine in the middle of the room is the table, adorned with a candle in a bottle. The coffee table is an upturned bucket and a slab of melamine. A red fridge-magnet photo frame on the washing machine table advertises *Rooi Rose* (Red

Roses), a popular Afrikaans women's magazine. There is no photo in the frame. There is also no fridge in the house. Nails against the wall to hang things on – a handbag, a toy guitar, a pot, two brightly coloured enamel mugs, a plastic clock. Lace curtains on the two small windows, a padlock on the outside of the wooden door. A single bulb in the middle of the ceiling. One plug point. The roof apparently has a leak – there is a bucket with dirty water to the left of the door. Gnats circle the surface of the water. Bathing seems to happen in a galvanised metal tub outside the house. Where the toilet is, I cannot figure out. I don't ask and we never find out.[5]

'*Hebban olla vogala nesten*' (Have all birds nests), my Afrikaans teacher, Jan Vermaak, wrote on the blackboard with his left hand when I was fourteen and in Standard 7.[6] The oldest known sentence in old western Dutch.

Eve Smit wears an almost permanent frown.

I am introduced to her and the infant that is being observed. I take the baby from Eve. The frown seems to soften, but it does not disappear. The baby stares at me, does not respond to my baby talk. '*Lekker onbeskof*' (Very rude), says Eve. I try to engage with the baby by dangling my car keys in front of her. She frowns like her mother. I hand her back to Eve.

I find it disconcerting to sit and watch the mother and baby. It is unbearably hot in the structure. I say goodbye to Eve and tell the infant-observing student that I will meet her at the car after her hour with the family is over. I walk over to the men at the fire. One man has left. The fire is dying. The men are eating the potatoes that were boiled in the pot. When I greet them, they are shy, but friendly. '*Goeiemore Mevrou*' (Good morning Madam). It is the middle of the week, the middle of the day. I wonder why three seemingly healthy young men are not working, but I don't ask. I tell them that I am a psychologist. I am interested in how things are with the people of Kylemore. 'How are they?'

'Us, *Mevrou*?'

'Yes, you.'

'But you can see, *Mevrou*, can't you?'

'What should I see?'

'Bad, *Mevrou*, bad. Since we're not living on the farm anymore, things are bad. We don't even have money for electricity. We just stay here with my aunt and mom and dad.'

I ask him what his name is. 'My name is Daantjie, Daantjie Dromer' (*Dromer* means 'dreamer'). 'And this is my little brother. His name is Dawid.' Dawid doesn't say a word. He doesn't look at me. He stirs the ash of the fire with the stick that was used to hold the pot.

I ask more about the people on the plot. They don't seem to be offended by my curiosity. Acquiescent, but not forthcoming. They give me facts. They don't tell stories.

Like many families in the valley, three generations of Dromers share one plot. The aunt, Diena, is 39 years old and works as a seasonal worker. Her partner is Patrick (41), a piano stripper. The couple has three children, Taslyn (19), Patricia (14) and Nicole (9). The other members of the household are Elize, who is a sister of Diena's mother and her husband Nicholas. They are known as Ma and Pa. Diena's intellectually disabled sister Rosie (33) also lives in the house, as well as the children of another sister, Pauleen: Nicoleen (27), Maria (26) and Jacob (19). The house has three bedrooms, a kitchen and a bathroom. Patrick, Diena and Nicole sleep in one bedroom. The other five cousins (Taslyn, Patricia, Nicoleen, Maria, Jacob) and their Aunt Rosie sleep in the second bedroom. Ma and Pa occupy the third bedroom. Lena, another sister of Diena's, lives in the back yard in a shack with her husband Willie and three children, Mervin (14), Danelle (5) and Britney (4). The two brothers, Daantjie (20) and Dawid (23) share a wooden Wendy house.[7]

Daantjie and Dawid have not had permanent jobs since they left the farm where they grew up. 'We just stand here next to the road where they pick up temporary workers. Sometimes we're lucky.' I gather that mostly they are not. Daantjie has a daughter who lives with her mother's family. 'They also struggle, because the mom doesn't work – she went back to school. And now I can't even help.' Before I can ask if Dawid has children, the infant-observer student appears.

'*Totsiens*' (Goodbye), I say to the Dromer brothers as I leave. '*Totsiens Mevrou*,' they say, waving politely. 'They don't seem so scary after all,' my student says. 'It is just that they always stand there, doing nothing.'

She laughs when she gets in the car. 'I think Eve was very surprised that you picked up the baby. You know that you're not supposed to? In proper infant observation you only watch, you are not allowed to interact. Mrs K will not be pleased.' Mrs K is her infant-observation supervisor. Fuck Mrs K, I think. Fuck infant observation. And for that matter, fuck psychology and fuck research.

'As if observing is not a form of interaction,' I say out loud and wave cheerily at my new friends at the dead fire.

'And all life long, you wait for that to mount up to a life'?[8]

I reverse onto the street, but have to brake for a toddler crossing the dirt road behind the car. I am in a rush to get back to my office, but as always, I get lost when I drive out of town. I have to retrace my route, back to the house, then take the detour that I always have to take if I don't want to end up in a dead-end street. Past the schools, past the clinic, down the road at the edge of town, along the river to the exit of the town, where the name of the town is displayed like the Hollywood sign on the Helshoogte Road, literally translated, 'The Height of Hell Road' or 'Hell's High Road'.

## Demographics

As psychologists and researchers working in the valley, we are challenged. We are used to starting our interviews with patients or research respondents by getting basic demographic details, or identifying information, as we call it.[9] Age, gender, race/ethnicity, religion, relationship status, living situation, parental status, job/studies, previous experience with therapy, current psychiatric diagnosis.

In the valley these basic demographic details become trickier. Who are we to decide to call a person 'coloured'? And what does it mean to be coloured? What is a family? Who is in the family? How do we describe household structure? Who is the mother? When is a parent a parent? Who counts as your children? How to decide on relationship status? What is relationship status if a couple lives together because they share a house or a child, but do not really care about each other? Or if they have a child together, don't share a house, don't co-parent, only sleep together when they are both drunk? What counts as a job? What if a job lasts only for a season or for a day? What if schooling is interrupted to give birth or join a gang? How do we describe the houses? We look at the different options in the census. House or concrete block structure on a separate stand or yard? Hut? Informal dwelling? Semi-detached house? Room? Other? Address is even harder. What if you live in a Wendy house, which is behind a brick house? What if you don't live on a street, but live in a shack next to the river? Why is there no space for dogs on the clinical evaluation forms? And how do we understand the dogs?

I realise that the particularities of the lives that I am working with are too complex for my forms. I realise that this is also true for the other contexts within which I work; I am just less likely to notice it. Working with those on the margins means that the problematic assumptions and limitations of our academic and clinical discourses become apparent.[10]

I taught a course in clinical evaluation as part of the Master's programme in clinical psychology for eighteen years. I would tell the students that the goal of a first interview is to obtain information and establish a relationship in order to understand the patient (by giving her · a diagnosis and formulating her central problem), so as to give her the support that she needs. My experience has taught me how fraught this process of getting to know a person is. In my classes I would quote from Wisława Szymborska's poem 'Writing a Resumé':

> . . .
> Concise, well-chosen facts are *de rigueur*.
> Landscapes are replaced by addresses,
> Shaky memories give way to unshakable dates.
>
> Of all your loves, mention only the marriage;
> of all your children, only those who were born.
>
> Who knows you matters more than whom you know.
> Trips only if taken abroad.
> Memberships in what but without why.
> Honours, but not how they were earned.
>
> Write as if you'd never talked to yourself
> and always kept yourself at arm's length.
>
> Pass over in silence your dogs, cats, birds,
> dusty keepsakes, friends, and dreams.

Price, not worth,
and title, not what's inside.
His shoe size, not where he's off to,
that one you pass off as yourself.

In addition, a photograph with one ear showing.
What matters is its shape, not what it hears.
What is there to hear, anyway?
The clatter of paper shredders.[11]

## Dwellings

> . . . all I ever wanted to paint was sunlight on the side of a house.
>
> — Edward Hopper, in Gail Levin, *The Complete*
> *Watercolors of Edward Hopper*

Where do you live? What is your address? Where is your home? When we ask our patients or research respondents these questions, the answer that is given and written down is typically an address. Something like '15 Sunflower Street' or 'Apartment 7, Aloe Heights' (the street names in Kylemore are all flower names).[12]

But what is a home really and what is it that we need to know when we ask about home? In her book *Homeless Wanderers* (2015), clinical psychologist Sally Swartz writes about the experience and treatment of mental illness at the turn of the twentieth century in South Africa. The concept of 'home' is central to the book: 'What constitutes "home" is necessarily defined by a semantic web, which links it to family, safety, enclosure and the co-operative use of available sources. In contrast is foreignness, unbounded space, the insertion of otherness and competition for resources.'[13] Amanda Kottler (another eminent South African psychologist) and Koichi Togashi write about the importance of 'feeling at home' – 'an extremely fine and frail experience, which, to varying degrees and depending on the relational contexts involved, every human being longs for'.[14] They add that in order to feel at home, 'individuals need emotional relationships with others, but, in these relationships, there is always a risk of being wounded by the discovery that this other who was initially trusted and appeared to be connected in the way the individual has yearned for, is a lie.'

In psychology then, we are not only interested in the physical reality of home, we are also interested in the psychic meaning of feeling at home. Home is not only where we start from in the physical sense of the word, it also refers to the original experience of being held or being contained, the experience that constitutes the beginning of our psychic development. The word 'home' conjures up images of reliability and consistency. The experience of feeling at home implies connection, but with boundaries. It suggests a space within which a person can safely rest and play, engage and disengage. Feeling at home is also associated with a sense of tranquil togetherness and co-operation. When we are not feeling at home or when we feel homeless, we may be feeling disconnected, unsafe, unboundaried, intruded upon, competed with or open to attack.

Psychologists typically think that the first place where the infant has this experience of being contained is in the arms of the mother. It is from this early experience of being held or being contained in the arms and the mind of the mother (physically and psychologically) that the individual develops her own capacity to hold and contain, not only herself, but also those that she will connect with.[15] While Western psychology has been criticised for its emphasis on the role of the mother, mothers are nonetheless mostly held responsible for providing their children with a psychological and physical home. This is also true in the valley.

If the idea is that 'a home in the mind', or a sense of internal containment, is necessary for an individual to become an independent yet connected person, the suggestion is that people who do not have the experience of safe containment will be in trouble and psychologically at risk later in life.[16] People who do not have the opportunity to develop the capacity to inhabit an inner space and feel an internal sense of safety are more likely to depend on others and their surroundings to contain them and soothe them. Also, when they have difficult feelings, they will not be able to name them, understand them or manage them, but will be likely to simply evacuate them, through violent action, projection or represssion.[17]

As psychologists we rarely visit the homes of our patients, but we listen for 'home' and 'homelessness' in their stories. On the one hand,

I listen for how the internal is being externalised. In the building, maintenance, decoration and adaptation of spaces one can see people 'making a definite "go" of things . . . one finds suggestions of human energy, determination, agency, innovation, enterprise, collaboration, presence, confidence and pride'.[18]

Willem Anker writes about eighteenth-century South Africa:

> Birds build nests without tools, it assumes shape from the inside, like a shell. The bird presses and stretches the material with her breast until it becomes pliable. The nest takes the shape of the bird's body. The female hollows out the nest and eases back the walls constantly until they become soft and warm. The house is her passion. Every blade of perfectly plaited grass in the nest has been pressed back innumerable times with laboured breath, with heartbeats. A pressure from inside, a physical, dominating intimacy. The nest is a burgeoning fruit challenging its limits.[19]

However, regardless of obvious attempts of some people in the valley to create safe homes, the hopelessness and despondency of others are reflected in their homes and their yards. 'Because this is the kind of place where the internal becomes external,' says Nathan Trantraal about his childhood on the Cape Flats, 'everything that is on the bottom comes up and people live within it. It is a very weird place. It makes you used to everything.'[20]

The students and I are not used to everything we experience. The student who did the infant observation with Eve Smit and her daughter reflected in a journal on how she responded to the environment:

> I once got a migraine from sitting in just the winter sun for an hour. Sometimes the seat I sat on was so cold that I thought it might be wet. Water dripped onto my boot and my bag from the roof. Once I sat on an upturned crate, which became very painful after an hour. I always went to the toilet at a garage in Stellenbosch before the observation, because I could not work out where the toilet might be [and did not ask], and in my mind, it was not a place that I would have wanted to visit. The stench

of the neighbourhood always assaulted my senses on arrival . . .
I sometimes felt disgusted by the poor hygiene, the dirt and the
flies . . . At times the proximity of scavenging dogs, the baby and
shared food unsettled me . . . I had a tuberculosis scare when after
an episode of bronchitis, I had a nagging cough that would not
go away and I felt very depleted. I had a chest X-ray. This may,
I think, to some degree have been about empathy, but possibly
equally about fear – that I would be contaminated, in many
ways, by what I was experiencing, and that I would never be able
to leave it behind. My desire to run away can possibly be seen
in the speeding fine I got when leaving a particularly difficult
observation called 'My grave'. The anxiety about not having
enough was contagious . . . It was very painful to witness great
need and not to be able to respond to it. I had many fantasies,
some of them wild, about assisting the family . . . Some sense of
fear pervaded the observation process for me until the end. My
fear was about being attacked violently, and specifically, of sexual
violence. I worried that my car would be stolen or damaged,
that my handbag would be snatched, and my car radio taken. I
worried that the family's dogs would attack me, I worried that
there could be a violent fight (I imagined a stabbing, in fact up
against my car) and that there was no visible police presence to
turn to.

    In summary, I often felt wretched, worried, helpless, afraid,
disgusted, stoical, relieved to escape, guilty, and in pain during
the observation process.[21]

The student's brutally honest reflection on the physical and psychological
impact of the environment is rare. Mostly the students do not talk about
how they feel about the abject poverty they are exposed to. We also seem
to avoid asking questions about how the women themselves feel about
the scarcity of space, food, medical care and work.

    In the houses, even if they are not small, space cannot be taken for
granted. Rose Fielies is 26 years old, has been married for six months,
has a ten-year-old daughter and is six months pregnant. She has just

discovered that her husband is having an affair with a married woman. This woman is also expecting Rose's husband's baby. Also a boy.

Rose coughs constantly throughout the session. She talks about how stressed she feels about her living situation; she lives in a free-standing house with ten other people: her mother-in-law, her husband, his two sisters, the husband of one sister and five children (including her daughter). The house is painted bright blue and is called 'Heaven'. It has three bedrooms, one occupied by the grandmother and three grandchildren. The second and third bedrooms are occupied by the husband's two sisters and their families, with Rose and her husband sleeping in the sitting room. She says, '*Ons slaap voorlopig in die sitkamer*' (We are sleeping in the lounge just for now). '*Voorlopig*' (just for now) in this case means for the last ten years. Two of the adults in the house work, the mother-in-law as a domestic worker and the one sister at Continental China, a crockery factory. The others are not working and stay at home with Rose.

Rose's first home was with her grandfather, her maternal aunt and her husband and their three sons, and her own mother. During her childhood her mother worked as a domestic worker and Rose remembers her as being drunk every weekend. When Rose was fifteen she fell pregnant with her first child and was thrown out of her maternal home. For a while she was homeless, wandering the streets with her husband-to-be, sleeping in empty houses. When she was seven months pregnant, the couple asked the boyfriend's mother to take her in, without telling her that Rose was pregnant. This house became her second home. 'Yes, because when I now, when I was expecting her [referring to her eldest daughter], then my people just threw me out. Then I didn't have a place to stay, then his mom and them took me in. That's how it is that I've been living here so long now . . . I wandered a lot in the beginning. I was seven months pregnant, only then his mom and them took me into the house. They never knew I was pregnant . . . Because, see, then of course it started to get winter. I wandered around a lot, so we slept outside, in empty houses, so . . . Yes, up to seven months then I said, I said to him . . . "We can't [live] like this now any longer. I can't take the cold anymore now, it's getting cold." He must tell his mom and them. Then he now went to tell them.'

Rose gave birth to a second child in this house, in the front room where she now sleeps with her husband, when she was seventeen years old. She had the baby seven months into the pregnancy, not realising that she was pregnant, as she was on contraception. She went to the hospital with the newborn child, but the nurses sent her home and kept the baby in the hospital. The hospital called her the same night to tell her that her one-day-old baby was dying and she should come back.

'I just dropped the phone, I had such a fright.' This detail she remembers more than ten years later.

She went back to the hospital. 'Then I got a lift with an ambulance driver again that evening. I was at the hospital the whole evening then. Yes, I sat there all the time. Until about just before nine. I can't remember the time anymore . . . It was about just before nine. Everything was so mixed up. I was so mixed up in my head, but it was about half-past eight, just before nine, then the child died.'

Now six months into her third pregnancy, she is home all the time. She had to stop working because of her cough. 'Um, I got, um, Dr Viljoen then, I got so sick at work one Saturday then I went to Dr Viljoen. And then she said but I had a bad infection. Now the workplace where we work is very wet. It's water all over and she said she thinks I should then not work any further because I already also had a miscarriage.'

Apart from the cough, Rose also complains of sleeplessness, headaches and inexplicable pains 'down there'. She is distressed about her husband, anxious about the birth and the baby. She drinks a little and smokes a lot. She is distressed and her distress manifests physically.

I see Rose again, six months later. She has given birth and is very down. Her living situation is unchanged, but her husband now openly has a relationship with the other woman. She speaks softly. Short sentences. She talks about the painfulness of her situation and uses phrases like '*Ek moet maar deurdruk*' (I must just push through) and '*Ek moet maar kop bo water hou*' (I must just keep my head above water). She has no one to talk to about her problems at the house. She tells me how her life seems to be a repetition of her mother's life: 'Like now, we are okay now. I also grew up like this. My mom and my dad and . . . I pushed through. But this isn't really what I wanted for them. I wanted to give them something better now.'

Rose's experience of home has always been conflicted and haphazard. In her first home she was abandoned by her father, lived with a drunken mother and was finally chased away. At fifteen she was a homeless wanderer, pregnant, squatting in desolate houses. She gave birth to a premature baby in the front room of her current home, she was sent home from the hospital and it was at home that she heard about the dying baby. She and her new baby still sleep with her unfaithful husband in the front room of her adopted home. For Rose, home is not associated with comfort and congeniality. It is a place of abandonment, trauma, competition, betrayal and death.

When I ask her, just before leaving, how she experiences the house, she replies without hesitation. The house is noisy, it drives her crazy: '*Dit maak my mal.*'

Can one feel at home in the psychological sense of the word when the physical space is compromised? It is difficult to imagine how a sense of psychologically feeling at home can be achieved in a context of physical homelessness. It is even harder to imagine how a mother who is not feeling at home, physically or psychologically, can provide her infant with containment or holding. In her last interview Rose tells me that the baby, whose name I never ask, is fine, but in his sleep he often has a startle response, wakes up and screams: 'All the stress that came with it . . . He just gets a fright sometimes, yes. I don't know, it's probably because I stress so much with him. It's not that bad now anymore, but he . . . he's often like that in his sleep. He wakes with a start. Hmm see, he cries like that.'

I don't know what Rose's response to her baby's fright was. I guess that the baby boy, so frightened in his sleep, was experiencing both his and his young mother's dread.[22]

Some students, when confronted with a lack of physical space, will often, but not always convincingly, try to reassure the women that the psychological home that mothers are able to provide is more important than the physical space.

Abigail, while being interviewed about motherhood, is asked if there is anything that bothers her. 'The only thing bothering me is my circumstances,' she says immediately. 'We struggle living in the bungalow.' The interviewer interrupts and tells her that it is good to have something to work on, good to have a goal. 'And as long as you look after them well, it does not matter. You know, Abigail, there are people who have huge houses who don't love their children,' she says, probably in an attempt to make the best of the situation. 'And that's much worse. Those children really don't have a home.'

Abigail replies, 'That's true.'

Abigail ostensibly agrees with the interviewer, but one wonders. For many women in the valley, a lack of physical space is a problem. As psychologists, we deal with psychological homelessness all the time, but we sometimes lose our ability to hear when someone talks to us about physical homelessness.

In a group therapy session with thirteen-year-old girls, it is also clear that there are dreams of other kinds of spaces. 'What do you do when you feel down?' asks the interviewer. Simone shares her dream, '*Sê nou maar my plak sak* [Say now I am in low spirits], I think about my garden and my tennis court. Swimming pool. Lie comfortably with a cocktail in the hand. "Yes, my lady".'

Their dreams about such spaces help them to defend against the *plak sak* (low spirits), but some of the girls do feel contained and held and have ways of creating soothing spaces in the here and now. 'Do you think it will be better when you're grown up?' asks the therapist.

One of the girls answers, 'Yes, it is nice to be a child. You get everything. You don't have to pay anything, you don't need to pay, pay for your house, you don't need to pay. Now, you can still after all always enjoy it. Plant things in your gardens, nice little things and then you breathe. Make yourself a fake tennis court. Yes, I can plant little flowers so long. Plant little trees so long. Pretty roses. And then I make a fake tennis court. You just put up a piece of rope. Then you breathe.'

Another girl in the same group writes in her group therapy diary:

Dear diary. We talked about jealousy. We also watched clips about mean girls. It was kind of fun. I really enjoyed it. There are problems at home. At the moment we are staying in the *plakkerskamp* [shanty town]. My mother and my auntie had a fight and my aunt accused my mother that she *tik* [was on methamphetamine]. I was very sad. We first lived with my auntie, then she put us out in the middle of the night and it was raining and we had to go and sleep with my mother's friend in the *plakkerskamp*. We each now sleep on a thin single mattress. Me, my mother, my brother, my sister. It is very cold and it feels very sad to me. Why should some children suffer while most children have good lives getting everything that they want? Life sometimes is not fair.

In the guest bathroom of my house (which has four bedrooms, three and a half bathrooms, and my daughter and I live there alone), there is a poster of a poem by the Dutch poet Koos Geerds:

*Einder, bedaar, ik heb een huis*
*dat mij bevrijdt; onder dit dak*
*ben ik een mens die adem krijgt.*[23]

## Boundaries

Hestia was the goddess of the fireplace ('focus' original Latin for hearth!) and Hermes the god of the threshold, the goddess of the centre point and the god of the boundary, of the hearth and the doorway, the one protects the living and the staying and the other shelters the coming and the going, the two poles between which our lives are lived, stasis and movement, rest and labour.

— Marlene van Niekerk and Adriaan van Zyl, *Memorandum*

The floor anchors your feet. It is the first mark we make on the earth. And look, the wall is a floor that is upright. The wall frames the window. Walls divide the floor, walls make rooms; when there are rooms time moves slower. The wall separates us from the world so it creates a new world, a framed world.

— Willem Anker, *Red Dog*

'There is no such thing as an infant,' says psychoanalyst Donald Winnicott. 'There only is an infant and a mother.'[24] While most psychoanalytic theory emphasises the importance of relationships within which we feel contained and held, it also asserts that central to human development is the idea of separation or individuation. Somewhere in his development, the infant must learn that despite his mother's ability to hold and contain him, she is a separate being. Even in the closest relationships, there must be a distinction between you and me. If boundaries are not in place, people do not own and manage their feelings, but project them onto others, thus defending themselves against painful feelings. As psychologists, we typically are concerned with psychological boundaries.

In the valley we are often confronted with a lack of physical boundaries.

The close proximities in the valley have to do with the number of people living in a single housing structure and the many structures on one plot. Boundaries between households and people are permeable. Pregnant fifteen-year-old Chantel describes the sleeping arrangements for when her baby arrives. For her, the important boundary is that she will have her own bed after the baby's birth. When the interviewer enquires about her living arrangements, she says that the baby will sleep in a room with her and her parents. She makes it clear, proudly, that 'it's not on one bed, I have my own bed.'

In the valley it is not always clear where one yard begins and another ends. Nandipha, a new resident in Kylemore, an *inkommer* (literally, an in-comer, a newcomer), tells us that people easily become overfamiliar in Kylemore, 'and then you must do it too. The people will – like, to give you a silly example: since we have been living here in this big house, people will just hang their washing on the line that is supposed to be ours. So, if I want to hang my washing, then there is already washing on the line and then it is frustrating.'

Everyone knows everything about everyone. One resident says, 'Look, we are a small community. You see how small Kylemore is. If a chicken stands at one end of town, the whole place is covered in feathers. So small is it. Everyone knows about everything.'

Competing radios and the constant commentary of people on each other's lives highlight the smallness of living spaces and the close proximities of people in the valley:

> Three radios are playing, one from the back house, and the other two from either neighbour. All three have different beats and moods. And they compete in a cacophony. There is music pumping on the radio in the adjacent room at the front . . . A

woman and a man come and go past the door; they seem to be living in what I thought last visit was the outhouse in the back yard. The woman calls to him, '*Jy hou so van kak luister, jou ore is al langs jou gat!*' [You like listening to shit so much, your ears are alongside your arse by now].[25]

Being entitled to comment on each other's lives and on each other's behaviour seems taken for granted.

Two spandexed and geared yuppies on a tandem bicycle passing through town, obviously a bit lost, cause two young boys to clutch each other in hysterical laughter: '*Hey. Jy. Kyk hoe naai hulle mekaar*' (Hey. You. Look how they are fucking each other). A colleague passes a group of school boys and hear them mumbling under their breath: '*Wit poes. Wit poes. Wit poes*' (White cunt. White cunt. White cunt).

'*Skel*' (yell at) and '*raas*' (scold) are not only instruments of social control. In psychological terms they also represent an example of an enactment of difficult or painful feelings that can't be tolerated or managed by the women. A student comments on this in a journal:

Meantime a woman in the left neighbours' yard is *skelling* [scolding] increasingly loudly. She starts by saying, yes, laugh, she is going to come over there and *klap daai gevreet* [smack that mug of a face] . . . She uses very violent language. '*Vandag maak ek haar vrek*' [Today I am going to kill her]. Something about how she is going to go and find someone and exactly how she will strike her through her face. '*Julle hou my vir 'n poes!*' (You think I am a cunt!) she says. Something about drinking beer, about why she drinks (and I suddenly think she must be drunk). '*Jou ma se poes!* [Your mother's cunt!] . . . *En die ergste van alles is dat julle kinders is, julle laaities wat so maak!*' [And the worst of all is that you're children, you're youngsters who do this!] she says in a slightly plaintive tone.

Good grief, I think, she is talking to a child like that.[26]

I don't think children – or anyone else – ever become used to the yelling and the scolding. In our clinical work with people in the valley, being yelled at by mothers, or having a history of being scolded by mothers, is often mentioned as a major cause of distress.[27] It creates a world that seems persecutory and dangerous, chaotic and noisy.[28]

'*Skel*' seems to be a way of connecting. In the words of Chantel, who is talking about her day: 'He sometimes yells at me,' she says.

'Why does he yell?' I ask.

Chantel answers immediately, 'Because he loves me.'

Another powerful form of communication and social control can be related to people not owning and managing their feelings. '*Skinner*' (gossip) in the community is accepted as a given; it is endured, but dreaded and despised. People in the valley report that they constantly feel as if they are under a certain kind of surveillance.[29] Gossip renders everyone in the community visible and everyone is conscious of possibly being talked about.[30] Nandipha, the '*inkommer*', complains: 'But it's so that people easily get overfamiliar and they just accept that you have to do it or that you can do it, or oh, it's . . . it's mine and I do it like this or so.' Nandipha says that the people in the community are more involved in each other's lives than she is used to. 'Actually, for my husband it is difficult, because he isn't, he isn't a guy who . . . someone else mustn't try to get involved in his private things or in his life. Or try to tell him what to do. It is actually quite frustrating for him because he isn't used to it. There are certain things that you discuss with your friends and that you speak about. But you don't speak about everything. Now, if you sometimes listen to what other people know about other people here, then it is actually frustrating, that people have so much say about other people's private lives.'

Sterretjie, a 54-year-old mother of four, also talks about gossip: 'And, like she said to me, like she saw, gossip is a big problem here. It is. People want to speak about your things and it works on you. See and you hear and you know, you know for a fact that it's not even true what the people say. But now, I am a person – I am not going to ask about it. I leave it. Now, it's things that work on your nerves, because you tell yourself: "I am not going to ask about that one", but you see him, it comes to you, he said this and that to you. It is not right.'

In a journal about a group therapy intervention, a student recalls that one of the group members describes the community as *7de Laan* (7th

Avenue), a place where everyone knows everyone and where everyone gossips about everyone else.[31] The same group member explained that she was happy when we discussed confidentiality at the outset of the programme because she does not believe in gossip, as this is not the way she was raised. The student observed: 'I noticed how guarded they were and how they really struggled to share their fears with the group.'

Gossip is not only a form of surveillance; it can also be understood as a form of envious attack, where the people who gossip project their uncomfortable feelings about themselves and their anxieties upon the other. Again, an unsafe and persecutory reality is created.[32]

Scolding and gossiping are powerful instruments of social control and important psychological enactments, utilised specifically by women to get rid of painful feelings.

The lack of boundaries does not only manifest as gossiping and verbal abuse. It also manifests as physical and sexual abuse. Paradoxically, in the community there is also a collusion to be silent about certain things, most notably about violence and sex. In the words of Zee, who talks about incest: 'How many people is here? They keep things in. They are ashamed to talk to other people. Even here in town, you don't know what's going on in the other people's houses. There's a man that lived next to me. We were neighbours for a long time. He abused his daughters. Beautiful daughters, too. People don't speak. And then there is all this hurt inside. It looks like nothing happened.'[33]

Following a group therapy session, thirteen-year-old Chestline writes in her journal. Her handwriting is childlike, she uses no punctuation:

It was the morning my mother went to town and my two big sisters were at home and my dad and I were also at home and they said that I should go outside because they wanted to clean the house and so I went and it was an hour later and I got really hungry and I came back to the house and I go into the house and it was quiet and I called my sisters but they were dead quiet I then went on the stairs and looked for them there.

The handwriting in the journal changes, the letters are now leaning to the right, the writing seems rushed:

And I then found them but I walked softly then when I got up there my father was busy with my sisters to *ryp* [rape] them but he did not see me they also did not see me they could also not talk because my dad said they *moet hulle monde hou* [must keep their mouths shut].

The student therapists read the journal entry that evening and call me, distraught. I struggle to sleep that night. We cancel our sessions for the next morning and drive to see Chestline. She is called out of her Maths class, seemingly pleased that we responded to her journal. 'Yes,' she says, 'I thought that you will want to come and hear.' I ask her where her dad is now, whether she is safe. 'Yes,' she says, 'he has been in jail for a long time now. That thing happened a long time ago. I was still small. Not even five.'

'And you have never told anyone?' I ask.

'No,' Chestline says, 'my dad said that we *moet ons monde hou* [not talk].'

We drive back. We are quiet. Glad, on the one hand, that the perpetrator is in jail and that it all happened long ago, but also devastated . by Chestline with the too-big school uniform and the eyes far too tired for her years, the secret much too big for that small body. What stays with me most, however, is her reply when I asked her how it is going at home now. She says, 'No, not so good, *Juffrou* [Afrikaans word for teacher, but also used to refer to older women]. My mother scolds a lot. She scolds me a lot. And sometimes then I think if my father wasn't in jail now, my mother wouldn't have scolded so much. Because he wouldn't have liked it. He liked me very much.' She tears up. 'Sometimes I just wish that he was at home again.'

In the mind of the thirteen-year-old girl, the house with the scolding mother felt more like a home with the rapist father present. The fantasy was that he could protect her against the intrusive scolding of her mother.

I think of the words of Javier Marias:

Talking, telling, saying, commenting, gossiping, passing on information, criticising, exchanging news, tittle-tattling, defaming, slandering and spreading rumours, describing and relating events, keeping up to date and putting others in the picture, and of course, joking and lying. That is the wheel that moves the world, Jacobo, more than anything else; that is the engine of life, the one that never becomes exhausted and never stops, that is its life's breath.[34]

## Identity

Our people ... us Coloureds are verskriklike snaakse [dreadfully strange] people.

— Chriszelda (research participant)

Many people take offense at being labelled coloured, for political and historical reasons. Others wear the tag proudly and to them it denotes a specific cultural identity or ethnic background. Still others use it as a means of endowing themselves with a false sense of superiority with regards to black people, as a way of disengaging themselves from being seen as and called black – to them black means inferior. We're very interested in the conflict engendered by and contained in the term, being coloured ourselves. Well, that's what our IDs say, anyway.

— André Trantraal, Charmaine Trantraal, Nathan Trantraal, *Coloureds*

There are, of course, other ways of belonging, of feeling at home, of having an identity, of separating oneself from others. In South Africa a dreaded form of separation has been, and still is, race.

In the valley most poor or low-income people are classified 'coloured' and will also identify themselves as such. In South Africa the category 'coloured' is used to refer to people who are said to be of diverse and mixed racial origins. The term is used to refer to an ethnic category of people who possess some degree of sub-Saharan ancestry, but not enough to be considered African.[35]

All of this I dutifully indicate in footnotes whenever I submit an academic paper to a journal. My standard footnote when referring to coloured people in academic papers is:

However, such categories are socially constructed and carry important social meanings. As such, we believe that it is impossible to conduct a meaningful analysis of our findings within the context of post-apartheid South Africa without making reference to previous racial classifications, since these still inform existing power relations. In this paper the category of 'coloured' will be used to refer to South Africans said to be of diverse and mixed racial origins; designated under apartheid racial classification as 'coloured'.[36]

When I deliver papers outside of South Africa my audiences typically cringe when I use the term 'coloured'. Watching the South African comedian Trevor Noah's talk show on television one evening, I heard that he also is questioned when he refers to himself as 'coloured' abroad:

Can you say 'coloured'? There is this whole debate going on. Can you say 'coloured'? Oooh. Some people say no, you should not say 'coloured', you should say 'black'. Overseas you can't say 'coloured'. You know overseas I was doing a few shows, working in London, backstage . . . Are you Zulu? No, close – I am actually coloured. Don't say that, that's racist. That's racist, Trevor. You don't call yourself coloured. That's racist and old school. The new kids are calling themselves 'nigger' now. But if you want to be PC [politically correct], you call yourself 'mixed race', mixed race. You are free here, brother, you are free.

'Mixed race' – that's the PC term worldwide for people like me.

Gotta be careful when I am in places like Cape Town, you know. Walking around, 'Excuse me, you are mixed race.' Knowing coloureds, they will probably be like, '*Jou ma se* mixed race, stupid *ga*' [Your mother's mixed race, stupid man]. Can't run around saying that . . .

In the Cape they call me a banana type. Yellow on the outside, white on the inside.[37]

As a white woman, I don't know how to write about being coloured, although I know how important race is, also and especially to me as a person classified as white.[38] I read what coloured people themselves write.[39] Hein Willemse, a prominent coloured literary scholar, writes about coloureds:

> The concept of 'Coloured', like '*Afrikaaner*' (in its usage before c.1850), '*hotnot*' (Hottentot), '*bruinmens*' (brown person), '*Kleurling*' (Coloured) . . . takes its place next to those terms originating from colonially structured societies to define the offspring born from sexual relationships between colonists/settlers and indigenous people. For example, in South America, the rest of Africa, Europe or Asia, common concepts such as mestis, mestizo and mulato/mulatto were used. This abundance of terminology gives an indication of the sometimes Social Darwinist-inspired efforts to describe these people and their degrees of 'admixture': bastard, cafuzo, catalo, eurafrican, eurasian, eurindian, fustee/fustie, griffe, griffo, guacho, halfblood, halfcaste, hybrid, cross, quadroon, quateroon, quinteroon, ladino, marabou, mestee, mestis, mestiso/mestisa, mixed race, mulatto, octoroon, sacatra zebrule, terseroon, zambo.[40]

Willemse writes how, in South Africa, where 'the colonist often declared that he knew his native, "[for] it is the settler who has brought the native into existence and who perpetuates his existence"', the 'Coloured was perceived as different, deficient, less than human and in need of guardianship'.[41] In reflecting on the portrayal of coloured people in literature, Jakes Gerwel articulates the 'paternalism of the master' as follows:

> Characteristic of this way of life was a childlike inability to make ethical decisions and hence a short-sighted carelessness, the abuse of liquor and merry-making, loose and loud cachectic lives, extremely large and poorly nurtured families, rough women abuse, naïve incomprehension of the contents of mimicked religious customs, and a general banality in almost all areas of life.[42]

Knowing his native, bringing his native into existence? In a Stellenbosch Master's thesis, written in 1933, the white writer declares: 'The Coloured was born in shame and in shame he continued his life and this to his own detriment and destruction.'[43]

Haji Mohamed Dawjee relates how being coloured necessitated a shamed demeanour in the apartheid years; she is angry that some coloured people are still forced to have this. She says:

> In order to survive and to get ahead, we sometimes find it necessary to live with our heads bowed. If we don't have the necessary insight, we think that this is a fulfilling way to get through life . . . And there is no pride and no sense of being brave. We cower in the face of this and we speak only when we are spoken to. And when I speak of pride, I am not speaking about arrogance; I mean your understanding and knowledge that you deserve to be somewhere, to belong. And that your existence has as much value as those of anyone else.[44]

In my work I don't want to be another colonist naming my native.[45] I don't want to write 'coloured' on a form. I want to understand what it means to people in the valley to classify themselves as 'coloured'.

But, of course, it is not something the women speak to us about spontaneously. Or maybe we don't ask.

Chriszelda is an exception. She is pregnant when I interview her and talks to me about naming her baby Chevron and how the naming is connected to her being coloured:

> Chevron? Hmm . . . I have a little book where I always write text verses at the church, and then I will always highlight it in my Bible. In the back, I made a column for me, daughters and sons and *linge* [short for twins (*tweelinge*) in Afrikaans], if it is now one of both, *linge* if it is only girls and *linge* if it is only boys. And . . . from when I was young, I was still at school, if I liked a name, then I wrote it down. Boys. Girls. The *linge* and all. And her name was also there, but there was many . . . that I now, specifically what I would have wanted to give her if it . . . Chevron was now the last name for me that sounded prettier, or sounded better . . . Us people do not pronounce a name as

it should be pronounced. And then I thought her name was going to be Tara. Then I thought Tara, because it was a coloured community. I am not going to keep it together if they say to her, 'Tara come here, and . . .'. For me, pronounce the things like it is, a thing like it is, don't wrap a *lap* [a piece of cloth] around a healthy finger. And . . . Chevron was the last. There was Tellie, there was Tarryn, there was Tayla, there was even Karen, I liked that. Erin I liked. Esna . . . but now Father also has something to say. Not Tara, and no . . . then I said, 'Let's decide on a name together.' Then I said to him, 'Chevron.' Then he said, 'Yes, Chevron.' He then drives a Chevrolette! Then I said, 'No, are the people going to think that's where it was made!' 'Let it go!' Then I anyway decided on Chevron. Yes. I decided on Chevron.

'That is a beautiful name,' I say, awkwardly, trying to be polite.

Oh, no, it's just . . . Us coloureds are *verskriklike snaakse* [dreadfully strange] people. But that's how I decided on her name. But Mother was also a little . . . Chevron? Then I said no, what will her names be now? I'm not going to . . . because my grandmother's name is Georgina, and the one daughter's name Georgina, and now the *meisiekind* [girlchild] of Georgina has to be Georgina, now how many *meisiekinders* are there? I said, no man, I don't like that! It's too much of one thing. Then I said Chevron is her name. Now what's her second name? Then I said Lelie. My mother said is it now together, is it now Chevron-Lee, or Chevron Lee or . . . then I said first name Chevron, second name Lee. Because she's not a dog, dogs have only one name. Then I put another *naampie* [Afrikaans diminutive of name]. Now she has two *naampies*. Yes, she's on my surname. Her dad's surname is . . . He wanted to have, then I said no, these days . . . the men just do what they want, and like they want, and if I say today, you are not going to see Chevron, then you run to the authorities, and the child is now on your surname, and then my child gets taken away from me. Then I said oh no, your male egos always get in the way, because you are now macho and big, it is my surname, because I am the man in the city. Then I said no, and if we marry, which can maybe happen next year, then I said to him, then you can go and pay, and then you put her name as Steyn. But for now, she is still an Alberts.

I try to make sense of this interview with Chriszelda (a 26-year-old single parent of one child, employed at a local accountancy firm). Her narrative of naming her child seems to evoke many of the issues that women struggle with in this community: race, gender, agency. There is an almost amused awareness of being part of a coloured community, a slightly ironic account of a man who wants to name his child after his car and a rather earnest determination to keep control over her child by naming the child herself and not giving the child the father's surname. Also, very clear here is the importance of the child, the anticipation, the planning, the hope – a certain kind of agency: 'And . . . from when I was young, I was still at school, if I liked a name, then I wrote it down.'

## A dog's life

I don't want to come back in another existence as a dog or a pig and have to live as dogs or pigs live under us.

— J.M. Coetzee, *Disgrace*

Outside the dogs are barking black.

— Tertius Kapp, 'Buite blaf die honde swart'

Across the border we are all Bastards, all runaway dogs.

— Willem Anker, *Red Dog*

Dogs do not feature on our clinical evaluation forms.

In the valley we all notice the dogs.

The dogs seem to be everywhere. Lean, light brown, short-haired, different sizes, typically very tame. Sometimes almost lethargic. In the journals of students, the dogs scavenge and slink and creep and cringe.

After a particularly depressing day, a student clinician has a strange encounter with a dog. She writes about it in her journal. A certain sense of unreality is palpable in the entry:

As I drove out of the community one day a dog stood in the middle of the road, staring blankly at my car, not sure whether he should move out of the way or wait to be hit by me. As I stopped a few inches before this dog and looked into his eyes I wondered what the point was indeed, of making any kind of move. He refused to walk any further so I made a dramatic manoeuvre onto the sidewalk to pass him by. As I looked in my rear-view mirror I wondered whether my dramatic moves had had any impact on this dog or the women of the community for that matter.[46]

There are the docile dogs, but there also are the pit bull terriers, the chains and open wounds reminding us that not all dogs in the valley have been tamed or trained.

In a therapy group with thirteen-year-old boys the topic is violence. The boys all indicate that they have been exposed to violence. When asked about violence at home they become very quiet. Inadvertently they changed the topic to dog fighting. The therapist writes in her journal:

The way they described these online fights sounded like they were extremely vulgar and cruel, with the dogs' dead bodies being cast to the side and houses filled with rooms that had blood splashes on the walls. I was quite shocked by this and found it very disheartening. But what really struck me was how invested and knowledgeable the boys seemed. I could tell they thought it wasn't okay what people were doing to the dogs, but it still seemed like they knew about and watched these 'fights' to some extent . . . Which makes me quite sad, really.

Anna Motz writes about how studying the conditions of household pets and treatment of animals in a home can be a useful guide to family disturbance: 'Through sensitive and thorough exploration of the treatment of all creatures within a household, human or animal, it is possible to glean a rich sense of brutality and sadism that operates within the home.'[47]

In a very disturbing group therapy session with unemployed women, a participant recalled how her dog stole her polony (cheap processed meat) and cheese sandwich from the table and she threw a knife at him. She left him with the knife in his back for the whole day. '*Hy sal nooit weer 'n polony sandwich steel nie*' (He will never steal a polony sandwich again), she says to the group.

Every now and then a student, used to middle-upper-class people's obsessive concern with caring for their pets, wonders why poor people have dogs. 'Why do "they" have dogs if they cannot take care of them properly?' the student might ask.

'Maybe for the same reasons we have dogs,' I hear myself saying sternly.

Having something vulnerable to take care of gives our lives meaning, but it also highlights our own vulnerabilities and therefore our humanity.[48] Dogs can make us more human. In the words of Tony Hoagland:

. . .

These barricades and bulwarks against human loneliness,

they used to fill me with disdain,
but that was before I found out my metaphysical needs
                                        could be so easily met

by the wet gaze of a brown-and-white retriever
with a slight infection of the outer ear
                        and a tail like a windshield wiper.

I did not guess that love would be returned to me
as simply as a stick returned when it was thrown
again and again and again –
in fact, I still don't exactly comprehend.

What could that possibly have to teach me
about being human?[49]

If dogs are indeed representative of our helplessness, our vulnerability and weakness, what happens to the dogs in particular contexts may suggest to us how extreme human vulnerabilities are dealt with in that place.

In our white suburbs we indulge our dogs, we spoil them.

I write about dogs and go to a restaurant for supper. I talk about my book. The steaks are huge and expensive, and my friend and I cannot finish our food. Piously we ask for doggy bags, discussing how much our dogs like the bones that go with this particular steak. Back on the topic of the psychology of poverty, doggy bags under our arms, we walk back to our cars. A *bergie* (homeless person) approaches us. He wants money. We don't give money, we say. He points to our doggy bags, 'I can do with some food.' Without thinking, my friend replies, 'We are so sorry, our dogs love these steaks and bones, it is for them.'

We walk on.

We stop.

'I can't believe what I just said,' my friend says and turns around to find the *bergie*, who has disappeared into the darkness.

In the valley the despondency of the dogs, their apparent listlessness, their captivity, their rage, may give us a clue about how it feels to be human and vulnerable in this place. How some of the dogs are loved and cared for, some neglected and tied up, others adopted, still others used for fighting perhaps give us an indication of how people in the valley feel their vulnerabilities are dealt with.

'All knowledge, the totality of all questions and answers,' Franz Kafka said, 'is contained in the dog.'[50]

Sometimes the dogs in the valley do bark.

They bark black.

# Birth

*'There is, of course, the wonder of birth (impossible to recollect) . . .'\**

Who shouted with glee when the colour blue was born?
— Pablo Neruda, *The Book of Questions*

The history of obstetrics is the history of civilisation itself.
— David Danforth, *Obstetrics and Gynecology*

First of May. Labour Day. My phone rings at 7.30 a.m. Fifteen-year-old Karesha Kleinbooi has gone into labour. She has asked me to be her birth attendant. I rush to the hospital when I get her call. I am met by the attending nurse, Sister Joubert, a sturdy blond woman with a no-nonsense haircut and attitude. She will hear nothing about birth attendants: 'Absolutely not,' she says. 'We cannot allow birth attendants at all. If I allow it for one of them, I will have to allow it for all of them. There are five of them now in the ward and can you imagine if I let you stay with one of them? Then they will all want you or someone.'

After a long negotiation, I am allowed to visit Karesha for a few minutes.

In the maternity ward there are six beds, three on each side. Karesha has a bed on the left side, furthest from the wall. When I enter, she is sitting on a chair, hands on her stomach, staring out the window. The

---

\* The quote in the subtitle of this chapter – 'There is, of course, the wonder of birth (impossible to recollect) . . .' – is from Sen, 2005: xi.

windows are large, with wooden frames, large oak trees outside. 'Nice view,' I say clumsily as I sit down on the metal-framed bed. I look around me. The ward is clean and neat. Four of the other beds are occupied. The other women are all lying down; I only see their hair and hospital gowns under the hospital sheets. The sheets are white, decorated with blue printed text, 'Property of the Provincial Administration' written in three languages. No one is interested in me or in anyone else. Every now and again one of the blue lumps under the sheets shudders and there is a groan or a whimper and then silence again. They all seem to be in the early stages of labour, five young women thrown together, each in their very private pod of pain. 'The *lekker spannetjie* [nice little team] of the provincial administration,' as Sister Joubert told me on my arrival.

I look at Karesha. She tries to smile, but her mouth gets distorted as she has another contraction. Her eyes are wide. Her skin is blotchy. She is wearing the light blue hospital gown, but underneath it she wears bright blue pyjama bottoms, blue with yellow bears and red balloons. I ask her about her contractions, how far they are apart. 'About five minutes,' she says. There is no clock in the ward. I try to time the contractions for her. They are erratic. Sometimes they are one minute apart, sometimes five. But they are very painful, she says. I don't know what to do with these pieces of information. I hear the sounds of the nurses lunching and laughing in the tearoom next door. With every contraction, I can see the little body and the brave face contorting. She never utters a sound. As I sit there, thinking of how to help her (water, ice, juice, cold cloths, a back rub?), Sister Joubert cheerfully enters with the food trolley. 'Now you probably don't want to eat,' she says to them all. 'Because you know what will happen then.' The trolley is noisy on the hospital floor. The women stir, but no one responds. 'I want to eat,' Karesha says. The sister looks at her with raised eyebrows and brings a plate of food. White rice, orange pumpkin and brown beans.

'Are you sure? Do you know what is going to happen if you eat? What will come out first? But, if that is what you want . . .' she shrugs. 'You know what they say, the first things that come out looks like the father. And the second thing that comes out looks like the mother.'[1] She laughs. Karesha does not respond. The sister leaves. I watch Karesha trying to eat, only to be interrupted time and again by a contraction.

'*Is jy klaar?*' (Are you finished?) asks the cleaning woman who comes to collect the plate. '*Hulle eet mos nie eintlik nie*' (They don't really eat), she says to me.

The sister returns with glasses of water for everyone. 'Ten more minutes,' she says to me. 'If you stay longer, the other girls will start to talk.' Karesha takes a sip of the water. She pulls a face. 'Yuk,' she says. I wish that I could take a sip from her glass, even if just to share something with her. The woman on the next bed gets up, bends over the bed and groans; deep, desiccated groans. The hospital gown is open at the back. I can see her bare back and buttocks. I look away quickly. Karesha is having another contraction, she stretches her body and then collapses again, small on the hospital chair. I do not know where to look. Sister Joubert puts her head around the door. 'Time to leave,' she says.

I leave.

## Conception and hope

When people find out that I work on motherhood and poverty, the standard question is: 'Why do "they" have so many children?' 'Why do "they" have children when they are still at school?' 'Why don't "they" just use contraception?'

'Why do *you* have children?' I typically reply.

There are many assumptions underlying the question about why poor people have children. The one moralistic assumption is that if you are poor you should not bring an expensive baby into the world. It is often assumed that poor mothers are either naive or irresponsible. Moreover, these assumptions often include the mistaken belief that women have control over reproductive decision-making and that if there is decision-making, it is a rational, conscious process.

As with all women in all contexts, the process of becoming and being pregnant is complex in the valley.[2] Sometimes the desire to have a child is overt, but often it is not spoken about or not conscious. Sometimes the desire has to do with what a partner wants or what a family prioritises. Sometimes women feel that falling pregnant is considered the inevitable fate of being a woman. Sometimes pregnancy is consciously sought or even obsessed about.

The statistics in the record books of the clinic seem to confirm patterns that emerged in our research and clinical interviews with pregnant women and mothers. Women in the valley typically do not have more than three children.[3] Most do not have second babies in the four years after their first babies are born. The spacing of children is mostly three or four years – it is rare for a woman to have babies in consecutive years. It is also rare for a woman, young or old, to be naïve about sex and pregnancy, and most women and girls we meet know about birth control. The statistics and the interviews suggest that motherhood is either consciously planned or unconsciously regulated.

In the valley women often have their first child in their teenage years, or at least before they turn twenty.[4] They typically have this *voorkind* (literal translation: before child) before they get married or even settle with a more permanent partner. In the therapy groups conducted with thirteen-year-old girls, the girls could easily delineate what the unspoken rules are about early pregnancy. In a group focused on pregnancy they speak loudly, interrupting each other. On the tape recording of the session it is difficult to hear who the speaker is:

'Miss, there are twelve pregnant girls in the school.'

'Before, when you're expecting, they say ugly things about you . . . but when the child comes people like you a lot, and the child too . . .'

'In the beginning, they hit you and so, but when the child comes, then it's "Come to Grandma".'

'My mother will say, "Take your things and get out of here please, you can go sleep under a bridge, but I won't be your parent." But as soon as the baby comes, then "Yay"! Yes, it's true, it's true.'

'. . . the church will at first gossip about your pregnancy, but afterwards, they will take in your child. And christen him.'

'They can *klap* [smack] you, but they can't *klap* the child away.'

Uproarious laughter follows this last comment.

While pregnancy is frowned upon if you are young, motherhood seems to elicit more ambivalent feelings, even if you are young. Girls and women seem to regard motherhood as pivotal in the life of a woman. In general, it seems that falling pregnant may initially lead to dismay (in the woman, in her family and in the larger community), but becoming a mother is associated with hope.

'This brings me to the question of hope – that sense that one may become more than one presently is or was fated to be,' writes anthropologist Michael Jackson.[5] He cites Ernst Bloch who 'makes pregnancy a metaphor for this yearning for the new, this heightened anticipation of what will surprise us, or give us a new lease on life'.[6]

Many women in the valley speak about hope and the conscious decision to become pregnant.

It is clear that such conscious decisions are informed by emotions. Twenty-seven-year-old Alice, who is married and already has two daughters, talks about her emotional longing for a child. 'You experience, so after a time when you now see your second-last or maybe your *jongstetjie* [diminutive of 'youngest'] is now already big and then you can . . . you now just want a little baby again or you just feel more or less, you now just feel jealous. One badly wants to be pregnant again, then you just feel that mother instinct – you just badly want to have a little baby again.'

She says that both she and her husband are religious and they regard the expected baby as a blessing, particularly because they recently heard that it will be their first boy. 'The day I told him that it's a little boy, then he said, "Thank you Lord." The Lord heard his heart's desire.'

Even though she is excited about having another child, Alice is clear that the pregnancy is not what makes her excited. 'I will definitely also not say it's just to brag with a big tummy or so. I am just waiting for the day that the baby now arrives in the hospital and the man comes to visit . you, or the day of the homecoming and everyone is happy.'

Pienkie is a 33-year-old unmarried waitress. Her salary is small. She is adamant that she wanted a child. 'I wanted to fall pregnant, because if I can tell you . . .'. She pauses. 'My first miscarriage that I had, the circumstances were exactly like it is now at the house. I said I'm not going to spite my parents by becoming pregnant, but I wanted to see how much better they are going to look after me if I am pregnant. Then I had the miscarriage.'

She pauses again. She pauses every time she mentions the miscarriage. 'And that was very hard for me. It was a day after my birthday.'

She now talks very slowly. 'This was the only solution that I now could think of. Go get yourself a little baby, your baby will give you more *troos* [consolation]. Because nobody else wants to . . . I feel like I am still looking forward to that baby.'

There is a desire to do things differently. She talks about being an unwanted child herself and her mother leaving her with her grandmother when she was a baby. 'My mother's exact words were, "I'm not sorry that I left you with your grandmother, you know?" She told me the story again, the story of leaving me with my grandmother. For me that was painful. She wasn't married to my dad, and my dad also didn't give her that support that she needed, but my mom will make more of her other *meisiekinders* [girl children] than she makes of me. There isn't communication between me and my mom. She'll be good to the one child, and the other child must just get himself a life. I want to be better than she was. I want to do what she did not do.'

Her desire for a child and her excitement about its arrival is infused with hope. Jackson writes about hope:

> All such aspirations have their origin in the sense that something is missing in our lives, and that there is more to life than what exists for us in the here and now . . . At times we imagine that the lost object was once in our possession . . . It was there before we realized what we had; it slipped from our grasp or was stolen, leaving us to hope that it might be restored to us, as well as to dread that it is irrecoverable. At times we imagine that what we need lies ahead, promised or owed, but as yet undelivered, unrevealed, or unpaid, not yet born. In this yearning for what is missing, but that we regard as rightfully ours, lies our sense of natural justice.[7]

In Pienkie's case the desire for a child is not only related to her own wish to be comforted, but also has to do with her own yearning to be a different kind of mother.[8] She is very open about her difficult relationship with her mother and how having a child is an attempt to have a different kind of relationship.

Similarly, many young women in the community also consciously decide to have children. Anthea (fifteen years old) talks about consciously deciding to have a child when she was fourteen. 'Fourteen? Okay,' the young white student psychologist says. 'And did you talk about it, or did it just happen?'

'Actually, we did talk about it,' Anthea says.

'Really?' the interviewer says, 'Is it something you wanted?'

'Yes, but everyone thinks, like my mother and them, that it just happened, but I don't want to tell them, no.'

The student asks about contraception. 'Condoms or the injection?'

'I was never on those things,' Anthea says.

'Nothing. Okay.' The student is a bit perplexed. 'Did you talk about what will happen, if, say, you get pregnant, or did you not think about it?'

Anthea says, 'No, I knew I would get pregnant and that.'

The student interrupts. 'And, was it, was it not a problem for you? Did you want to get pregnant?'

'Yes,' Anthea says. 'Yes.'

'Did you ever tell your boyfriend you want a child?'

'Yes, I told him when his sister had a child. Now, he is older than his sister. Then he said he should have made a child first and then his sister. When his sister had a child, I was really into his sister's child and then I also wanted a child.'

The student resorts to her 'Really?' again. 'That's happy,' she continues. 'Okay, so you did not talk about contraception or so?'

Anthea does not waiver. 'He once told me to go on that stuff, then I said no, I am not going on that stuff. He told me the whole time to go to the clinic because I felt sick, so then he said I could also go for the contraception. Then I said no, I won't go. Every time I said that I won't go.'

The interview now moves on to Anthea's desire to get pregnant and her conscious attempts to get pregnant.

'So, you wanted to get pregnant?' The student is incredulous.

'We kept on once, then I went and then they told me I am not. Then we tried again and again and then it was like that.'

The student, now openly surprised, asks about the father. 'Did he know you were trying? And did he agree, he said that he also wanted a baby?'

Anthea, as young as she was, knew what she wanted. 'He first said, but what will my mother and them say, and am I convinced of this, won't I be sorry? Then I said I won't be sorry.'

In this interview the student explicitly checks all the usual assumptions about teenage pregnancy: that becoming pregnant was not talked about, that it just happened, that it was something not wanted, that it was not a decision or a joint decision to become pregnant, that contraception was not considered or discussed, that the consequences of becoming pregnant were not considered, that women have no agency in sexual matters, that young motherhood is undesirable, that falling pregnant is not a conscious and deliberate effort.[9]

Anthea introduces another narrative, one that defies the usual assumptions.[10] 'Actually, we did talk about it . . . I don't want to tell them now . . . I was never on those things . . . No, I knew I would get pregnant and that . . . I told him when his sister had a child. I was really into his sister's child and then I also wanted a child . . . He once told me to go on that stuff, then I said no, I am not going on that stuff . . . Then I said no, I won't go. Every time I said that I won't go . . . We kept on once . . . Then we tried again and again and then it was like that . . . Then I said I won't be sorry.'

While many women plan their pregnancies, other women describe pregnancies that may not have been consciously chosen or planned, but are not necessarily unwanted. This may mean that there is an unconscious wish or desire to have a baby.[11] These wishes are often complex.

Twenty-six-year-old Janine is university graduate who had her daughter, an only child, when she was thirteen years old.[12] She lives with her mother and father, her sister, her sister's thirteen-year-old son and her own thirteen-year-old daughter. The partner whom she has been with for the last year and a half has also recently moved into the house. She referred herself to therapy and is seen by a clinical Master's student in training. The therapy is initiated with the question that psychologists typically ask at the beginning of a first session.

'Um, but first, Janine, if you can tell me what brought you here?'

Janine is extremely articulate and emotionally reflective. 'Um,' she says, 'basically the feeling of restlessness, uneasiness and lately more anger than depression. It used to be more depression. It used to be anger, then sadness, and now more anger again – yes, more anger than sadness, ja. And basically, just the feeling of not being able to let go of stuff, of stuff, and ja, and not having a life. Living too much in my head.'[13]

She giggles slightly.

When asked about what causes her to feel like this, she says that there are many things. 'I think just a combination of a lot of stuff. I don't think there's only one thing. So, a lot of stuff from the past, a lot of stuff from the present, so.' She pauses. 'So, I don't think it's just one specific thing.'

'Look,' she leans forward in her chair, 'I had a baby when I was thirteen years old, so she's now also thirteen years old. Which I think might be part of the problem, um, she's growing up pretty fast.'

'Now,' Janine smiles. 'Um, ja, basically my parents gave me the option of either keeping the baby or giving her up for adoption because they only found out that I was pregnant the day that I was about to give birth. And, ja, so I guess all of that . . .'

She pauses, laughs again, nervously this time. 'All of that which is still a problem, ja, it's still a problem. I think more of me having a baby then and my parents finding out that I had a baby, but mostly me having a baby. But the baby herself is not a problem. I think anything related to that, like not telling my parents that I was pregnant and ja, also up to now they don't know who the father is. So, up to now basically my parents is helping me raise the child, and ja, so. Ja, I am . . .'

She does not finish the sentence, then goes on. 'So, ja. And then, then I guess work. Work sucks. I have a boyfriend who irritates me more than anything else, which I can't seem to get rid of. Ja, quite a lot. But I recall last year I was quite depressed, more depressed than angry. And now I feel more angry.'

She immediately links the anger to her childhood and the loss of her father's special attention. 'Um, I guess I was an angry child. I was angry at everybody always and ja. I don't know why though. When I was a kid I used to get everything I wanted and needed, so I guess all of this related to me having a child. I recall my half-brother came to stay with us. About a year or two before I had my child and I think it started then. I was about ten then. I think I used to have a happy childhood. I can't remember much about being a child, except being a tomboy. I used to play with all the boys, um ja, I don't remember much else. I think I was fine, I think more to getting a teen was more a problem for me than being a child. Ja. I just, like when I think about being a child and being a teenager, I can't really remember being a child or having difficulty then. But when I was a teen I can recall a lot of difficult stuff. Mainly my half-brother moving in. I think that was the beginning of all, of all my problems. And, ja, so I didn't know about him, so I went with my dad to go and pick him up and so all of a sudden there was just this stranger coming to stay with us. I was the baby then, so it was kind of like someone else was taking my place. It's probably not knowing about his existence and him coming to stay there. He was poor and dirty and so everyone felt pity for him and so ja. And also, I didn't know he was coming to stay then.'

Janine gets a bit tearful. 'I didn't know who he was, I think of all that sort of . . . Ja, and I don't think anyone discussed it with me, so, I suddenly started getting upset.'

Janine is now crying bitterly; she takes a tissue before continuing. 'I know I'm much older now, but it still irritates me. I don't even think it's just him – it's my dad, he had two children before the marriage and then two more in the marriage, so that's it.'

Not being the baby of the family anymore, she explains, she spent more time at her cousin's house and started a sexual relationship with him.

'Oh, back then,' she says, 'I used to spend more time back at their house than at my own house. Like the baby, like before my half-brother came to stay. Ja, and so even when he came to stay there I spent even more time there because I don't want to go home with him there, and, ja, it's kind of like he's my boyfriend, but not really, it's secret. Um, he was eighteen at the time. I was still stupid, so I didn't think of that it's wrong or, ja . . .'

She also almost immediately links her mood to losing her father's special affection when she was thirteen. Because she was not the baby anymore, she had her own baby, who immediately became the baby in the house.

Although Janine did not plan to have a child at thirteen, the baby, when she arrived, was not unwanted. After having the child, Janine settled down, stopped the relationship with her cousin, finished matric and got a university degree, the first member of her family ever to do so. Understanding that her disappointment in her father and the loss of his affection indirectly led to her becoming pregnant, she is concerned about her daughter. She again becomes tearful when she talks about this. 'So I do wish she was a little bit different to who I am, but she is much the same as I am. Ja, I definitely want it to be different for her because I don't want her going through the same stuff I did, or, ja, feeling in some way similar to how I am feeling or was feeling.'[14]

Acutely aware of the danger of history repeating itself or the 'compulsion to repeat', as we call it in psychology, Janine comes for psychological help.[15] She is clear that the root of her problem is anger, anger that she already felt before she had her child.[16]

Can we, in this case, talk about an unconscious wish for a child?

Britney is a fifteen-year-old young woman who feels ambivalent about being pregnant. While she did not consciously plan to get pregnant, she consciously stopped the contraception, ostensibly to please her boyfriend and to avoid having the cramps that she ascribed to the contraception. When asked how she is doing, she is quite straightforward. '*Spyt* [regret], on the one hand, I feel regret; on the other hand I am pleased.'

'Really? Why do you feel regret?'

'I don't want to have a baby yet,' Britney says.

The student psychologist makes the usual assumptions: 'Why? Was it an accident? And why are you happy?'

Britney is clear about her reasons for being happy. 'Because this is my first time and my grandparents and them have now accepted that I am pregnant.'

While there are many cases of babies that are not consciously planned, but were wanted, there are also cases where women do not want to fall pregnant, but it was something they had to accept.

Dewey is a highly intelligent and ambitious 21-year-old woman. Dewey is able to talk about her career plans, her decisions and actions. She was not on contraception, but still expresses that she was *verbaas* (amazed) when she found out that she was pregnant. While Dewey herself, like many women, does not see her inaction with regard to contraceptives as a certain kind of agency, it seems clear that not to do something is also, sometimes, a form of action.[17] There is power in passivity.

'We were really *verbaas*,' Dewey says laughingly. 'I don't know what I thought. Probably not that quickly . . . I did not think it will happen that quickly. Because we did not . . . it was not long after we started being sexually active that I became pregnant. It was probably a month, then I found out I was pregnant. I actually hoped that it would take longer to get pregnant. My mother told me that she got pregnant with me the first time she had sex. So, I hoped it would not happen to me like this.'

Pregnant Pauline is also 21 years old, a bit oblivious about her pregnancy. In a two-year relationship with the father of the baby, she shares a room with her mother, her three siblings (all younger than 21) and her nephew and niece, now toddlers. Her brother gets a weekly salary and she helps out in the vineyard now and again. There is no other income. She knows about rearing a child; she has helped to take care of nephews and nieces and cousins. Although a bit annoyed that her younger sister had a baby before her, she did not consciously try to get pregnant. Her mother told her it will happen when it will.

Pauline is interviewed by a 21-year-old coloured graduate student. The interview is punctuated with lots of laughter, a bit raucous at times. However, the student writes in her journal that she was quite shocked about Pauline's attitude. 'She was,' she writes, 'almost *rustig* [tranquil] about the baby's arrival. It is almost as if she did not want the baby, but that she knew that she had to get pregnant sooner or later. Her sister had a baby at fifteen.' The interviewer also writes that she is shocked about the house in which the baby will be raised: 'For me it was a shock to see that a baby must be born in such circumstances, a shock also that it really does not bother them. That is what they are used to; the baby will also get used to it.'

Pauline was initially unaware that she was pregnant, even though she went through her sister's pregnancy and childbirth (her sister is now eighteen). It was her twelve-year-old brother who convinced her to go to the clinic when she was about three months pregnant. She tells a story that makes her and the interviewer laugh. 'And one day I now sat here and I hear the children say to me, "But you now are getting really fat." I say, "No, what fat? I don't even have a lot of fat." Now they just say, "No, you are getting fat." Now I am wearing a little miniskirt. My mother says, "You look *darem baie snaaks* [really very funny]." I say, "No, I don't look funny." But I feel my breasts, they feel as if they are out. Then I think, goodness, maybe my mother is right. But then my sister also says to me, "You really are getting fatter. I am not wrong, you who always were so skinny." I say, "*Nee, jong, julle almal lieg vir my* [No, man, you are all lying to me]." I have a little brother, in Grade 6 now. He said to me, "Nana, I look now at Nana so, but the nipples of Nana's breasts look now different." Now I ask, "Now what does it look like now?" He says, "It is black now." I say, "But Nana does not know why it is black." Now he says, "Nana has to go to the clinic." Now I am scared of the clinic. I don't like things like that. He says he will take me to the clinic in the morning.'

She says that her little brother and boyfriend took her to the clinic the next day. 'The sister tested me then and she puts that *klop ding* [heart monitor] here on my stomach. My little brother then says, "Do you hear now, Nana, I told you that you are pregnant, because there is the heart beating." Then only did I understand that the sister is saying that I am pregnant. Then I asked her, but how can the people see it now? Then she said sometimes one can see it on your nipples and on your shape, your body gets swollen. Then it also came to me, but now I can't even say how it happened.'

Pauline's apparent denial of her pregnancy is not unique. We often come across women who only disclose their pregnancies to partners, friends, health-care workers and employers in the last months of pregnancy, often claiming that they themselves only became aware of their pregnancies at this time. This failure to disclose pregnancy is so common that there is a saying in the region '*langs die pad kraam*' – this literally means 'giving birth next to the road' – referring to a woman who gives birth unexpectedly, without anyone knowing that she was in labour.[18]

In the psychological literature, this phenomenon is called undisclosed pregnancy.[19] Psychologists have speculated a great deal about the possible reasons women may have for obscuring pregnancies,[20] with feminists emphasising that what is 'kept at bay' by pregnant women who do not acknowledge their pregnancies is knowledge of the female body.[21]

In the valley many of the women who did not acknowledge being pregnant to themselves or others, retrospectively said that being pregnant is a problem and a burden, an anxiety-provoking experience that elicited feelings of guilt and shame. They emphasise societal attitudes and responses to pregnancy, with their own subjective experiences of pregnancy being subsumed by their expectations of how their significant others and employers would respond.

The women in the valley, like so many people who are socially and politically disempowered, are often forced to make use of very rigid defence mechanisms in their efforts to keep a job, a partner, church membership and sometimes even a home.[22] For disempowered people it may become necessary to deny, cut off or split off parts of themselves that do not fit the expectations of their communities or society.[23] In the valley, the necessity to obscure might be related to different factors: a long history of political disempowerment, the community's position in the economic system (poor or economically disempowered) and/or their position in a patriarchal society (the maternal body being experienced as threatening to a neat and rational social order).[24] This is especially true for young women in a context where their sexuality is denied and their submissiveness to adult authority is expected and assumed.

If low-income women's position in society and their subsequent need to deny and repress certain feelings are highlighted during pregnancy, this is even more the case when anticipating childbirth and during labour.

## Pregnancy and dread

Every woman partakes in the chain of guardianship and transmission . . . Tell me and let me tell my hearers what I have heard from you who heard it from your mother and your grandmother, so that what is said may be guarded and unfailingly transmitted to the women of tomorrow, who will be our children and the children of our children.

— Trinh T. Minh-Ha, *Woman, Native, Other:*
*Writing Postcoloniality and Feminism*

Therefore my loins
Are seized with trembling;
I am gripped by pangs
Like a woman in travail,
Too anguished to hear,
Too frightened to see.
My mind is confused,
I shudder in panic.
My night of pleasure
He has turned to terror.
— Isaiah 21:3–4

Over the years, I have heard detailed stories of pregnancy and childbirth from many women in the valley. These stories capture many of the issues prominent in becoming a mother when you are poor. There are hints of how the practices, rituals and myths related to pregnancy, birth and motherhood are not only extremely personal and very local, but also profoundly ideological. Their stories show how, when women become mothers, 'these seemingly natural processes of swelling, bearing and suckling, the flows of blood, semen and milk are constituted and fixed not just by the force of cultural conception but by the coagulation of power'.[25] During pregnancy and childbirth, human attempts, human rituals and human language are used to gain control over an embodied process that seems to be regarded as chaotic and fragmented.[26]

In the valley, while motherhood is mostly anticipated with excitement and joy, childbirth is commonly anticipated with dread, fear and apprehension. The inevitability of suffering and pain seems to be accepted. Notions such as maternal satisfaction and birth planning are notably absent from the narratives.[27] There are no rosy fantasies about childbirth in this community.

If you are poor in the valley, life begins in the maternity ward of the local provincial hospital. In our interviews with mothers we become aware of the fact that the wonder of birth certainly is not obvious to our research participants. The maternity ward is mostly depicted as a kind of torture chamber. In an interview, one young woman described the delivery room as '*die kamer met die skêre en die messe en al daai dinge*' (the room with the scissors and the knives and all those things).[28]

Pregnant Millicent is nineteen. She is a slight girl with big eyes and talks about how she dreads labour. It is all about what 'they' say. 'They tell you what happens when you don't dress yourself warmly if you are pregnant.' She laughs. 'Because they say if you are barefoot, then you get, they call it dry cramps or pains that you get. But it is terrible. It is very terrible. And they don't want me to get such pains and so . . . one friend of mine was pregnant for nine months, nine months she was pregnant and then she walked another month. She should have given birth in the ninth month, but then it was the tenth month with the baby and then she just let the hospital give her the pains. And then they said those pains that they give you are worse than the ordinary pains that you get, so I have to be careful. I have to be careful of a caesarean.'

She speaks louder. 'And I have already had a *voorsmakie* [literally: little fore-taste] of this with my miscarriage, my threatening miscarriage.' She now pauses after every phrase. 'It was the needles and the drip and it was very painful. And I did not eat, just through the drip, and I was very nauseous and I had to have intravenous feeding and I can't eat a lot if I am under pressure. And for those two days I did not eat. My face was kind of pale.' She laughs. 'Of hunger.' Another laugh. 'And all the people eat and drink tea in front of you. And I, I just pulled the blanket over my head.'

In anticipating labour, Millicent provides a catalogue of anticipated ordeals: pain, cramps, aches, nausea, hunger, isolation, injections, nurses, needles, drips. She states that one must be careful and offers a whole list of admonitions and advice, from how to dress (dress warmly and don't go barefoot) to how to be (staying calm and tranquil, don't act out and don't be nervous). She says that with her *voorsmakie* when she was hospitalised with a threatening miscarriage, she dealt with the dread by pulling a blanket over her head, maybe suggesting that the best way to cope is to repress the dread.

When the women of the valley talk about their anticipation of birth, they depict it with very much the same anticipation of horror that we hear in the depictions of childbirth from the prophets of the Old Testament.[29]

I remember, as a child, listening with terror to the Dutch Reformed *dominee* (preacher) reading Genesis 3:16: 'To the woman he said, "I will make your pains in childbearing very severe; with painful labour you will give birth to children. Your desire will be for your husband, and he will rule over you."'[30]

In this community, the labouring woman is associated with physical and emotional vulnerability. The women anticipate childbirth with horror,[31] expecting pain and panic, fear and helplessness, chaos and confusion.[32] In the words of one valley woman, Abigail, who is anticipating that her partner will not be with her during childbirth: 'But now that I really need him, and he wanted to be with me, he can't be with me, but like my mom says what is written in the Bible, the woman will have pain and the man will go and work.'

When talking about their anticipation of labour, the women speak about being afraid. It seems that what they fear most is the pain. Alice says, 'It is only the pain, the pain is all, yes.' Makeila says that this time she is feeling nervous. 'It feels so long ago. It is just the pains that one has that are so sore.' Thirty-one-year-old Sonblom is pregnant with her second child. 'I am a bit scared . . . Now after twelve years. I don't know. We will see. The pain.' She laughs nervously. Ria also is scared: 'I get scared, myself . . . now that it is closer to the time, I am just so very scared.' Jean also talks about fear: 'I am a little scared. No, no. My friends, those who already have children, they say, oh, it is sore, and this and that, and they talk me into being scared.' When asked how she feels about giving birth, Shireen says, 'A little scared. They just say that it is very painful.' Elize is also a frightened. 'It is the first time,' she says.

Fear seems to be pervasive when talking about childbirth. The term '*bietjie bang*' (a little scared) seems to be the standard way of expressing the fear. It is okay to present the fear, but only if the qualifier '*bietjie*' (a little) is also there. Some of the women, however, acknowledge that they were more than a *bietjie bang*. Young pregnant women articulate more intense anxieties.

Pauline is tall, lean and muscular, but has images of being broken: 'I am already so scared if I think *ek moet nou . . . nate breek* [I must now . . . tear seams] and so and I am very *saggeaard* [sensitive]. *Vir my lyk dit ek gaan seker dood as ek moet geboorte gee* [To me it looks as if I am surely going to die if I have to give birth].' She laughs, a little anxiously. 'But then I went to the sister at the clinic and I told her I was *bietjie bang* [a little scared]. Then she told me no, it is your first baby, you must just trust in the Lord and say to him that he should put his strong hand in your weak hand and then you will see, you will go through it yourself. And she says, she says I must just give my co-operation there at the hospital. Then I will not suffer so.'

Jenna, one of the youngest pregnant women we encounter, is fourteen years old and excited to have a baby, as it means she will get a bed in the two-roomed house, not merely the couch. She also says that she fears the day of giving birth: 'of having pain. I know people talk, it is very . . . it is very sore and you tear and all those things. And sometimes they cut you. It scares me!' She continues, 'I don't know how bad it is, but I know they say it is sore. I don't know . . . My mother said about the blood and stuff and I don't know pain.'

Dewey, resigned to having fallen pregnant so quickly, is also anxious about what is going to happen. 'I am really scared,' she says, 'of the pain.' She pauses. 'And if I can cope with everything and so. The people that talk. They make me scared the most. The pain.' She pauses again. 'And all the stuff. I am not someone who likes pain. I can't bear pain. I am very *kleinserig* [have a low pain threshold]. The people say it is very sore if you tear. And if they work on you. If they close you up. They do it without you being asleep or so. My mother does not talk so much. She just once said it is sore, it is bitter pain with one foot in the grave and the other one on the other side. I told her not tell me about how sore it is. The stories scare me, I said to her.'

Dewey lost her baby at seven months.

Part of the local talk about childbirth is the phrase '*een voet in die graf en die ander voet buite die graf*' (one foot inside the grave and the other foot outside the grave) – in other words, it is said that childbirth is a matter of life and death. One foot in the grave seems to be a common image. Eighteen-year-old Nathalie also uses this image, saying that she knows about childbirth because her two friends went through it. She laughs, 'They say you will make it or you won't.'

There also is a pervasive theme of '*die mense vertel*' (the people tell), '*hulle sê*' (they say) and '*hulle praat*' (they speak), suggesting that there is a general tendency for people to talk about childbirth and to frighten expectant mothers. It is clearly women (friends and mothers) who are the tellers of these frightening stories. It is not clear why women tell such stories to each other. The women themselves speculate about the impact of the stories. Pauline says that she is annoyed with people who scare her: 'I just thought by myself, *hulle praat jou nou mos bang* [their stories make you scared]. And now, now I don't pay attention anymore because I came back from my friends and asked my mother how it is. And I can't listen to stories or show fear, now that my sister who is younger than me beat me by pushing out that bigger child of hers. No, I can't. Then my mother said I don't have to be scared, it is not as sore as people say.'

Not everyone is so scared. Feisty twenty-year-old Suzanne resignedly says that it will be a lot of pain. 'Then I say, no, I am looking forward more to it coming. If the pain comes at that time, I hope I can take it. The pain I can take. If the pain comes, it has to come. Other women go through it, so what does it matter? I look forward to when they give the baby to me. Otherwise I am not afraid or fearful.'

Sana, a 28-year-old domestic worker, is expecting her third child and is one of the few (if not the only) women we come across who does not feel affected by all the stories. However, even this rather resilient and confident woman eventually felt disempowered in the process of childbirth. For instance, she was not allowed to have her husband with her, even though she planned to have him there.

In the women's conversations prior to birth, vulnerability – rather than control – is highlighted.[33] While there is a huge emphasis on birthing plans in the psychological and popular literature about childbirth, the women of the valley seldom explicitly talk about birth plans. However, there is a clear understanding that the best way to cope with childbirth is to hand over control to the medical staff. Paradoxically, rumour has it that if you are scared and nervous, you should try to appear calm and peaceful, so as to ensure that unwanted medical procedures are not inflicted upon you. The advice is that it is best to be acquiescent, compliant, obedient and co-operative.

Millicent says that she especially worries about the nurses. 'They say I must keep myself calm. I should not go on like the other women when they work on me. I must keep myself *rustig* [tranquil]. But if I am going to go on and if I am nervous, then I can just forget. *Then,*' she stresses the word, '*then* they will do things to me that I don't want.' She pauses. 'Don't be *hardgebak* [stubborn] if they work on you. The best is to work with them. If I give my co-operation, then everything will go well. You must just do what they say.'

Rumours about the nurses are rife. Dewey talks about the one girl that told her that when she tore, 'they just sewed her up like that'. The girl said that the sister worked very roughly, but was nice to her, 'which is better, sometimes they are rough and they are nasty'. Dewey also has been told by her mother that one should not be *hardgebak* [stubborn] when they work roughly.

Punishment, according to Bianca, is inevitable if you don't co-operate. 'They say if you don't lie still, then they will strap you up . . . You must just do what they say.'

Wilmien, an older married farmworker with two children, seems to summarise the general attitude to childbirth. 'Childbirth is heavy, but every woman has to go through it. To give birth is the cross that every woman must bear, but she must listen and learn and do what the doctors say, then everything will go well.'

It seems that there is an underlying but quite profound mistrust of medical personnel and medical procedures. Thus, even before the women actually enter the ward, there is a set-up in which the patient is the lone victim; she has to be compliant, obedient, acquiescent. The nurse is not an accomplice or collaborator, but potentially a cruel persecutor or a benign torturer. Medical procedures are anticipated with dread. Strikingly, there is no anticipation of care.[34]

Of course, one wonders what the impact of the fear and dread are on the actual experience of labour. Pregnant Ankie is annoyed by the rumours and their impact. 'The things they tell you,' she says, 'the things they tell you make you *nogal bietjie bang* [just a little bit afraid]. I think one should just experience it for yourself. One should not let other people make you anxious with their talk. Because if people make you anxious, then you of course go into it *bang-bang* [scared-scared]. Then you also can't help yourself.'

The fear is paralysing and disempowering.

## Childbirth and vulnerability

> Who gives [birth]? And to whom is it given?[35] Certainly, it doesn't feel
> like giving, which implies a flow, a gentle handing over, no coercion
> . . . Maybe the phrase was made by someone viewing the results only
> . . . Yet one more thing that needs to be renamed.
>
> — Margaret Atwood, 'Giving Birth'

Clinic statistics seem to suggest that the beginning of life in the valley
is not life threatening. Babies are mostly healthy at birth; there are
relatively few babies of low birth weight.[36] Most births are vaginal.
Caesareans are rare.[37] There seem to be relatively few infant deaths and
miscarriages. Most mothers seem to breastfeed for a year or longer. When
talking about childbirth, most prominent for women is the physical
pain, the feelings of disempowerment and humiliation, and a profound
sense of loneliness.

### *Pain and vulnerability*

When women in the valley talk about childbirth, they mostly speak about
pain and how they tried to defend against the pain while in labour.[38] They
describe giving birth as a moment of profound physical and emotional
vulnerability. While all birth stories are unique, it is striking how the
words women use to describe the experience are similar.

'I won't say, um, yes, it was – how can I say? – nothing that I expected.
Many people told me that every woman experiences her own pain and
everyone's birth is different. I thought I would be so strong, that I can
make it. But I came through it. For me it was very bad. I never realised,
I always said, nothing is more painful than toothache, and wow, it was
much more. I always thought why would people go for birth if it's that
bad? That is why I thought it's just a very easy process. I never realised it's
so bad, but like I feel now I'll probably never give birth again.'

In trying to write about the pain that the women experience, I
lose their names. Inadvertently I make them lose their identities, their
individuality, their humanity. I feel like the conductor of a macabre
speech chorus.

Despite the fact that most of the women anticipated pain, many
of them emphasised the fact that nothing could prepare them for the

severity of the pain and that they had no idea how painful birth would be.

'I never knew it was so sore. I didn't know it would be so *vrek seer* [damn sore]. I didn't know it would be so sore.'

'I thought everyone just talks you into being scared and so on . . .'

'I didn't know it would be that bad.'

'No. I thought it would be easy, but it was difficult.'

In trying to describe the pain, many of the women remarked that the pain was beyond description, beyond words, beyond comprehension.[39]

'Nobody will understand how sore it is.'

'It's very sore yes. You can't tell anybody how sore it is. You must rather go through that yourself.'

After childbirth, many women relate that the pain was so severe that they thought that they were going to die.

'The birth I will tell you is *vrek seer* [damn sore]. I almost died.'

'It was one foot in the grave. It's very sore.'

'Now, at four centimetres it already feels as if you want to die.'

Others said that it felt as if they were going to faint, to go crazy or as if they were moving into a state of total regression. They said that they were losing touch with reality.

'At first it was a light tummy pain, but then it felt as if I was going to faint.'

'She promised that I would faint because it is was so bad. But the pain just went on. So sore.

'It was just different, the pain, it seems you can go crazy.'

'Because at a time then it felt to me I can now go off my head.'

'I sat naked. I rolled naked on the ground just for that cold because it is so sore. It is almost like hot flushes that come over you.'

To describe the intensity of the pain the women use words like *seer* (sore), *bitter seer* (bitterly sore), *vrek seer* (damn sore), *brandpyn* (burning pain), *skietpyn* (shooting pain), *erg* (terrible), *anderster* (different), *rooi* (red) and *baie seer* (very sore).[40]

Very few of the women (if any) said that it is a pain that one forgets. In a community where secrets are rife,[41] and suppression and repression are standard defences, the severity of birth pains is something that most women remember.

'I can never forget it, it is worse than a *vuishou* [punch with a fist].'

'Many people say, you forget about the pain quickly and then you go on. But I don't believe in that. Because if I have pain, I remember it for a very long time.'

While some women do try to describe the pain, they mostly claim that it is beyond description. When talking about the pain, they therefore frequently describe it in terms of how they responded to the pain. The women are remarkably forthcoming in relating these moments of extreme vulnerability and powerlessness and there are many instances of women simply abandoning themselves to the pain. In the background of these accounts the maternity ward lurks as a desolate place where the disorder of pain and few attempts to manage it render the would-be mothers temporarily helpless and hopeless.

The response to pain that is the most prevalent in the descriptions is screaming (*skree, skreeu, raas*).

'And I did. I screamed. I began to scream . . .'

'Then when I came there and then they said to me, "*Jy kom nog raas-raas aan hierso* [You arrive here making a noise]."'

'And then later when I couldn't anymore, I just screamed at the sisters.'

'I now didn't want to make terrible noise, but I now screamed *voluit* [at the top the voice].'

'My mom ran out because I screamed too much.'

'After a time, then I went to lie down again and so my mother woke up, because then I started to scream, because the pain is now really bad.'

Some women remember that they cried rather than screamed – and for some this distinction is important:

'You can't do otherwise, you want to cry.'

'I cried, but I didn't scream.'

Because the pain in the moment seems to be beyond words, it is often expressed physically.

'You can climb up the roof, climb the wall or something. Just want to walk, jump off the steps!'

'So all the time when that pain came I maybe held onto the chair or I started pulling my hair or something like that.'

'Because I got hold of them their hands and their fingers and twisted everything because it is sore, it was too sore.'

'I grabbed everything that was close to me.'

'It went difficult, because when the pain comes, then I pull at someone.'

'I bit my lips but they got so swollen so.'

'I started pulling my hair.'

The women describe some of the urges they feel and the things they do during childbirth as them being 'difficult' or 'resistant' or 'disobeying instructions'.

'I was just, I became difficult because the pain was so bad.'

'Yes, they put on the heart machine and so, and that I also wanted to rip off.'

While most accounts of childbirth are of physical abandonment and helplessness, some women do talk about trying to take control, despite the fact that preparation for childbirth seems non-existent.[42]

'Then I said to my mom, "Mommy, I'm going to push now."'

'And began to let my breath go in and out like that, lightly in and out. Blow out and draw in and so I made it easier for myself.'

'But the pain was very bad, I breathed a lot, they said I must breathe hard and so.'

'And the breathing also helped. He dropped down, he dropped, he dropped lower. Like some people just lie and nothing happens, and they now sit all the time with the pain. To help yourself it is very good.'

It is rare that a woman actually talks about getting support for addressing the pain.

'Then she rubbed my back. I began to throw up. Then she rubbed my back until my godmother came. Then my godmother rubbed my back the whole time and then my *ouma* [grandmother] came and my mom. *Ouma* washed me.'

Some of the women relate the fact that during labour the pain renders one hopeless; there is no comfortable place left.

'It was very long. It is pain that you can't stand. It feels you want to tear your hair out of your head and so. You don't know how to stand, how to lie. You can't walk, you can't lie down. I was on the toilet later.

I didn't even care about the dirt and the germs. It was so sore I just collapsed on the toilet.'

'Then I couldn't anymore. They waited for my water to break. Usually a woman's water breaks. Then I couldn't anymore. I was about eight centimetres far, then they felt up in me again.'

'I can't anymore, I can't anymore. They still wanted me to walk then my mom said they must now do something for me, they must do something now, because I was screaming then. I was screaming that I can't anymore.'

'And then later, then I couldn't anymore, then I was tired, then I couldn't anymore. Then I couldn't anymore.'

'Then I couldn't anymore.'

'What I said, but Lord, help me!'

Most of the women, just after giving birth, are quite sure that they don't want a baby again, or certainly not soon again.

'Then I said, no, I will never go fetch a little baby again. It is too sore. It is terribly sore. This is why I say I'm never going to fetch a little baby again. It's very sore. I don't know, maybe I'll feel different in ten years time, for now, I feel now because the memories of the pain are there, I will say not again, not again, yes. Because it is too sore. The pains are too sore. It was very sore, yes.'

'But the way I feel now, I will probably never give birth again.'

Despite the obvious severity of the pain and the declared intention not to go through it again, mothers, almost to a person, see the pain as an inevitable and even natural part of childbirth, an experience that is not avoidable. In other words, pain should be endured, confronted, tolerated and accepted as part of becoming a mother: 'n vrou moet daar deur gaan (a woman has to go through it).[43]

'Then I had to just now accept pains, just now accept it just like that. Because it is . . . you can't do anything about it, you have to accept it.'

'I could just go on with it, in a way. Nobody's really going to help. The sister also tells you that you must push through.'

'You must just stand your man.'

'I suppose it's also natural, every woman must probably just go through it.'

"But everyone must go through it, every woman must go through it.'

'No, every woman must go through it.'

'You must just accept the pains, just like . . . You can't do anything about it. You must just accept it.'

Sometimes it was apparent that birth was regarded as a kind of endurance test, a competition between women about how much could be endured and tolerated.

'People told me . . . some people said it hurts if they think back, others said no, it's a good feeling. You feel like a woman, while you go through that pain. But I have, like I say, I felt I'll make it. I'm strong enough to make it, pain isn't that bad for me.'

'Then I think my little sister did it and she is younger.'

'Then you think about your friends who also lay here. And then you know, you must just push through, yes.'

'Yes, and um, how can you say, the best of all is I kept my pain in. I didn't go on like the other women. They say you have to work with the pain.'

In their birth narratives, the women describe a loss of control and a moment of profound vulnerability. They talk about losing touch with the self, with reality and with others. Childbirth is described as a moment of dissociation or of near-death. This loss of control is maybe also suggested in the fact that the pain leaves the women wordless during birth, but also without language or narrative when trying to talk about it.[44]

My research assistant, a gutsy and clever 22-year-old, works through the manuscript of the book and writes me an email. '*Ek het elke hoofstuk geskei en maak nou Labour netjies. En het besluit ek gaan nooit geboorte gee nie*' (I have separated each chapter and am now tidying up Labour. And I've decided that I'm never giving birth).

## Regulation and control

While most of the birth narratives that we hear are stories of disorder and loss of control, the focus of medical staff working in hospitals is typically to control the process. In obstetric textbooks, the process of labour and delivery is typically broken up into stages and phases, with a partogram being used to graphically evaluate the progress of labour at each stage.[45] According to the principle of active management of labour, the maternal body and the process of labour undergo a reconceptualisation and a functional redesign, according to a universal standard. The ideal childbirth is considered ordered, surveillant, technocratic and risk averse.[46]

In the public hospital where the women of the valley typically give birth, there also seems to be four stages of labour: the stage of walking the corridors, the stage of ringing bells and screaming, actually giving birth and then the loneliness.

### Walking the corridors: The absence of the gaze

Pregnant women from the valley are usually dropped off at the hospital by a friend or a neighbour who has a car. This typically seems to be the only 'planning' that happens – 'How will I get to the hospital?' The process of giving birth seems to start with the instruction from nursing staff to walk the hospital corridors. What 'they' (the nurses) want seems to be incontestable and irrefutable. When 'the kid's head is out', the nurses are alerted by the patient screaming or ringing the bell above her bed. An older mother of three, Lea's experience is quite typical: 'I went in to the hospital and when I got there they saw that the baby is only four centimetres still, too far. So, I had to walk up and down in the corridors. And the sisters said to me, if I feel it coming, then I have to go and lie on the labour bed . . . [47] And when they saw that the baby is still too far, I just had to walk up and down the corridors.'

Pienkie talks about a similar experience: 'You must walk the corridors and you can't lie down.'

Alice comments on the notable absence of nurses in the early stages of birth. 'No, they're not with you. They go their own ways until you ring the bell or scream. Then only do they come. Because I pushed until the kid's head was out and then I rang the bell. Because they don't want you to push beforehand.'

The women talk about feeling forgotten, lost and lonely in their pacing of the corridors.[48] Patients report that without the nursing staff's attention, they experience a sense of isolation and loneliness.[49] Wilmien's recollection seems to indicate a profound sense of being alone during the birth process. 'The sister, they only said to me, "Look here, it is like this. You must help yourself now."'

Rose says, 'I was actually on my own, helped myself and he's so small, I so struggled with him. She simply said if the pains come I should push. And I shouldn't push like this, I should push like that. She did not really help me . . . I wouldn't say she was nasty, just, you're almost on your own.'

Suzanne also expresses this sentiment. 'No one will understand how sore it is and I walk with the pain and you have to walk like that until ten centimetres. That is how it works – until ten centimetres, you must walk with your pains. Now, by four centimetres, it already feels as if you are dying. Then you still have to do those six before they do something to you. You have to walk up and down in the corridors and you can't lie down. Nothing is done. You feel as if no one worries. But they do not give you anything, they can give you nothing. You simply have to walk until the pains come. And then I could not any longer, then I was about eight centimetres and then they felt up in me again. Then I said, "Oh I can't anymore, I can't anymore". They still wanted to make me walk, but my mother said they should do something for me now because by then I was screaming. They do not care about you.'

Despite the fact that women often said that they feel abandoned and neglected during this stage of labour, this 'procedure' of pacing is understood by both staff and nurses to be to the benefit of the women in labour. The patients themselves think of this as a procedure – it is thought to accelerate the labour and relieve the pain.[50]

'I just walked up and down in the corridor. It loosens things. It makes things move down. Down and more down. Towards the vagina.'

'They gave me nothing for the pain. I just walked, up and down . . . if one sits still then the pain gets worse, but if you walk.'

'No. No. They didn't want to give me medicine. They said that they don't have . . . I got on to the bed and then again off when the pain came. I couldn't walk, but when I lay down the pain came. Then I got up and then I go on like this, but I didn't walk. Then they said, "Oh, *ja-nee* [yes-no], just get up every time when the pain comes."'

*Summoning the medical gaze: Screams and bells*
The implicit routine of the hospital dictates that the nurses can be summoned once the baby's head has emerged.[51]

'You know the story of when you must push and when you shouldn't. And then I just screamed at the sister and then she came and asked me if I am ready to give birth.'

'I screamed, and when they got to me, then the head was emerging, and they told me to push.'

Often the women's appeals for attention (whether they are ringing the bell, screaming or asking) are not taken seriously. 'I screamed for them. They didn't want to help me. I told them that I want to make a poo. The poo could not come out, so I went to the toilet. They told me to wait and wait. Then I went to the toilet and the cleaner came and fetched the doctor . . . It was the child who wanted to come. And then, only then did they help me, they did not want to help me immediately . . . they did not worry when I told them I had a poo . . . And then his head was already out. And then I went to lie down and then the sisters came immediately. There was a young girl, she was about eighteen or something . . . the nurse cursed and screamed at that girl. She was in the ward and then she said that she can see the baby coming. She was sitting on her bed with her legs pulled up. I said, "I can see the head from my bed" and the bell at her bed was broken. I then rang my bell and the same sister screamed at me because I rang my bell. And I then said to her, "But there is the head of the baby." . . . Then they made that girl walk to the theatre. And I said, "What if the baby fell out in the corridor, what would she have done then?"'

Ilse had to struggle to convince the nurses that it was time to lie down on a bed – the bed that would guarantee her the right to the gaze (surveillance and intervention). 'I told the sister, I can't last any longer, the pains are stronger. She says to me, "No, but the child lies only six centimetres far." I say, "But it does not feel as if he lies six centimetres far, he feels quite close already" . . . They say I must walk in the corridor. I say, "I can't walk anymore." Now if it comes it feels as if you have a pee or a poo . . . I say, "I can feel the child is coming." And I went to lie down and when I pushed, I felt something exploding . . . I felt a warmth coming . . . I felt, I felt, but here, here is his head coming and there is not a nurse, no one with me. And I tell them, "But I am going to push now," and I did and when I pushed he came. When they got to me he was pushed out already. They only had to cut the umbilical cord . . . I had a normal labour.'

But even on the bed, the domain from which she can demand the gaze, she still cannot rely on the gaze being there. Her loneliness during the labour seems to be almost taken for granted when she states, 'I had a normal labour.'

There are many accounts of women going through the final moments of birth by themselves – when the bell was broken, the screams not followed up or the appeals not attended to.

Thirty-year-old Lea already has a five-year-old daughter. She lives in a house with only her husband and daughter, shares a bedroom with her husband and could afford to stop working, as her husband's income was sufficient. She clearly planned this pregnancy and is clear that she does not plan to have another child. She has more agency than many women of the valley. Her stories are laced with a wicked and even macabre sense of humour. She is indignant about being left alone by the nurses during labour. 'The nurses all went to lunch. They said to me that if I feel it coming, I should scream to them for help because you just ring a bell and then they come. But then I thought, you are having a nice lunch and I must lie here. You can't leave a person alone on a labour bed.'

Laughingly, she recalls how she decided to play a trick on the nurses, to only call them after the baby was born. 'You go almost three rooms away and if you ring the bell and they don't hear you, you have to jump up and scream for them to come and help you. So, I thought, today I want to show you a nasty thing, so when I screamed for help and they got to me they all ran around the bed, because the baby, the baby's head was already out, then the worst was over . . . Because there you lie and you lie wide open. And I said to her, "But you told me that I should help myself and when I feel something coming, I should scream for you." Now the sisters laugh with me and I said, "You said I should scream for help. I told you I wanted to show you a thing."'

However, even Lea is less humorous when she talks about the feeling of being abandoned that she experienced after the birth. '*Jy kom nou huis toe, dan voel jy net soos hulle jou daar gelos het*' (You now come home, then you feel just like they left you there).[52]

The nursing staff's absence often is experienced as a punishment. 'She turned her back on me and walked out, that is all she did, was turning her back on me. And I felt terrible.'

'They told me that he should be born by five o'clock. Yes, they said that if he wasn't born by five o'clock, then they will leave me. Oh, so I pushed. And then ten past they said to me, "No, you gave birth well."'

When we ask the nurses working in the maternity ward about this, they are clear that while leaving the patient to be on her own during the early stages of labour is standard procedure, leaving patients during the second stage of labour is used and experienced as a type of sanction or punishment.[53]

Over the years, I have heard endless accounts of verbal violence in which women reported incidents of sarcasm, scolding, shouting, being ridiculed, being blamed and seemingly intentional humiliation. Women talk about being blamed for their behaviour during labour (for being messy, for acting like savages, for being disobedient), but it seems that female sexuality is attacked in crude and aggressive ways.[54] 'They told me to lie down, but I could not. I could not hold it anymore. So, I sat up straight. Then the sister came and told me to lie down, because I am messing everything up.'

'If the people perhaps cry or scream, then they tell you they did not tell you to get pregnant – you have to accept your pains. "*In soos 'n piesang, uit soos 'n pynappel* [In like a banana, out like a pineapple]" is what they say.'

'And the nurses are all right, but some of them are very strict. They shout at you: "Open your *boude* [buttocks]." And okay, they did not say this to me, but many of them are very rude, because this is any woman's struggle. It is not necessary to hurt them. Like in "Yes, open your legs. You had no problems opening your legs when you slept with a man." It hurts me a little . . . many women, it touches them, man. It hurts them, it hurts them emotionally. I heard them doing that to another girl because before I went into labour, I walked down the corridor. Then I heard at the door.'

In this public hospital in South Africa '*skel*' (harsh scolding) seems to be standard maternity ward procedure for the controlling and managing of the patient in labour.[55] 'Yes, I've often seen that, seen a sister scold a patient. And then, I'm unhappy about it, but I don't talk about it, I keep it to myself.'

However, it seems that even those who do think it is problematic tend to normalise the scolding of the nursing staff. 'And I've often seen that, she should have known what's coming.'

'So I will tell her, don't worry, the sister only scolded you because your baby is so important. Because if the sister didn't try to deliver your baby, the baby could've died, or something could've happened to him. So, the sister didn't want that to happen, that's why she was a bit rude to you.'

Harsh language is often used in a light or joking way and is often not found offensive by the labouring women. The jokes seem to be a form of managing or controlling the birth process. In the words of one of the nurses, disturbed by how young patients are treated by a sister: 'We get many that are sixteen, seventeen, eighteen. "Why did you not listen to what your mother said to you?" They throw words at them, say things that hurt them. And one actually needs support during that time. They are in pain, they cannot help what happened. Last year there were such cases, where children came in and the sister didn't speak to them nicely. One doesn't feel good about that and then you say to the sister, she shouldn't be so serious with them. Tell them what they should know, but not, do it in a proper way, don't be rude to the patients.'

The violence is not only verbal. Physical violence is also witnessed or experienced in the maternity ward. Patients are slapped and pinched or simply handled quite roughly. 'Because they work very badly with the girls. Very poorly. Especially if you are a girl and you are not married, and you arrive there. Then they are rough with you. And especially the black girls. They are hit, if they do not want to open their buttocks or if they don't want to push, then they're hit between the buttocks. This they do. Now who wants to be hit if they already are in pain? You can't do it like that.'

'The sister takes her fingers and pushes them up in you, then she feels, she is practically digging – sorry that I tell it to you like this. Then it is so painful. But they were not too bad. They just, they just are, it almost is, it is sore, and you have to stand your man. I mean if I keep my legs closed then they will dig, then I keep closed and then it is "Open your legs." Now, not nasty, but they also are not the friendliest people.

"Open your legs. You knew it would be painful and it must finish now."
And I have to open my legs so that the process can begin.'

'But it was just, they did, one of them really pushed me in very
painful ways on the inside, the after pains were very sore.'

Even the nurses admit that patients are sometimes handled quite
roughly. They talk about getting so angry or frustrated that they have
violent feelings towards the patients. 'Sometimes if, then the patients are
difficult, they don't want to co-operate, then you just feel – you're not
allowed to assault a patient, but sometimes you just feel like, then you
think, oh, you just want to assault that patient, if the patient won't push
and so on.'

Patients seem to know that if they do the right things and follow
instructions, they will not be scolded or treated badly. 'I got very scared.
The sisters said that I should keep calm, not go on like other pregnant
woman and I should keep myself tranquil, but if I carry on and am
nervous, then I can forget, then they will do things to me that I don't
want.'

## After birth: The wavering of the gaze

After birth, it seems that women are mostly left alone. Women rarely
talk about this 'stage' of labour. If surveillance and intervention are
sometimes feared, women also dread being left.

Many women comment on the fact that no pain relief was offered
after labour. Anna talks about trembling with pain. 'By Friday it was
different nurses that were on, but they did not give you your pain pills
every three or four hours as you need them. Now the cut starts to come
alive and I tremble with pain. By the time that you go and ask them
whether there is not a pain pill, it is already too late, because look, that
pill still has to work through your body and later I felt so miserable that
I thought to myself, wait, my fever is not too high, I will ask the doctor
if I can't go home, because of the nurses who didn't give me pills. I would
rather get it at the pharmacy or so. Then the doctor gave me pills and
then I thought to myself: Why do the nurses not give it to me every
three hours? Why should I go and ask for the pills? Save the energy, is my
feeling. They are strange. I feel it is better to go home.'

In general, pain relief procedures seem to be almost non-existent in this hospital, with most women going through labour without being given anything for pain. It seems that the standard way to approach labour is 'all women have to go through it' or 'you must stand your man'.

There are several accounts of women suffering after having given birth. There are many stories of powerlessness and humiliation.

Suzanne talks about the sadness and pain that she experienced after having given birth. 'I was very sad, because I did not know that it would be that painful and I was cut. I was too small down there. So, I was cut, and it was still alive when they cut me down there. Then it was very painful, you understand. Then I couldn't walk, and I couldn't lie down, and I had to breastfeed her and then I was very down and tearful, understand? And she's also teary because she's not being fed. And I can't and they all have to come and help me, because it is too painful, and I had twelve stitches and they also became alive . . . You have to doctor yourself. Salt water you have to put there, but no pain pills. They gave nothing.'

Abigail, a twenty-year-old college student, is well supported by her parents and boyfriend, but very disappointed by her hospital experience, even though she was a private patient. 'The doctor then left and the sister took the baby. Then they told me I should go for a bath in a salt bath. I told them then that I won't be able to because I can't get up . . . the evening I screamed for the sister because my stomach went, it was loose, out of control, but I could not because I had the baby on me, I could not get off the bed and put him in his own bed. I can't leave him . . . I screamed for the sister to just come and take the baby. I did not expect her to clean me up. Just to come and take the baby. But no one came. I had to struggle by myself. And then I went to clean myself.'

Her baby got jaundice and she was readmitted to the hospital. 'When I came to the hospital on Wednesday, with jaundice, I have pain and was so emotional. I was so sad because it feels to me the baby cries, but I cannot be a good mother for him. I can't do anything. I have pain. I cannot stand up. I had backache and I cannot pick him up and I keep my hand on him, but he doesn't want to stop crying. I wasn't so . . . and the nurse – I told them I had a lot of pain, I'm going to bath. It was so dirty the bathrooms. Then I said to the nurses it feels as if I am going to get an infection – I'm not even well yet, I still have stitches. Then the one nurse took me to their bathrooms in their place. And I had salt in the water, gave salt water, lay in the salt, and then I felt a *bietjie* [a little] better again, there was, luckily it wasn't infection. It feels so, it was very *grillerig* [gruesome] there, and, I still had the pain all the time. I couldn't lift my legs. I sat there, they brought me a chair and I just sat there, I could really do nothing. If I wanted something, I had to ask someone to bring it.'

Abigail's baby also was not very happy in the hospital. 'He cried there in the hospital, all day long, and the nurses say he mustn't cry because his little tummy isn't strong, he's too small, and then I just had to be strong, and then I said to them, they see I struggle. But few really help me. The nurses said I should just have asked the girl next to me.'

Abigail was exhausted and fell asleep with her baby. 'Then there was a sister, she came immediately, and then she said to me . . . I, I couldn't sleep. For me it feels, I sit on pain, I have pain, now I sit on top of it, sit and sleep. Sit there and then I had the baby on me. Now I know it was very irresponsible – he drank and then he lay on me, but then I just nodded off, and um, I have so, my eyes were just closed. I didn't really sleep. She comes along, and screams, she says, "It's irresponsible and you don't do that, you don't sleep with the baby. Put the baby down." Then I said to her, "I'm sorry." I then kissed the baby because I now feel that I was irresponsible, but I was tired, everyone sees I don't sleep at night, the sisters sit and sleep in their room. Now, I mean I was tired, then they said to me I must go home.'

She did not want to leave the baby, however and decided to take a bath with him. 'Then they said that I didn't wrap him correctly. I wrapped him my style, like I now could wrap him, there where he lay. I feel no, the little baby is still small, as long as he is just warm, as long as he is just covered, the sister then carries on, and she tells me no, I can go to jail for what I do and she scolds me. And then I sit still. I think maybe she is right, in, in, in a way to say that to me. I am irresponsible, but I now again felt, how can you wrap the baby? Maybe I didn't wrap him the right way, like she felt he should be wrapped. This that I did, I did like I did it. I feel it's my baby. I mean, every mom does things in their way, and um, I felt very hurt and I cried, then she said to me that I must cry, cry, because um, I will feel better and then it just felt and then I felt I, I don't want to be sad anymore, and this hurt me very much this that she said and then I said to her, "But I just want to go home." I was very sad, then I said to my mom this is how she feels, she doesn't know what pain you have.'

While all the main tenets of a medicalised childbirth can be clearly discerned in the accounts of patients and nurses (order, surveillance, intervention, risk aversion),[56] the accounts of the nurses and patients are not of medical encounters that are precisely ordered and meticulously controlled.[57] The birth narratives that we hear sound like the exact opposite of the ideal clinical encounter: they describe disorganised, dysfunctional, noisy, messy and even violent encounters between women. There are empty hospital beds and crowded corridors; missing nurses and scolding sisters; broken bells and no medicine; screams and slaps; threats and jokes. It seems as if in the face of the impossibility of a pure medical encounter, both patients and nurses in their furious and desperate accusations of each other ('not human', 'barbarian', 'not right', 'not nice', 'not pretty') invoke each other's humanity, remembering that the other (and the self) is a person that is supposed to care, to do her duty, to do the right thing, to be obedient, to be good. It may be exactly because the impossibility of the 'ideal medical birth' is so clear in this context that the nurses and patients seem to feel frustrated, disappointed, resentful and even enraged.[58] Both patients and nurses can talk about these disappointments when confiding in psychologists, but in the maternity ward they act out with and against one another, rather than talking to one another.[59]

Women's dread of the maternity ward may lead to an active decision to have their babies at home. Carina Truyts, an anthropologist who did her fieldwork under my supervision in the valley, writes about one such chosen homebirth:

Jessica Arendse sits in a large armchair in Stellenbosch public hospital. A red and black chequered blanket is tucked around her waist. Her newborn son lies sleeping on his back in a mobile crib beside her, bundled up in blankets and a babygrow. His arms are crooked at the elbow, both palms facing upward. The three of us are alone in the small room.

Jessica gave birth to her baby in her and Elvis's room in her adopted hometown of Kylemore at about 2 a.m. The only other person present in the room was her boyfriend, Elvis. Neighbours gathered outside. When the bleeding continued postpartum, the emergency services were called . . . Jessica explains how the nurse admonished her for choosing to give birth at home, alone, explaining, 'This morning the nurse came and said to me: "Do you know how dangerous it is to give birth at home?" Then I said, "I *know* what happened the first time," you see? She won't tell me what to do.'

I ask Jessica why she wanted to give birth at home.

'I wanted to have him at home, Carina. It's family-less [at the hospital], people-less. It's not for me. And I told them at home: "Don't interfere. Don't phone the ambulance. And [to Elvis] don't call your mother. Just leave it. It's better for me to give birth at home." It was really painful. But it was worth it.'

She seems to be in mild shock. 'I lost so much blood, Carina. I lost so much blood.'

Jessica wants to go home desperately. So desperately that she smeared icing from a cake her mother brought onto her newborn's lips. She hoped this would raise his blood sugar: the magic spell that would grant her exit rights.

The nurse takes the baby away for the blood glucose test.[60]

Family-less. People-less. And home-less?
Don't call the ambulance. Don't call your mother.
While the anthropologist is still pondering this, they hear a baby crying.

Jessica reacts quickly, she sits up, hastens to the door. 'Is that my child crying like that?' she asks a passing nurse. The nurse ignores her. Jessica hovers in the doorway until the nurse brings him back. He had been crying. 'As soon as they release me and my child I won't walk out of here. I will run.'[61]

## Abandonment and loneliness

This utter desolation and sense of abandonment in the birth narratives is what is most intense: women seem mostly to be alone when they give birth. Almost none of them have birth companions (a family member, a partner or a friend). While the presence of nurses and health-care workers seems to be quite unpredictable, more standard is that many (if not most) women give birth without having a birth companion present. This is quite startling because the literature is so clear that women who have a birth attendant and feel supported during labour are much more likely to have a satisfying birth experience.[62]

Tina is a 29-year-old college-educated woman who tells the story of giving birth to her second child. There is ambivalence in her story. While she says that she told her husband that she did not want to give birth by herself again, she also seems to think it may be a good thing that he was not present.

'I gave birth the Friday afternoon,' she says. 'Um, the Friday night [my husband's family] came too late, then they didn't allow them. They didn't allow them at all. Then they had to turn back. It was very bad. I didn't really know they were there. Because you must enter through emergencies. And security stood there. The Saturday morning, very early they told me but they were there the Friday evening and then they didn't want to let them in.' She laughs, seemingly a bit embarrassed. 'Actually, I wanted it like that. I don't know how I would ha- . . .' She interrupts herself with another laugh. 'If someone was now with me, I – like my boyfriend now told me last night, he really wanted a little boy. Then it was a little girl again. Then he said to me yesterday evening that we are going to try again. Then I said, I said to him: "No, man, you are then never here when I give birth." Then he said: "No, man you can take the pain. You can do it alone."' She laughs again. 'Then I said, but it, it, it's not about me not coping with the pain. You want that, that um, support. You just want it. But actually, I was, am, glad that he wasn't there. He would have made me mad when I carried on! I think he would have done it when I now carried on about the pain and so.'

From Tina's story, it is clear that there are many factors that may have led to her ending up in the maternity ward on her own. However, we don't know whether her giving birth by herself was her choice or her boyfriend's choice or whether it was a simple consequence of hospital procedures. Implicit in Tina's narrative is the matter of agency – to what extent she (and women in general) can control who is with them during this event and how they cope with this apparent lack of control.

Blondie, seventeen years old, laughingly describes how she gave birth with only two nursing sisters attending. Interestingly, despite the sisters being present, Blondie's sense is that she was alone. Blondie was abandoned by her boyfriend after he found out that she was pregnant and she was very able to talk about how angry she was with him. She does not express any anger about her mother and sister leaving her alone in the hospital; she seems to accept that they had no choice and she had no other options.

'Before the time my mom was with me. That's now when they dropped me at the hospital. And my little sister. And she actually did scold the dad. Because the dad had never been with me. Because he now works. And after a while then I said because my mom still had to go and work the morning and my sister had to go to school and my little brother must still be prepared. Then my mom said that she is now also going home because it now depends on me today. And then she said to me she holds her thumbs and she will pray that the child is healthy and that both of us come off well.' She laughs resignedly. 'And yes, then she went home . . . When I gave birth two of the sisters were there. Just the two *sustertjies* [diminutive for 'sisters'], the sister who now caught the baby and so on. It's only them. But the whole time I was alone.'

The fact that women use the word 'alone' seems to suggest that even though they typically don't plan on having a birth attendant, they still have a subjective feeling of being alone when no one familiar is in attendance. The presence of the nurses did not alleviate this sense of loneliness.

Petunia, a 22-year-old married woman, is able to express the sadness associated with being on her own. Petunia's husband had to work and had to look after their first son while she was in labour. 'Look here, this is just how it is, you must help yourself now. The nurse will do nothing for you. They have nothing to do with you, unless they now see the baby is coming, then they come. They have nothing to do with you before then. You must just fight on your own there. You are on your own; they are just there for delivery, for the birth, then they now came to help, but further you are alone there you must just help yourself.'

In these accounts of labour the loneliness and sense of isolation is acute, but these feelings also go with a resignation and a certain kind of acquiescence. In the cases of some individual women, such as Lea, a more defiant or resistant tone can be discerned. This, however, is the exception rather than the rule.

Given this tendency to be left alone or to choose to be alone in the birthing room, the women seemed to experience loneliness in its most extreme forms while they were giving birth. It is a loneliness that is the result of a sense of being abandoned: abandoned by partners, mothers, aunts, friends and the nursing staff. It is a loneliness that seems to be anticipated and expected.

Giving birth is then a moment of profound vulnerability. After giving birth on her own, nineteen-year-old Anthea articulates something that I hear from many new mothers. 'I feel like a woman,' she says, 'but mostly like a child. And less like a woman, but meanwhile I'm still the same. Then I feel a little bit womanish, but still a child. For me I still feel like I usually felt, but is just so – how can I now say? – I am now in a way one side that I feel like a parent, but I feel myself still like a child. And for me it is, if I now were over twenty then I would now have felt like a grown woman, but I am still a child, even though I now have a child. So on the one side I feel like a mother, but not completely.'

## Maternal love and bonding

Childbirth, characterised by pain, vulnerability, loss of control and loneliness, is not the end of the story.

Maternal reverie is.

Fifteen-year-old Jenna is sitting with her three-month-old smiling baby on her lap while I interview her. He faces her, watching her as she speaks. When I ask her what motherhood is like, she says that it is wonderful. 'Wonderful,' she repeats. She laughs a shy little laugh. '*Ek kan dit nie eintlik beskryf nie* [I can't actually describe it]. *Alles* [Everything]!'

She returns the baby's gaze, holding his hands. 'Like in the mornings when I get up, he's awake before me and then, then he bullies me and he pulls my hair or he pinches me, just to wake me up. And if I perhaps sleep and he wakes up, and sees there's nobody around him, he cries. Cries!'

She emphasises the word 'cries', almost as if she is in wonder.

'And he's already used to faces around him. Always wants someone close to him. *Dan moet ek nou wakker word* [Then I must now wake up].' With mock indignation, she says, 'This morning, three o' clock he wanted to wake up, then I also had to.'

She laughs another seemingly pleased laugh.

'I'm a bit tired at that time, but then I have to sit and play with him.' She looks smilingly at the baby. 'I sit up with him, talk to him, tickle him when I feel so.' She demonstrates how she tickles him. The baby laughs and gurgles. 'I ask him,' and now she says in a baby voice, '"*Wil jy nie slaap nie* [Don't you want to sleep]?" or "*Hoe kan jy dan so vroeg wakker wees* [How can you be awake so early]?" And then I play, I tickle him a bit again.' She shows me how. 'And then if he laughs, I say, "*O kry jy lekker nou* [Oh, are you enjoying it now]?" Then I play a bit again. And I pinch him here between the *boudjies*.' She playfully pinches the baby's bottom. The baby laughs more. 'Very *verlief* [in love] with his ma.'

The interaction between young mother and baby moves me profoundly. I know I'm seeing something. I don't know exactly what.

The interaction that I observe and am told about is very much the mother-infant interaction that Donald Winnicott refers to as holding and playing.[63] The mother's loving attention to the baby manifests in her physical handling of the child, how she holds him, dresses him, feeds and bathes him. Winnicott also emphasises the importance of play. The child's ability to play is seen as a developmental achievement and a symbol of his trust in his mother.

Sanna also talks about her playful interactions with her newborn baby. 'Then everything is okay, then the two of us get along well, then we chat and carry on. He likes chatting very much and he can chat non-stop. If you keep quiet, then he just looks at you like that. You can't keep your mouth shut, he just wants to hear your voice and when he sees you again, then he now wants to see that you move [laughs]. "What is it . . . my *kindjie* [diminutive of 'child']? Let's drive, brrrrr brrrr, brrrrr" [laughs]. When he drives, then he makes little little bubbles with his mouth.'

She demonstrates how they play at driving. She continues to express how she feels about her baby. 'I feel good about him and I love him very much. We two are very close. Together we are everything. I breastfeed him and he is very close to me. In the evenings when I come in and he hears my voice, they are now maybe giving him bottle, then he immediately leaves that bottle and then he looks up at me. And in the mornings, when he now knows I'm going to work and I will be away for the day, then he now sees me, then it looks to me as if he wants to cry. Because now in the mornings, when he wakes, then I must make him sleep before I take him to my mom, before I go to work.'

Sonneblommetjie talks about her preoccupation with the baby after birth.[64] 'Just after the birth I went to bath myself. To get rid of old blood that bottled up for nine months. I went to take a bath then already, he slept right through. I didn't close an eye. Not because I had pain. I was tired, but not tired like I now have to go and rest. I lay awake all night and watched him. Even when he slept, I picked him up and let him lie next to me. I rubbed his little hand, then I lay him down again. Then I sat up next to his little baby bed. Then I pick him up again and then I hold him tight and then I talk to him. Oh, for me it was something.'

Millicent describes how giving birth changed her as a person. She talks about a certain kind of crazy love and a fierce wish to protect: 'About him, I am, I'm – how can you say? – I am very mad about him.' She laughs. 'He, he made a big difference in my life, because, um – how can you say? – um, I'm a completely different person. I'm almost just on the defence, I just want to protect him. I am almost like a lion or a little dog, a dog that looks after her *kleintjies* [little ones] that want to protect her *kleintjies*. Yes, if someone comes close to him, I growl. I am like that.' She laughs again.

Twenty-one-year-old Robena has had a baby against the wishes of her parents and was abandoned by the father of her baby. Despite her dire circumstances, she tenderly describes the interactions between her and her child. 'He had so many facial expressions in the beginning. He pulled his face in all sorts of ways that made me laugh. Or he did other things that made me laugh. Nowadays, if I perhaps sing for him or I'm still busy with a thing, then I let him sit in his pram, and now I sing, to now just keep him quiet, out of the blue then he also gives a scream and then I think now he's going to cry and if I look at him, then he sits and laughs or sits and smiles at me. These are the things that I maybe would have missed if I left him with someone else, if I had left him with other people. If I was not around, these are all things that I would have missed. And I really don't want to miss it.'

Robena also describes how the baby is on her mind, even when she is away from the baby. She is asked whether it felt difficult for her to go back to work. She answers the question indirectly. 'I can't say that one moment passes that I don't think of him. But while I am at work, I wonder: Is he naughty? Is he crying? Is he sleeping now? Do they have problems with him? Is he hungry yet? It is like that all the time. And then, even when I am talking to, say, my boss, in the end then, it also is about that, because my thoughts are there all the time. So, I don't know how it happens that we talk about the children, about his children and about my children. But, it always happens because they stay somewhere in your thoughts, in your unconscious. You always think about them and then it just happens. It's not that you planned it or that you wanted it badly, but it just happens.'

She is the quintessential self-sacrificing mother.[65] 'It's something that I didn't understand. I understand it now. You will rather give up everything. You will rather give your child a piece of bread than eat a piece of bread yourself. You will always check that he has what he needs, even if you don't have it. So, he will always always have. You will rather give things to your child, rather than take things for yourself.' She speaks about her feelings for the baby in almost poetic terms:

'Because the feeling that
it awakens in you
is something indescribable.
Your friends make you feel happy,
they make you feel excited
even your family,
your mom or dad make you feel happy
or they make you feel special,
but the feeling that a child awakens in you
is something that you don't just get anywhere.'

Profound connection.
And love.

# Love

*'. . . the affection of relatives (often thoroughly disrupted) . . .'\**

It is bad to live without a hell: aren't we able to reconstruct it?
> — Pablo Neruda, *The Book of Questions*

I am, of course, speaking of the way of life which makes love the centre of everything, which looks for all satisfaction in loving and being loved . . . It is that we are never so defenceless against suffering as when we love, never so helplessly unhappy as when we have lost our love object or its love.
> — Sigmund Freud, *The Freud Reader*

In a murderous time
the heart breaks and breaks
and lives by breaking.
It is necessary to go
through dark and deeper dark
and not to turn.
I am looking for the trail.
> — Stanley Kunitz, *The Collected Poems*

June. Early winter's day. Mahler and the mountains in my car. The fields are white with *varklelies* (literally, 'lilies of pigs', arum lilies). Muddy

---

\* The quote in the subtitle of this chapter – '. . . the affection of relatives (often thoroughly disrupted) . . .' is from Sen, 2005: xi.

parking lot. Crisp air. My morning is almost fully booked. Some old cases. A few new ones.

Patricia Solms is my first case of the day. She and her husband recently lost their ten-year-old daughter to cancer. Five years ago their baby son died of meningitis. My next client, pregnant Desire Williams, is fourteen years old and severely depressed. She wants to have an abortion. The pastor at her church has forbidden it. Worryingly, ten-year-old Desmonique Pieterse, molested by her father, does not show for her weekly session. She is still living with her mother, her father (*that* father) and younger brother in one room in her uncle's house. Paulette Verdriet is twelve years old and lives with her mother, father and two sisters in a shack. Her father drinks every day, frequents the *smokkelhuis* (illegal tavern). He has a girlfriend. He screams at Paulette's mother: '*Jou naai, jou ma se poes. Ek maak jou vrek*' (You fuck, your mother's cunt. I will kill you). Her foster sister of two died in a shack fire the week before. Paulette heard the crying and then eventual silence. She has bad dreams.

The clinic nurse also has new patients for me. The first case is a sixteen-year-old boy who is afraid of his anger: he is angry with his alcoholic father who almost killed his mother and is now in jail. The other is a boy also of sixteen who got two girls pregnant. 'Is there nothing to do in this town, but *stoot* [have sex]? Why don't you rather kick a ball?' says the nurse when she introduces me to him.

On the desk next to me is an open box of condoms and a life-size erect wooden penis, used for sex education classes. In small print on the penis, it says, 'Only for external use.' I struggle to focus on the boy.

Delize Plesier is my last patient of the day; this is her third session. She is a 33-year-old seasonal farmworker with a Grade 7 education. At the time of the session, she has a fourteen-year-old boy, a nine-year-old girl and a six-month-old baby girl. The Protestant church group that she joined just before the baby's birth insisted that Delize marry her long-time partner, Piet. Before that they had been living together for about thirteen years. The couple live with their three children and Delize's mother on a farm in a small house with two rooms, a kitchen, a small living area and a bathroom. In the first session Delize already told me that her husband is a heavy drinker and a womaniser and he beats her regularly. She is soft-spoken and seems very sad.

Delize starts the session by saying somewhat apologetically that she always talks about herself when she sees me. 'But I want to ask,' she says shyly, 'is it good, should I . . . It feels to me that I complain, that I only complain to you about my problems. Can I talk about them? It feels to me, yes, as if it is about my problems that I come and talk about and that is not the actual thing that you really want to talk about? If maybe it is only about the baby?'

I tell her that the sessions really are about her. Reassured for the moment, she continues. 'Yes, there were many times that I thought, wow, with whom? Is there not someone to whom I can open my heart? Can take my problems to? Because you can't with everyone.'

Now she goes on to talk about her husband Piet: his womanising, his drinking, his spending, his sexual demands and his violence. She also reveals that she is worried about contracting diseases because Piet sleeps with women who are rumoured to have diseases: 'Like the two of us, we sleep together, I'm careful of that. I'm scared. Maybe I can't get the germ, but my baby can get a germ by his sleeping around.'

Her biggest worry is about transmitting a virus to her baby through breastfeeding. I ask her whether she is still intimate with her husband. 'Ja,' she says, '*nie eintlik nie*' (not really). She pauses frequently as she speaks. 'It feels as if when he moves in that direction I get *grillings* [shudders] through my body. I don't know whether he's clean or not. Because a man that walks around so much at night, you know what type of person he is. Because the actual thing is he doesn't come for me, he doesn't act correctly like other men react to their their wives. But with other women, as we now work, I can see in the house he won't just talk to me, as soon as he [sees] other women outside the door . . . then he enjoys talking to them. Laughs and talks. Now when we maybe have an argument here in the house and I tell him those things, he will always tell me I'm jealous. Then I tell him, "But I'm not jealous. It just things that hurt me. I see how you talk nicely to other *vroumense* [derogatory word for 'women'] and when they ask you to do something you'll quickly do it for them, but for me, you'll never – if I ask you, you'll never do it, or you won't give a good face."'

'The heart breaks and breaks / and lives by breaking.'[1]

Delize now speaks more slowly, with longer pauses. 'The attitude he has in the house is not that good towards me or my children. Actually, my biggest worry is about my kids. See, it seems he doesn't give them attention, he doesn't give them love. The only thing he does is to *raas* [scold] and *skree* [shout] at them. Or they must now just do a job like he wants now.'

She feels lonely and frustrated as a parent and is aware that she tends to take out this frustration on her children. 'At the Apostolic Church they just say you – like the teachers now teach the Sunday-school kids – that you may not smack your child. You must take the child, then you must make him sit down and talk nicely. So that he can understand you, because if you *raas* [scold] and *skree* [shout] at her, then you just make the child worse than he is. The children are so stubborn. Many times I just feel like taking a thing and smacking the child, but then it comes to me again, it's wrong to smack my child. Because I take it, the problem lies with us as parents. Now if the father can just support me with the children, then things will come right. When he is sober, not when he is drunk. Now, the moment I need him with the children, then he isn't there.'

Delize tells me that she recently had a violent confrontation with her husband. Telling this story, her demeanour is still sad, rather than angry. Her speech is slow, not belligerent at all. 'Actually,' she says, 'we had a *lelike* [ugly] confrontation last week and I almost had him burned, burned with boiling water . . . He lost it totally the other night, while I was writing up my groceries for the Friday and Saturday. I felt him hitting me on my mouth, my jaw hurt. Then I thought there is only one way – because before that I boiled water for the child's bottle, so I took the water and he realised and he followed me and he took my chair to throw it at me, but then I took the kettle just like that with the water and I gave him a shot of the water. That water then broke him down. He had a fright and he made a noise so that my sister-in-law came running. Then I told her that I just burned him. That was the only way in which I could defend myself. But he did not really burn, the water was not of a strong heat because then he would have had blisters, his skin would have burned. He only got a fright. But now I am quite cautious, now after I did this. I think that he can try it with me too and then the water is boiling. And maybe I have the child on my arm. I really don't know what to do with the man.'

She talks about the church and her frustration with not being able to participate fully in church activities, as her husband does not support her. 'He should be working with me, but he doesn't. It feels as if there is very little interest from his side in me and my children. I accept and accept. Most days I think this is probably the way it should be. They say if there is not a struggle, there is not victory.'

When asked about the possibility of leaving her husband (a fantasy that she expressed in a previous session), Delize says, 'The church people, the priests, they say if you are married, only death, only death can set us apart. It does not exist with them, the possibility that you can get divorced, then death should separate you. Now, they say, if they pray, they pray the Lord should take that person away, so that I can get rid of him. Look, he is, they say he stands in my way. I want to continue with things, the work of the Lord, but he stands in my way.'

Her disillusionment and sadness are palpable, but also her resignation. 'And the thing is, I now thought the man will now improve after he had a little baby because he has now already seen the child. The child is there, so he must now improve. But nothing changed, the time in the hospital was, the interest, the little interest that he had and so on. Nothing went well in the time I was in the hospital, where he now had to stand in my place for me.'

Then, suddenly, startled, interrupting her own story, she looks at me, panicking. 'As I sit here now, the worry grabs me. What's the time? One o'clock?'

'Yes,' I say. 'It is one o'clock. Are you in a hurry?'

'Ja,' she says, 'because he can now also maybe get difficult and I didn't really leave them something to eat this morning. And he is now . . . so I must put everything in his hands myself.'

I apologise for not having watched the time. We agree about a next appointment and she leaves in a rush, but still moving slowly, with hanging shoulders. Her clothes are loose on her slight body. 'The breastfeeding takes its toll,' she said earlier.

Outside it is bright and cold. The streets smell of rain. The children wear track suits and walk and play on the wet tar road outside the clinic. The scrawny dogs, as always, are everywhere.

I stop to pick some arum lilies. It is against the law. It starts raining. I drive too fast. I want to get home. Get the lilies into water.

## Guilt and power

On that day in the clinic I was confronted with 'family' and clear evidence of how 'an unhappy family is unhappy after its own fashion'.[2] In these families, there are two dead children, a raping father, a pregnant schoolgirl, a devastating household fire, a fornicating, fertile schoolboy, a boy furious with his father. However, somehow, on this day it is Delize who stays with me while I place the glass vase with arum lilies next to the clock and the tissue box of my private practice office. Gentle Delize who stays and stays while her heart breaks and breaks, her silent rage overshadowed by the longing to be heard and the hope for change. Through the dark and deeper dark, I am aware of her exaggerated sense of responsibility and her almost invisible power.

I think of Victoria Sweet and her book *God's Hotel: A Doctor, a Hospital, and a Pilgrimage to the Heart of Medicine*:

> When I looked into Mr. Hickman's open wound and saw that, exposed and vulnerable, nestled in the hollow that the surgeons had created, was Mr. Hickman's beating heart.
>
> It was extraordinary.
>
> I could see the fine, delicate film of the pericardial sac glisten as it pulsed and caught the light. Woven through it – I could just make out – were tiny veins and arteries. It was so alive, that beating heart! It was as alive as Mr. Baker's body at my first autopsy had been dead.[3]

So many broken hearts in the valley.

The arteries of the broken heart remind me of the arteries of the wooden penis on the desk of the consulting office of the clinic office. '*Wat maak hierdie houtpiel hier?*' (What is this wooden cock doing here?) one of the boys said angrily, after being ushered in by the nurse. 'I can't concentrate with that here.' Remembering this, defensively distracted once again, I google 'arteries of the penis' and find out that when something is wrong with the arteries of the penis, it typically implies problems with arteries of the heart. The penis, a journal article says, is like a barometer, a canary in the coal mine, for impending problems in the coronary arteries.[4]

'*Kanarie, klikvoëltjie*' (Canary, telltale bird), says my friend Pieter when I tell him the story.

Delize began her session by apologising to me for talking too much about herself. She ends the session, realising that she might be late for making her husband his lunch, worried that he will be upset. I feel terrible when I rush back to my private practice on the other side of the mountain. I have taken on her guilty sense of responsibility. I feel worse for picking the arum lilies. A cheap and easy attempt to escape from my middle-class guilt and the pain.

As a psychotherapist I know that the feelings I have about patients after sessions often is my most important source of information about the patient. We call it 'countertransference'.[5]

Delize, like many women in the valley (and elsewhere), endures a violent relationship, seemingly selfless in her submission and suffering.[6] She is hurt by her husband's betrayal and abuse, but also protests against her fate (usually silently, but in this case with a kettle of hot water), hoping for a good outcome eventually. She knows that the suffering she has endured is unjust and undeserved, but endures it in the hope, conscious or unconscious, for some eventual greater good.[7]

'I have to put everything in his hands myself.'

'There is no victory without struggle.'

'Only death can set us apart.'

'Then I took the kettle just like that.'

Despite occasionally fighting back (maybe unconsciously nudging fate in the direction of death and victory), in general, Delize remains faithful to the cultural and religious rules of the nuclear family, rules that compel her to stay, to serve, to be submissive and to endure.

How can terrible aspects of experience be incorporated into daily life and kept alive when people need to survive and tend to their ordinary activities? Those aspects of unbearable reality tend to be banished . . . the need for loved ones to stay close is so deep, and the need to maintain the status quo so ingrained . . . the hope of change and feelings of forgiveness are powerful forces that lead people to remain in dangerous places, with violent partners, working frantically to make them safer or trying not to provoke their rage.[8]

Delize's staying in a relationship where her role is that of service, submission and selflessness, in her eyes, is neither in vain nor pointless. She tolerates the suffering both to accomplish a goal (to maintain the relationship, to be a good woman) and to avert the more painful eventuality (to lose the relationship, to be a bad woman). In her eyes, her suffering is thus justified.[9]

Delize's husband, Piet, when we interview him, is very clear that womanhood is synonomous with *swaarkry* (suffering) and care. 'No, when I found out I'm a man . . . was the time I now started going to school . . . was Sub A or B that I started noticing. We always took a piss next to the road, for example, and there I thought, why can I then stand and pee? And the little girl children must sit and pee. Then I now asked that question to my cousin who walked with me. Then I asked him, and he said, "It's a girl child that one, we are boys." Then I asked him, "Why does a boy stand and pee then, and a girl sit?" Then he said, "Girls can't stand." So that's when I discovered I'm a man.'

'So there I started to understand, my manhood . . . See, it was like this for me, with the peeing, I pee faster than a girl now . . . the efforts she must put in, I can just stand just here and pee, and so it was for me. Life is better for a man.'

'Men,' he says, 'have more freedom. See, in general, a person is then so . . . I can take off my clothes when I'm warm and walk around with a bare chest when I'm warm. If she is warm, a woman can't take off her clothes and be without a top. Or, how can I now say . . . For me, it's better to be a man than to be a woman. A woman, I think, has the most hardest life, harder than a man.'

He continues, 'Men have easier lives than women. A man always has the easiest life, than a woman. Now see . . . for a woman it is difficult. See, the first thing that a person thinks, if you now see a woman like today, is she, hmm, today now already washed and dressed and, and tomorrow she now wears that which she put on today, again. The day after tomorrow she wears that again, then you start, hmm, thinking bad of her. But a man can walk with clothes two to three days. See what I mean? Those people don't get those wrong ideas of the man in them that same time. But a *vroumens* [woman], you always think bad of her. Look, the woman must always be on her neatness, like I now just talked about.

The man sits outside chatting with other men. Here, inside the woman must look for food for that man who is standing outside chatting, so that he can eat just now. She can't chat all the time. She must manage the house. She must manage the children. She must manage everybody. Just now she must be at her job. Children must go to school.'

In Delize's narratives about herself we see someone who consciously and unconsciously lives according to powerful societal scripts such as those described by her husband, but also someone who has internalised her abusive relationships by experiencing herself as dependent, powerless and shameful. According to Anna Motz:

> [Those] who were abused in early life and carry a sense of shame in relation to this, will find this shame reactivated in their violent adult relationships, and this makes it a familiar pain that, in a perverse way, confirms their fears about themselves: they are confirmed as worthless, deserving of pain.[10]

Delize feels that there is no other option but to be submissive and subservient, selfless and suffering. Her responsibility is to stay. As a poor, coloured woman living in post-apartheid South Africa, leaving seems impossible.

However, there is another subtle emotional thread that runs through her narrative. There is anger and indignation, a moral outrage, an insistence on justice and also hope. She is not simply resigned to accept the injustice of the abuse, she endures it and can complain about it, hoping that things will change or that she will be saved.[11] Mostly, however, she feels guilty about her outrage.[12]

Delize's story of staying is one that I am familiar with. As a psychotherapist I hear versions of it on a daily basis in the valley, but also in my private practice.

Take, for instance, stay-at-home mother Cara, whom I also see on the afternoon of the arum lilies. As always, she arrives a few minutes late for her session, the tyres of her huge white 4×4 screeching when she stops on the pavement outside my office. She is anxious, a bit breathless – with lists of things that she has to do this afternoon, a list she got from her husband, Johan, a very successful businessman, when he came home for his lunch and afternoon nap. The to-do list is impossible as always (getting the swimming pool pump fixed, having his favourite coffee roasted at the Deluxe coffee shop in a part of town where there is no parking, picking up his latest cycling gadget at the bike shop, making sure that his ten-year-old whisky is in stock, booking the ticket for his upcoming hunting trip, walking the dog, renewing his gym membership and, of course, keeping the three children (a toddler and two primary school kids) and their stuff out of his way.

Johan has not beaten Cara (yet), but burnt toast drives him to shouting and swearing; her car left in the driveway between errands will make him pound on his car horn; an open door or drawer is grounds for a kid getting '*n goeie pak slae*' (a good hiding) and serving dinner in a track suit may produce a week-long sulk. Should one of the kids crumple a paper on the back seat of the car, he will accelerate and drive too fast, scaring the whole family, thus avenging the unforgivable onslaught on his tinnitus. Johan checks the wetness of Cara's vagina after they have male visitors, so as to make sure that other men do not excite her. Cleaning his car once, she found a condom under the seat. They never use condoms in their infrequent, functional, faceless and dry sexual encounters.

In the session, Cara comments on her shortcomings, sarcastically. 'I know I'm not perfect – Johan has thoroughly informed me of how far and on how many levels of my humanness I fall short. I probably should have tried harder.'

Cara has not (yet) thrown boiling water at Johan, but deliberately overspends on everything that he does not approve of, frequently bumps her expensive car, drives too fast and gets numerous parking tickets. She secretly plays violent video games for hours on end. She has (once), when he (once again) said to her that she is like a child without any sense of responsibility, told him to go fuck himself. He then smashed his precious glass of whisky against the wall, went to bed without speaking to her and did not allow her to go to church with him for a month, which felt like some kind of victory.

Both Delize and Cara insist on staying on as the caretakers of their husbands and families.[13] They stay because they have learned that women are defined by relationships and that it is their responsibility to care for and maintain their relationships.

However, although women like Delize and Cara seem trapped, they are not totally without power. While they may not have overt power, they are often acutely aware of the vulnerability and dependence of their violent partners.[14] Sometimes they do not leave because, consciously or unconsciously, they understand that the violence of their partners is a male way of expressing need and fear. If this is understood, it seems possible to forgive and to stay – rather than to further humiliate a man who already feels ashamed. 'Shame,' Motz says, 'is a powerful force in maintaining violent relationships.'[15]

## Shame and dependence

Surprisingly, Piet, Delize's husband, when I meet him, does not fit my stereotype of a violent, abusive husband at all. Somehow the seemingly scary men never do.

Piet is a small man, has a limp hand and smiles all the time, incessantly. His eyes are watery, although he never cries. Piet is seen by a 30-year-old male graduate student and has a different story about his relationship with Delize. According to him, the disagreements and arguments in the household are few and they are typically solved amicably, behind closed doors. He describes the ideal husband. 'The two of them like each other. He's not the man who'll actually lift his hands against his wife. They love one another and the children also love them. There's no arguing among them.'

He talks about the joys of fatherhood. 'There are things that make me feel good. Because you know the – how can I now say? – always when you come into the house, they respect you. It makes you feel you are here the highest in the house. The main person in the house. Look, you get that feeling. It's a good feeling. They're not rude to me or so. Always nice talking, good company.'

Piet is also quite clear about what a bad husband is. '*Meneer* [Mister], there's just many around. Always arguing, always wanting to fight, always saying bad words, such horrible bad words, and in public. Fighting in public.'

He lifts his one hand in a threatening way and says loudly, 'I'll give you a *helse klap* [hell of a smack] now, or I'll kick you.'

He drops his hand, his voice softer, but he seems upset. 'Like that, in public. So that sort of life they now have. They just chase the kids around. So, that poor little kid, you already make him scared of you, wild for you. Now, in that time that you chase him around like that, you already teach him how he should chase people, fight and so.'

Piet links the feeling of being respected to being a loving husband and portrays himself as such. The therapist, frustrated, writes in his journal that he thinks that Piet just told him what he thought would be the right thing to say. 'Also,' he says, 'Piet clearly did not think that he could have refused to come for a session and tellingly said at the beginning of the interview: "*Meneer* can ask questions, I will reply."'

*Meneer* is ten years Piet's junior.

This kind of obedience or acquiescence is something Piet learned as a child. He loved his parents, he says, and he did what they told him to do. 'There's not actually something for me against my parents, in the house. I always did as they said.' He describes a childhood dominated by rules, discipline and punishment, with a clear ground rule that children should not be seen or heard. 'That time, in the olden days, it was like that . . . when I come from school in the afternoons . . . when we finished eating, take school clothes off, school work, if you got homework from school, finish. And first finish your afternoon chores, then you have to ask, may you go and play now. Now, you maybe have an evening chore too that you have to finish before dark. Collect wood and bring wood into the house, and maybe fetch water or so. Now maybe you played out late there with the *chommies* [chums] and you forgot that chore. My parents were like that, if you didn't do it, the sjambok always hung there against the wall. I got many hidings.'

He feels it was good that his parents were strict. 'So I began to understand my life from there, understand, understand how life goes. Look, if *Meneer* and I made an appointment for today now. *Meneer* came now, and I have, I'm not here. Then *Meneer* would have felt bad and afterwards I would have remembered, I had another appointment. It will now have stayed in my thoughts, it will now bug and bug and bug me.'

In the session there is little sign of the violent husband, the enraged father, the man who spent almost three years in jail for *messteek* (stabbing someone with a knife) and another two years (so he says) in hospital for stab wounds that he obtained in a subsequent fight.

By the end of the session Piet appears to be exhausted and reluctantly admits that he sometimes drinks one beer too many. 'I can't actually . . . my wife does not really want me to drink. Now I go drinking and I come back, then she always talks to me in such a kind of *rowwe manier* [rough manner]. And those are things that I also don't like. It is not good if she talks such things with me. I like it if we always talk to each other properly.'

The consequences of his drinking, he says, are not good. He lowers his head and looks down. 'I think wrong things, I do wrong things and so. I scold and swear. Wrong things. Always the wrong things. And if you then become sober, then you feel bad about it. Ashamed, I am ashamed. Ashamed, that's how I feel.'

His replies now are brief, his sentences short. The most prominent emotion of the wife-beater seems to be shame.

On the depression questionnaire, administered at the end of the session, Piet scores 'severely depressed', despite saying to the interviewer at the beginning of the session: 'Today I feel happy *Meneer*. I'm a person who never has many worries. I, like my parents taught me, I must accept all people, as I accept myself.'

Reflecting on Piet's words about violent fathers – 'Now, in that time that you chase him [the child] around like that, you already teach him how he should chase people, fight and so' – I wonder where Piet himself learned to fight. Earlier on in the interview he talked about the worst hiding he ever received as a child. 'One morning I got a big hiding from my father. I did, before I went to school now, I peed in the *kooi* [vernacular for 'bed']. Peed in the *kooi* while I was sleeping. And that my father never liked. I was like eight, *daar rond* [approximately]. My father hit me all the way to the school, the school was not far from us. All the way to the school. And in front of the teacher he also hit me. *Lyfhoue en sterre-houe en bene-houe, so* [blows to my my body, blows to my bum, blows to my legs] . . . Thick blows so with the sjambok, those. It was actually for me, that morning, the worst hiding that I got from my parents. It was two weeks, two weeks before I could sit. My parents didn't know doctors. They made their own stuff to heal sores and so. *Stukkende plekke* [literally, 'broken places', injuries caused by blows in which the skin is cut or broken] everywhere. On my bum. All over my body. At night when I sleep, I lie now on my tummy, because the other side with *stukkende plekke* hurts.'

Piet's painful story about a hiding in which his bed-wetting was punished in a very public way is again a story of shame.[16]

In the valley many violent interactions start with the sentence '*Moenie my vir 'n poes vat nie*' (Don't take me for a cunt), meaning, 'Don't underestimate me, don't disrespect me.' American psychiatrist James Gilligan, who worked with violent criminals for decades, is convinced that the most powerful way to provoke anyone into committing violence is by shaming him. Think Cain and Abel, the Trojan War, the Second World War and the Weimar. Violent interactions always start with someone or something being shamed. Also, Gilligan says, people resort to violence when they feel that they can wipe out shame only by shaming those whom they feel have shamed them. Ironically, however, the most powerful way to shame anyone, Gilligan says, is by means of violence.[17]

This vicious cycle is clear in Piet's story of rough times. '*Daai tydjie* [that short little time] that I now started getting rough, at that age that I was not going to be told by anyone, lots of arguments. *Ligte bakleitjies* [Light little fights]. I used a knife once, in that time. Then I stab one chappie, eight gashes with the knife. And they charged me by the law. He survived, he's still alive. Charged by the law and the law punished me. I went to jail. That is now because of the gashes. Got two years and six months.'

Jail, however, was not the end of his punishment. 'After that, when I now came out of the jail, then I went to my sister and them's house, that my parents left for us. Now one day, it was so half cold in the winter then. Now we stand outside in the yard round the fire that we now made, now we stand around the fire like that. Now that one, that I now stabbed, the one with the eight gashes, his nephew stabbed me, a *betrek-hou* [a blow given by taking hold of someone]. He pulls me toward him and he stabs me here in the head.' He touches his temple. 'So that the knife's blade comes out here.' He indicates the back of his head. 'Through my head. I just saw him stab – he lifts his hand and he comes with the knife. This is the last thing I knew. When I woke up, then I was lying in the Cape in Tygerberg Hospital. I lay in the Cape in Tygerberg Hospital for a year and six months.'

The person who has been shamed can be thought of as having been killed psychologically.[18] The self has died. People are psychologically killed (their humanity is taken away) if they are treated with contempt or disrespect, as though they are unimportant or insignificant, if they are not recognised as human beings.[19] Gilligan says:

> One after another of the most violent men I have worked with over the years have described to me how they had been humiliated repeatedly throughout their childhoods, verbally, emotionally, and psychologically (taunted, teased, ridiculed, rejected, insulted). They had also been physically humiliated by means of violent physical abuse, sexual abuse, and life-threatening degrees of neglect (such as being starved by their parents, or simply and totally abandoned, as in coming home to find that their parents had absconded from the family's apartment, leaving them behind).[20]

Shame, Gilligan says, can be understood as a defence against both an unbearable longing and a ghastly fear. The need is to be taken care of and loved:

> Shame can be [understood as a defence] against wishes to be loved and taken care of by others . . . When people . . . find themselves wanting to be loved and taken care of by others, they experience an upsurge of shame, which typically motivates them to move in the opposite direction by becoming active and aggressive, independent and ambitious. If they do not perceive themselves as having nonviolent means for becoming independent and being able to take care of themselves (such as skills, education, and employment), the activity and aggressiveness stimulated by shame can manifest itself in violent, sadistic, even homicidal behavior.[21]

The fear is of being abandoned, rejected or ignored:

> The fear that underlies and stimulates feelings of shame is the fear that one will be abandoned, rejected, or ignored and

will therefore die because one is so weak, helpless, dependent, unskilled, and incompetent that one cannot take care of oneself, because of which one is also so inferior, unloveable, and unworthy of love that one probably will be abandoned. This is implied, and entailed, by the fact that the self-image that stimulates shame is the image of oneself as a helpless, dependent infant who would die of starvation if abandoned by a parent-figure.[22]

Of course, Piet's desire to be recognised was also thwarted by apartheid and the racism of post-apartheid South Africa. South African psychologist Wahbie Long cites Nancy Fraser on the problem of misrecognition: 'I want to reframe the question of misrecognition as a question of justice – because misrecognition involves 'an institutionalized relation of subordination,' a relation that prevents South Africans from participating as peers in a dignified social life.'[23]

Piet, the ashamed wife-beater, despite the shameful hidings, has also loved and had opportunities for love. He remembers his father with tenderness, certainly someone he liked to be seen with and spoiled by: 'And we children loved to go to my dad's car, or to the bakkie [pick-up truck]. We were there. So I . . . and we grew to love my dad. Loved them now, as they give us the opportunity now, so we also got used to the opportunity now, and do as they want it . . . I always loved walking with him to church, Sundays . . . Chat, and I always get sweets from my dad, or my dad buys me a sucker, or so. You now walk past the shop. Shop that he now walks past. So I came to love . . .'

Piet remembers his mother as caring and conscientious: 'My mom was a good mom for us. *Kleertjies* [diminutive for 'clothes'] always clean and *kossies* [diminutive for 'food'] was always on time for us . . . I felt very close to my parents. The day that my mom died . . . *Meneer*, that day we cried.'

A man like Piet thrives when he gets respect and recognition, the opposite of disrespect and contempt.[24] In psychology we talk about the curative power of being seen, being attended to.[25] The danger with men like Piet is that instead of being admired and respected by the women in their lives, they will be detested and despised, also leading to their being disrespected by their children.

However, to explain the intricacy of the shame it is crucial to embed individual biography in the larger matrix of culture, history and political economy.[26]

A violent person's venture into psychotherapy may be one attempt to be seen, to be recognised and respected. Punishment may take guilt away, but may, simultaneously, increase feelings of shame. Gilligan says: 'That is the basic psychological reason why punishment – that is, revenge – far from deterring or preventing violence, is the most powerful stimulant or cause of violence that we have yet discovered.'[27]

If a young man who exhibits a potential for violence should be further shamed on a continuous basis, and the shame and humiliation become so intense that it is overwhelming, he may become unable to see the other options for self-respect and resort to the violence of gang life as a way to get self-respect. The danger of this happening in a context where he is part of a demographic group that, in post-apartheid South Africa, is still subjected to systematic shaming is great. Race is still a huge issue. Uneven development has also ensured that young people may have even fewer opportunities than their parents. Neo-liberalism will make their escape from the cycle of shame and violence their own individual responsibility. A dominant patriarchal culture, where violence is often seen as a way of maintaining one's masculinity or a sense of masculine sexual identity, will certainly also serve to make it difficult for young men to escape the cycle.[28] In South Africa in general, but in the valley in particular, violence has become a way of communicating and is often honoured, while non-violence is shamed.

Young men's potential problem with shame and violence is, therefore, not simply an individual problem caused by abandoning parents and an angry wife. It also has to do with the fact that in contemporary society there is 'a general sense that very little respect is to be had'.[29] This is particularly true when people are poor and do not have jobs that pay a living wage and where racial discrimination is still determining who shall be respected and who not.

In a society like this, it is as if 'everyone competes to get what affirmation he can from what is available'.[30] People are needy, angry and aggressive. In such an unequal society, Gilligan says, 'for the severely alienated and desperate a gun can become like a bank card – "an equalizer" in the contest for respect, and for the material status symbols that are among the main bases of respect'.[31]

The challenge, therefore, is to try to take into account the inner world and the outer world simultaneously. When psychoanalyst Donald Winnicott, famous for his statement that there is no such thing as an infant, there is only an infant and his mother, discusses his concept of holding,[32] he says: 'One can discern a series – the mother's body, the mother's arms, the parental relationship, the home, the family including cousins and near relations, the school, the locality with its police stations, the country with its laws.'[33] What shapes a person is all their caretakers and caring institutions: the larger family, the community, the schools, the hospitals, the psychologist, the police, the government and even larger societal institutions and processes.

Says Willem Anker in the novel *Buys*: '*Elke seun met 'n geweer of 'n spies of 'n piel in sy hand het 'n moeder*' (Every son with a gun or a spear or a prick in his hand has a mother).[34]

## Care and rage

> Woman of stone, heart of iron,
> Disconsolate woman, ready to kill.
> The seed of your hands with the hand that tilled.
> — Euripides, *Medea*

How did it happen that I, who, as a researcher and clinician, wanted to focus on motherhood and caring, have ended up writing mostly about vulnerability, shame and violence? I should not be surprised. Depictions of the violent side of caring, specifically of mothering, are old and everywhere.

While writing this book, I go to Prague to deliver a paper on murderous mothers. I visit the Franz Kafka Museum. The first exhibit is a letter Kafka wrote about the complex relationship he had with both his mother and his mother city, in which he says, 'Prague never lets you go . . . this dear little mother has sharp claws.' I read Zadie Smith's *The Autograph Man*, in which she writes about a Jewish mother as 'a violent tea cozy'.[35] I tell my daughter the story of Snow White. It is the stepmother who poisons the sensual Snow White by combing her hair and dressing her up in lace, finally killing her by feeding her a poisoned red apple – her father strangely absent. My daughter notices that it is also Cinderella's stepmother who keeps her from going to the ball. It is the spinning wheel of Sleeping Beauty's godmother that puts her to sleep for a hundred years.

Stonewoman. Ironheart.

This is how Euripides, in the year 341BC, describes the epic and maybe most notorious violent mother of all times, Medea. In his play Medea kills her two sons when she hears about the infidelity of her husband, Jason. Euripedes, who certainly had empathy with his notorious heroine, describes her emotional state as 'disconsolate'; she was hopelessly unhappy and unable to be comforted. He also provides a reason for her distress and her act of murder. He lets her say: 'Of all creatures that can feel and think, we women are the worst treated things alive.'[36]

One of the biggest challenges of post-apartheid South Africa is to understand why, almost systematically, the institutions that are supposed to be caring have become violent and cruel. We have to try to understand why this is so.

One such institution is the institution of motherhood.[37]

There is a lullaby that many Afrikaans-speaking children grow up with, myself included. I don't know whether it is sung to children in the valley. The song rather ominously depicts the dynamic life cycle of a man's ambivalent relationship with his mother. The mother sweetly lulls the baby to sleep on her lap, protects him against looming dangers, but she also abuses, abandons and kills. Even when he is a grown man, the mother is intrusive and she keeps the man small, a baby forever, '*tot hul dood*' – until they die.

Siembamba, mama's little lamb,
Siembamba, mama's little lamb,
Wring his neck, dump him in the ditch,
Step on his head, then he's dead.

Siembamba, I'm a baby now,
Siembamba, I'm a baby now

Keep me safe in my need,
Lull me gently in your lap.

Siembamba, I'm mama's little boy,
Siembamba, I'm mama's little boy.
But you will see I'll be grown up just now,
Killing pesky guys dead.

Siembamba, I'm mama's young man now,
Siembamba, I'm mama's young man now,
You can let me go from your warm lap now;
I'll kill the guys dead myself.

Siembamba, I'm a married man now,
Siembamba, I'm a married man now,
But mama thinks I'm mama's boy still,
Won't believe I'm grown up now.

Siembamba, all are mama's boys,
Siembamba, all are mama's boys,
All the men so grown up, so they say –
All are babies until they die.[38]

The line between nurturing and poisoning, giving life and killing, is
indeed a fine one:

she was my mom
and she taught me
how not to love
myself.[39]

Yet she was also:

the woman that
kept her sick leave
for when someone
else in the house fell ill.[40]

Although many women hurt others, such violence is often ignored.[41] As with women's anger and hostility, violence among women is still not expected or accepted, as it is not in line with traditional gender beliefs. Violent mothers, in particular, present a challenge.[42]

While many of the women we encounter in the valley present like Delize,[43] that is, with symptoms typically associated with a diagnosis of depression, for many so-called depressed women feelings of hostility and anger are actually more prominent.[44] However, anger and hostility are not acknowledged as a symptom of depression in formal diagnostic systems.[45]

Constructions of femininity dictate that 'good' women are calm, in control and self-sacrificing in relationships and that they engage in self-silencing feelings or behaviours in order to conform to these ideals.[46] 'Good' women should not experience, much less express, anger.[47]

The idealisation of the early mother-baby bond as the 'most perfect, the most free from ambivalence of all human relationships' has led psychologists to pay little attention to the anger of mothers.[48] As Joan Raphael-Leff writes, even feminist psychologists have failed to explore 'painful maternal experiences of ambivalence, persecution and hatred'.[49]

In the valley feelings of anger and hostility manifest in different ways. Aggressive fantasies are frequent. Scolding, swearing, shouting and yelling are often reverted to. Sterretjie, a woman diagnosed with depression, talks about her anger and how it manifests: 'Because I shout at my children a lot. I shout and just swear because then I am very angry. I get hugely upset and now . . . then I can't get rest. Oh, I can't. I am now going to scold, on and on and on.' She claps her hands.

Cathy, another woman diagnosed with depression, is as angry. 'Yes, I yell at them [her children] a lot – really, I yell a lot,' she says. 'I yell at them about anything they do. If they make a small mistake, I will yell at them.'

In the valley women often talk about how their anger leads to violence. They are mostly violent in their households, with partners and children as the targets. The violence we hear about sounds quite extreme. However, it is quite common for South African mothers to use corporal punishment.[50]

Leila describes her anger: 'Rage within me that wants to come out. It is like a thunderstorm. Nothing and nobody should lie in front of me, nothing is right for me. And then the rage pushes up in me and then no one should be in my way because then I simply am that angry bear. I would say if I have to describe my depression, I am just pissed off today. Today, today, no one should mess with me.'

She continues, 'Then I ask God silently to make me calm, tranquil, because I [hate] the way when they [her children] made me angry to attack them with the fists or I strangled them or threw things at them to get my way. I later on thought that is why my children are like this because I keep on scolding.'

Why are the women so angry and aggressive?[51]

Unsurprisingly, women's reasons for being angry are typically related to relational experiences and their disappointments in relationships. Women are angry about relationships and their deficits.[52] Women are distressed that their children are not living up to their expectations, not fulfilling their hopes and dreams. Most women know the feeling. Antjie Krog writes as a middle-class, white mother:

> and I go crazy
> my children assault me with their rowdiness
> > selfishness
> > cheekiness
> > destructiveness
> their fears complexes insecurities threats needs
> beat my 'image as mother' into soft steak on the wooden floor.[53]

The mothers in the valley also often relate their anger and violence to pain and disappointments associated with not being the mothers they wanted to be. Middle-class mothers often feel the same:

> I smell of vomit and shit and sweat
> . . .
> I sulk like a flour bag
> I am chipped like a jug
> my hands drier and older than yesterday's toast
> give half-hearted slaps against the clamour.[54]

Ideal mothers and ideal children seemed to be implicit in all the anger narratives.[55]

Twela talks about the type of person she wants to be: 'I don't want to be that person, that bad person, like swearing and whatever. And I don't want to be impatient. It isn't right to swear to express your feeling, to be impatient to express your feeling. It isn't right.' She continues: 'Yes and I don't want that angry. It's . . . it's frightening. I don't want that angry. And, and, and it isn't good because we can do anything wrong – you can, for instance, can make somebody hurt or you can hurt yourself. I don't want that kind of angry. I want to talk with a kind voice, but I don't want to shout back and ignore them or whatever. I don't want to do that.'

'And then we just argue and I'm so scared that . . . that I might . . . that I might do the thing to my child or if I, just, that feeling that I have – *hoe kan ek nou sê* [how can I say]? – that, that, that feeling what I had inside me, that, that, that bitterness and all that dark things that I had – *hoe kan ek nou sê*? – that I can give it to him.'

It is difficult to be a mother.

I go outside and sit on the step this Sunday morning
neither sober nor embarrassed
wondering
how and with what does one survive this?[56]

We might not.

## Repetition and ambivalence

The whole of our culture in the west depends on the murder of the mother.

— Luce Irigaray, in Margaret Whitford, *Luce Irigaray:
Philosophy in the Feminine*

I learned from you
To define myself
Through your denials.
— Audre Lorde, *From a Land Where Other People Live*

In the valley it is not only the boys and the men who have learned the language of violence. The girls know early on that relationships and families are dangerous places. Heterosexual relationships are almost automatically equated with betrayal and violence, even by very young women.

The students in clinical training run an empowerment group with thirteen-year-old young women, girls. The topic is 'Your Dreams' and the girls are boisterous. They talk loudly, interrupting each other and underlining their words with gestures and movement. In the group they are asked what they see as the biggest potential problem they will have to face in life.

'*Outjie* problems' (Boy problems), says Sandra without hesitation. 'He . . . he cheats on you with someone else . . . he beats you. My mother says if a boy beats me like that one day, he will always beat me, and then I should leave him.'

Rodine is adamant that she will fight back: 'No, my auntie told me if the *boytjie* [diminutive of 'boy'] hits me, I should hit him back. *My houe is in* (My blows are in)'.

Sandra is still convinced one has to leave: 'But I will still leave him, even though I gave him a *lekker* [good] beating.'

Wildene agrees: 'I will first hit him and then I will leave him. Then he will know he won't mess with me again.'

Sandra can see it: 'Then his eyes are swollen . . .'

Wildene elaborates: 'I will throw boiling water at him . . .'

Sandra explains how she will do it: 'I will hit him with the pan . . .'

The young therapist is nervous. '*Sjoe, jong* [Wow, man], that is a lot of rage.'

Chestline says: '*Ek sal vir hom warm knyp met 'n tweezer*' (I will pinch him with a tweezer so that he burns).

The student therapist asks the quiet girl what she will do. 'She, she will run away,' Sandra quickly answers.

The quiet girl, Jessame, answers slowly: 'I will burn him with a hot iron.'

Boiling water. A pan. A hot iron. Tweezers. A different take on the concept of domestic violence?

While the girls boisterously explain how they will fight back, they are also aware that women tend to stay in violent relationships – some might be fighting back, but some might be suffering in silence.

Maria brings this up as a problem: 'On the TV then you see how the men beat their wives and the women do nothing. They keep quiet.'

The therapist asks why they think women remain silent about violence and do nothing. Maria is clear: '*Want hulle is bang . . .*' (Because they are scared . . .).

Tina completes the sentence: '*hulle verloor die man*' (they lose the man).

Simone adds: '*Bang . . . hulle liefde maak hulle blind*' (Scared . . . their love makes them blind).

Wise Maria states emphatically: '*Dis hoekom ek altyd sê liefde maak blind*' (that's why I always say that love makes you blind).

The other girls echo her. 'Love makes you blind,' they all repeat.

Tina says: '*Miskien is sy nog baie lief vir die man en sy is nou bang om hom te verloor*' (Maybe she still loves the man very much and she is also afraid to lose him).

Wildene adds: 'And sometimes the man threatens them . . .'

They discuss a few examples of violence in vivid detail. Then they try to be wise again, understanding the acquiescence of the battered women.

'*Die liefde*' (Love), Wildene says resignedly.

'Yup,' Sandra says. 'Doesn't matter what he does, they just forgive them easily.'

'He just gives her a *soentjie* [diminutuve for 'kiss'], then she is happy again.' This is Simone.

'Happy,' almost a chant from Maria.

Wildene repeats: 'He kisses her.'

Well aware of the fact that women tend to stay in abusive relationships, the young women now turn to how dangerous men can be. '*'n Man kan jou lelik verongeluk*' (a man can harm you in nasty ways), says Sandra.

The therapist asks them how they feel when their mothers get beaten.

'Too much. It's just too much,' says Maria. 'Just don't beat my mom like that. That is just my mom. It's just my mom. No, no, no. It doesn't work like that.'

'We love them,' Sandra says, 'and we want to protect them.'

Some of the girls, however, feel that their mothers deserve to be beaten.

Maria excitedly says, fist in the air, 'Then sometimes you say, "It's right. Beat her! Beat her! Beat her!" Because she doesn't want to hear.'

'No, I never say that,' Sandra says.

Maria says: 'Your mom sometimes doesn't want to hear.'

Rodine explains: 'Your mom now beats you, now your dad comes, now your dad beats your mom. Then you say, "It is right, it is right." She then beats me.'

'No,' says Sandra, 'I will say, "Daddy, leave Mommy. It is right that she beats me."'

Thoughtful Sandra now suddenly turns to the group with a question: 'Now why when a man and a woman fight, you must now answer me, nè [not so]? When a man and a woman fight, why does the child always take the mom's side and never the dad's?'

The group seriously engages with the question, talking over each other.

'We don't know,' Maria says, 'because the dad is often wrong.'

'Now say,' Sandra is persistent, 'the mother comes home drunk and say, klap [beats] the man all over the place and the man now beats the mom. Why do you always take the mom's side?'

'No,' Rodine says, 'because I say "No, Mommy is wrong."'

Maria is adamant: 'No, I sal saamklap [will join in with the hitting].' She thinks for a moment, then changes her mind. 'No I'll just sit there and watch and say, "Klap each other, hit each other!"'

Sandra stays confused and says to the therapist. 'It's not true. They just say so. You always take the mom's side.' She stresses the always.

Wildene has a different answer. 'Because you feel a mom cares more about you. A mom really cares more about you. A mom looks after you.'

The girls' animated conversation about their beaten-up mothers is fraught with ambivalence: mother cares about you, mother takes care of you, your mother hits you, Mommy is wrong, your dad hits your mother, that's right. Implicit in this conversation is a very familiar story, that caring can be cruel and violent and that mothers are both loved and hated. This story is not only one that we often hear in the valley, it is also a dominant story in psychoanalytic developmental theory and feminist psychoanalytic theory – the inevitability of the murder of the mother.[57]

Much has been written about the conflict between love and hate, specifically the love-hate relationship children have with their carers. Girls typically have very strong and intense bonds with their mothers, but these bonds are often characterised by conflict, anger and fury.[58] The struggle with the mother is often articulated by girls and women as a wish to be the opposite of their mothers: they are critical of their mothers, focus on the qualities of their mothers that they most dislike and struggle against showing any such qualities in themselves.

Feminist psychologists have written about how in Western culture, 'the mother's fall from grace' is the major source of anger in the mother-daughter relationship.[59] While boys and girls typically are devastated when their mothers are devalued and treated with contempt, harshness and cruelty, for girls this is a double blow: their attachment to their mother is also identification – this is the person they are going to become. The devaluation of the mother necessarily also implies their own devaluation.

Marguerite Duras, in her novel *The Lover*, talks about the metaphorical murder of the mother in contemporary society:

> We're united in a fundamental shame at having to live. It's here we are at the heart of our common fate, the fact that [we] are our mothers' children, the children of a candid creature murdered by society. We're on the side of society which has reduced her to despair. Because of what's been done to our mother . . . we hate life, we hate ourselves.[60]

Adrienne Rich introduces the term 'matrophobia' and claims that all daughters perform radical surgery to get rid of the victim mother in themselves:

> Matrophobia can be be seen as a womanly splitting of the self in the desire to become purged once and for all of our mother's bondage, to become individuated and free. The mother stands for the victim in ourselves, the unfree woman, the martyr. Our personalities seem dangerously to blur and overlap with our mothers; and in a desperate attempt to know where mother ends and daughter begins, we perform radical surgery.[61]

For women in Western culture, their mothers represent powerlessness, regression, passivity and dependence.[62] Interestingly enough, while the girls in this group talk about how their battered mothers are powerless to leave, weak in their dependence, they also present their mothers as fighters, as being violent, aggressive and often intrusive. Similarly, many of the adult women we work with are diagnosed with depression and link their distress as adult women to their relationships with their mothers, relationships characterised by intensity, but often also by anger and violence.

Corrie is a 62-year-old pensioner and still remembers the hidings she got from her mother, with the imperative to be silent: 'I knew that if I cried, Mom gave me a hiding and I would cry more. I mustn't talk back or I will get hit . . . They were very strict . . . It was very bad . . . Then she would say, "You hold your mouth now!" Now my pain becomes worse, now I must bury it because I will still get more hidings if I carry on. Now this is all stuff that I have held back inside'. Corrie starts crying and says, 'For all these years . . . that dark blood in the rooms of my heart.'

Julia Kristeva in the valley?

Kristeva writes about how girls and women desperately try to identify with their powerful fathers, but when they become mothers, they inevitably reconnect with their mothers and become them:

> For a woman, the call of the mother . . . troubles the word: it generates hallucinations, voice, 'madness' . . . It is a fragile envelope, incapable of staving off the irruption of this conflict, of the love which had bound the little girl to her mother, and which then, like black lava, had lain in wait for her all along the path of her desperate attempts to identify with the symbolic paternal order.[63]

Strikingly, many of the women explicitly articulate how they don't want to be like their mothers. For example, Liza says, 'I want to have an open relationship with him [her son]. I want to give him what I didn't have. So I want to be a better parent than what my parents could be for me.'

Dabbie echoes this sentiment: 'Yes, I don't want what happened between my mother and me to happen again between my daughter and me.'

It is clear that the violence in their households and the subsequent hurting and humiliation of their mothers disturb the teenage girls in the group session deeply and they talk about how they literally try to block their ears and put blankets over their heads, so as not hear the fighting. They now talk over each other.

'I won't say anything. I'll put my earphones in my ears and when they *skel* [scold]. Then I listen like that. *O jinne* [Oh God], I can't take it.'

'When our people almost always *skel* in our house like that, then I'm busy with my phone. Or I pull the blankets over my head and I cover my ears.'

'I cry, *jong* [man] that time.'

'I, when I pull down the blankets then, I'll now hear the one now beating the other. Hear one of the kids crying. Their clothes full of snot as they cry.'

'Just say someone now fights, my mom and my dad now fight, now just say I know and I hear them *skel*? I switch the TV on very loud and then I watch TV.'

The girls are clear, however, that there are dangers in not being aware of what is going on. 'While you are here in another world, then your mom lies dead.'

The ensuing discussion about what can happen during a fight is heartbreaking.

'No,' says Sandra,' my dad won't go that far.'

'Oh yes,' says another one, 'my dad will.'

A third one says, 'You don't know, your dad will. They will do it. If the mom makes the dad angry, *dan sal hy daai ma doodslaan* [then he'll beat that mother to death].'

Sandra, the girl who is clear that her father won't kill her mother, makes a little speech. 'I always say, one day I want a husband like my dad. He never beats my mom and if they argue they are okay again with each other later. And if they argue I know he won't beat her because he's not like that. I want a husband like my dad. My mom said in the church the minister said a girl must say she wants a husband like her dad and a boy must say he wants a wife like his mom. My dad does not beat me. He works hard. In the sun. My dad is a builder.'

Not everyone is as lucky. One of the girls describes her very violent father and how her emotions shift during the violent fights: 'My dad – I don't want to call him "Dad" – almost everyone knows him, they know my dad is a strong man. If my mom and dad *skel* [fight], I get a little tear and it is a *bang traantjie* [scared little tear]. Because when my dad starts with her, *hy sal mens lewendig in die grond in doodklap* [he will beat her to death, into the ground while she is alive]. And then I think: *o jirre* [oh God], he is going to kill that woman. And it will take like a whole army to get my dad calm again because he's too much on it, too much in it. She makes him very angry and sometimes then *kry ek ook lekker* [it also gives me pleasure], then I think: beat her, beat her, beat her. My cousin says my dad's hands must be chopped off if he beats my mom like that. I say if he kills her, *ek maak hom net daar vrek* [I'll kill him dead right there].'

I will kill him dead right there.

She is thirteen years old, school uniform adorned with a class captain badge.

The mood in the group is sombre now, the feistiness has been subdued. In the conversation there is the clear wish not to hear and not to be exposed to the violent love they inadvertently have to witness. There is the profound ambivalence: the terrible fear that the caring mother will be murdered if there is no vigilance, the longing to protect the mother and to take away the power of the father: '*My pa se hande moet afgekap word . . .*' (My dad's hands must be chopped off). Always present, however, is the hate for the mother and the feelings of complicity with the murderer: '*Dan kry ek ook lekker, dan dink ek: slaan haar, slaan haar*' (then it also gives me pleasure, then I think: beat her, beat her, beat her).

Sandra, the girl with the good father (the father who works hard in the sun), starts to collect the cups in which Coke was served. She puts the screw top on the almost empty bottle and tightens it, her lips pursed. '*Dis nou soos 'n begrafnis hier*' (It's now like a funeral here), she says.

The other girls giggle and put the remaining muffins in their jacket pockets.

The therapists pack up the crayons and the dream sheets, throw out the empty Coke bottles and leave. The quiet girl's dream sheet lies on top of the pile in the back of the car. She dreams of becoming a lawyer. Her mother is a domestic worker. 'My biggest dream is that my mom and my mom's children live alone on an island in a big house. We must be rich. We must be a happy family.'

The dark blood of the rooms of the heart. Black lava. The call of the mother.

# Labour

*'. . . perhaps some schooling (mostly not) . . .'**

But is it true that the vests are preparing to revolt?
— Pablo Neruda, *The Book of Questions*

The word 'labour' can be a noun, a verb and an adjective. It carries multiple meanings, it is associated with capitalism and reproduction.
— Mary West, 'Speaking with a Forked Tongue'

Where do people earn the Per Capita Income? More than one poor starving soul would like to know.

In our countries, numbers live better than people. How many people prosper in times of prosperity? How many people find their lives developed by development?
— Eduardo Galeano, *The Book of Embraces*

July. Snow on the mountains.

Wilmien Wilders is 43 years old. The nurses at the clinic referred her to me because she is severely depressed. Her file is very fat with medical ailments. '*10 April: Vaginale afskeiding. Swelsel in lies. Afspraak vir Papsmeer. 16 April: Pyn op die bors. Afspraak by Stellenbosch Hospitaal. 3 Mei: Papsmeer. Amatryptiline. Afspraak gemaak met Lou-Marié* (10 April: Vaginal discharge. Swelling in groin. Appointment for a Pap

---

* The quote in the subtitle of this chapter – '. . . perhaps some schooling (mostly not) . . .' is from Sen, 2005: xi.

smear. 16 April: Pain in the chest. Appointment at Stellenbosch Hospital. 3 May: Pap smear. Amatryptiline. Appointment made with Lou-Marié). 'Appointment made with Lou-Marié' means that the nurses don't know what to do with her.

Wilmien walks into the consultation room, sits down and cries. Big tears. 'I am hungry. Very, very hungry,' she says. I wait. 'And me and my husband, we are separated from bed and table. I don't have a feeling for him anymore.'

As a psychologist I deal with bad relationships all the time. But I do not know what to do with hunger.

I ask about the relationship first. The couple got married on 28 September, twenty years ago. They have two children, not close to each other in age. Two sons, a twenty-year-old and an eleven-year-old. Wilmien says that it will be nothing for her to divorce her husband. He drinks and he smokes *dagga* (marijuana) and he does not give her any money. '*Ek wil op my eie gaan*' (I want to go on my own), she says. '*Ek weet nie wat ek vanaand gaan eet nie. Ek sal maar die kleintjie na die skoonmense stuur. Hulle gee altyd vir hom kos. Hulle is erg oor hom*' (I don't know what I am going to eat tonight. I'll just send the baby to the in-laws. They always give him food. They are fond of him).

On the wall of the consultation room are instructions for inserting a female condom. Cheerfully coloured pictures of how you can get the HIV virus and how not. A handwritten note from the nurse to herself: '*Josie, hoe populêr is Jesus in JOU lewe?*' (Josie, how popular is Jesus in YOUR life?)

I ask about work. Wilmien lost her job as a factory worker a few years ago. She had the job for twelve years. '*Ek weet nie eintlik wat gebeur het nie. Dinge het begin sleg gaan en ek het eendag vir my supervisor gesê: "As jy vir my 'n gat grawe, sal jy self daarin val." Toe laat hulle my gaan.*' (I don't really know what happened. Things started going badly and one day I said to my supervisor: 'If you dig a hole for me, you will fall in it yourself.' Then they let me go.) She has not worked since: '*Wie gaan nou vir 'n 43-jarige werk gee?*' (Who is going to give a 43-year-old work?) I look at her. She looks much older than 43. She is wearing a few layers of clothes. She lifts up her jacket to show me how loose her clothes are. Her body is bony and small and scarred. But tough. Her face is crinkly, with slanting eyes and high cheekbones. The laughing lines of her eyes make her seem amused, even though her mouth stays sad. '*En in daai jaar is my ma ook dood. My steunpilaar*' (And in that year my mother also died. My pillar of strength). She tells me that she also has '*hoë bloed en 'n hart* (high blood pressure and a heart problem). I look at the fat clinic file. '*Ek sien nie meer kans nie*' (I can't see a way forward anymore; I give up), she says.

I ask about her history. (Does hunger have a history? Does it matter?) Wilmien is the oldest child and has three brothers (Paul, Jacobus and Patrick). All four children are from the same parents. When Wilmien was still very young, her father lost his eye while pruning trees and received compensation from the government. With this money, he bought a plot in Treurwilgerstraat (Weeping Willow Street) and this is where the family lived for most of Wilmien's childhood. Her father died when she was fourteen or fifteen and the family lost the house.

I have my history, but Wilmien Wilders is still hungry. The only thing I can do is to make an appointment for the next week.

In the next few weeks we talk about empowerment, without ever using the word. After our first session, she comes weekly, always on time, always with the amused tears, telling me how hungry she is, how angry she is, how sad she is. Together we make plans. We agree that her biggest priority is to get a job. She cannot divorce her husband if she is not independent. She does not want to go back to the factory. We decide that she should go to Bergzicht Training to take a house management course.[1] We have to figure out how she will get money for the taxi fare (R10) for the initial appointment at Bergzicht. Psychologists do not give their patients taxi fares.

She gets the fare somewhere and enrols for the six-week course. When I see her again, six weeks later, she is in the waiting room when I arrive. She runs to me with wide-open arms, soap opera style. I say 'Wilmien' in soap opera style. She laughs the deepest laugh as she hugs me. The crowd in the waiting room stares at us. 'I finished my course,' she says. '*Ons het gister diplomas gekry*' (We got diplomas yesterday).

In the kitchen of the clinic (no consultation rooms available on this day) I ask, 'What have you learned, Wilmien?'

'Everything,' she says.

'I learned that a mop actually is a *dweil* [Afrikaans for 'mop']. A mop is just a mop in English. And I learned to do washing – all the white stuff go together and all the coloured stuff together. And how to iron and how to bake a chocolate cake. I baked a chocolate cake for the first time in my life on Monday, but then my *groot klong* [big boy] ate it all. Then I was very angry. We learned how to cook. Not only food, but also macaroni and lasagne. I met a lot of new people and I got along well with the teachers. Most of all I struggled with making the bed. It is very difficult to make a bed. If I get a job, I will take my book with me and always check in the book how to make the bed. But for my ironing I got 30 out of 30. And I was in school 22 years ago. I think I am also going to do the frail care course in January. The farewell yesterday was just very difficult. I even shed some tears. I couldn't wait to tell Lou-Marié.'

All in one breath.

*'n Koek, 'n kooi, 'n klong en 'n dweil* (A cake, a bed, a boy and a mop).

On the way home, I also shed some tears.

Our sessions end because soon after her report-back Wilmien gets a job. Weeks later I drive home with my daughter and, at the corner of my street in Stellenbosch, I see Wilmien. I stop and call her. She seems delighted to see me. She explains that she got a job in this street, a few blocks up from my house. *'Ek sukkel net want ek mag nie op die mense se stoele sit nie, so ek raak moeg. Maar ek sukkel darem nie meer met die kooi opmaak nie.'* (I just struggle because I am not allowed to sit on the people's chairs, so I get tired. But at least I do not struggle to make the bed anymore).

*'Wie is dit?'* (Who is that?), my daughter asks when we drive away. I do not know how to begin to answer the question.

## Surveillance and exclusion

Today on the WhatsApp group of my neighbourhood (Watch Neighbourhood X):

07:58    Suspicious vehicle at Flower Street CL11111
07:59    Security: On our way
08:01    Security: Silver Hyundai. Not stolen
08:03    Security: Gardener of Flower Street 1

| | |
|---|---|
| 08:09 | Security: J1 reported he also confirms he works at nr. 1, will be monitored |
| 10:26 | Two brown chickens on morning walk in Shiraz Street |
| 10:50 | I'll adopt them!!? |
| 10:51 | They belong to our neighbours, we have them safely back in their coop |
| 10:52 | Oh, *ek sa hulle gaps* [I will snatch them]. *Te oulik* [Too cute] |
| 12:58 | Big group of people in Shiraz Street moving in direction houses/neighbourhood. Actions unknown |
| 12:58 | Security: Sending vehicle |
| 12:59 | Security: Vehicle on its way |
| 12:59 | Security: On our way |
| 13:04 | Security: People doing construction work in the area and it is their lunchtime now |
| 14:12 | Children busy ringing door bells in Pinotage Road again |
| 14:12 | Security: On our way |
| 14:28 | Security: See no children so far |
| 14:31 | Security: J1, 2 removed the children and warned them |
| 14:32 | Security: J3 also found children in front of 52 Cabernet Street. Removed |
| 15:08 | Will you please come and have a look at Riesling Street a suspicious man |
| 15:09 | Security: On our way |
| 15:09 | Security: Description of clothing? |
| 15:09 | I didn't pay that much attention. Walking with child |
| 15:10 | You will know when you see him |
| 16:06 | Security: Man is monitored out of area |
| 16:06 | Thank you very much |

One member leaves the group.

The rules of Neigbourhood X.

*Kinders moet gesien word maar nie gehoor word nie* (Children should be seen but not heard).

Children should not be seen or heard.

We also prefer not to see or hear builders, gardeners, domestic workers.

Brown chickens are okay.

What are we doing when we, the privileged, are watching, identifying, monitoring, warning, removing? What does it mean when a security guard messages the neighbourhood that 'man has been monitored out of area' and someone (presumably one of my nice neighbours) says, 'Thank you'? What does it mean when someone else leaves the group, wordlessly?

'Monitoring someone out of area' seems to resemble Michel Foucault's notion of surveillance of the panopticon.[2] The neighbourhood watch becomes a system of normalising power that is based on the total surveillance of individuals by an invisible power that has the ability to see all. To maintain social and political order what does not fit in must be rejected, removed, expelled.[3] As such, parts of a culture and maybe even parts of the self are disowned – those parts seemingly connected with shame, humiliation, degradation, powerlessness, insecurity, dependence, danger, fear, desperation, vulnerability, impulsivity, anger, neglect and sadness.[4] Each voice from the margin can be seen to represent the potential for an encounter with lost parts of ourselves – and therefore is excluded.[5] These techniques and procedures of exclusion can be regarded as a personal or cultural survival strategy, excluding what we cannot bear to know about ourselves and what we cannot bear to acknowledge about the Other.[6]

The cute chickens can be adopted. The dangerous-looking men, the needy beggar, the unkempt stranger and the unruly children cannot be tolerated.

In the case of the neighbourhood watch, the 'monitoring out', exclusion or expelling is quite literal, but techniques of exclusion can also involve psychological strategies (states of splitting, amnesia, repression, dissociation).

I think of the hairwasher at the hairdresser that I have been going to for ten years. Her name is Marion; she is a coloured woman. Even though she has held my head in her hands, put her fingers in my hair for years, I don't allow myself to really see her as a person. I do this by making polite small talk and then closing my eyes.

I don't engage.

'What was hardest was not just that white people saw me,' says African-American feminist lawyer Patricia Williams, 'but that they looked through me, that they treated me as though I were transparent. By itself, seeing into me would be to see my substance, my anger, my vulnerability, and my wild raging despair.'[7] Audre Lorde, a prominent African-American feminist protests: 'I find I am constantly being encouraged to pluck out some aspect of myself and present it as the meaningful whole, eclipsing or denying the other parts of self. But this is a destructive and fragmenting way to live.'[8]

While in the process of working on an academic paper on childbirth, I go for a haircut.[9] I put on the black plastic cloak and lie down on the chair at the basin, ready to become just a brainless head. Starting my usual small talk, with my reading ready on my lap, I ask Marion how long she has worked at this salon. I think I ask her this every time she washes my hair and I never remember. 'Nine years,' she says. 'Is the temperature of the water okay? *Is Mevrou seker*? [Is Madam sure?] But now I want to leave. I have never had a raise. I can't come out on my money.' It is unusual for her replies to be more than one sentence. I close my eyes and ask her what she wants to do. 'Anything,' she says. 'Before this I was a chef for seven years. But I will do anything: housework, office cleaning, anything. But only Monday to Friday. I can do anything. *Ek sê mos altyd* (I always say), if you can do hair and food, you can do anything. I am now 46 years old and my youngest child just turned one. I want to be at home on Saturdays.'

The shampoo is cool on my scalp.

It is Friday.

If you can do hair and food, you can do anything.

But something else interests me. I am, after all, the expert on motherhood. If she has a one-year-old, she has been pregnant and has given birth recently. And I do remember that she is from the valley. Voyeuristically, I say '*Sjoe* [Wow], you had a baby a year ago?' (I turn over the printed-out paper on my lap, 'Childbirth, Complications and the Illusion of "Choice": A Case Study', a recent article in a so-called high-impact feminist journal, *Feminism and Psychology*).[10]

She starts massaging my head with slow, expert movements.

'Yes, no one wanted to believe me that I am pregnant. I was 45 then. They told me it is just hormones. But one knows one's body. I knew I was pregnant. At seven months I took a home pregnancy test and when it was positive, I went back to the clinic. They still did not want to believe it, but when they did the test, it was also positive. So it was only at seven months that I went for an ultrasound. In the waiting room there were only pregnant black girls who wanted abortions. Many of them. The woman of the ultrasound told me after the ultrasound that everything seems okay, but they can't guarantee it because I am so old. I said, "No, I trust my body. Everything will be fine." And I worked up to the day I gave birth.'

Her hands on my head are wonderful.

'That was a Saturday. When I left work, I said to them, "Today is the day" and I walked and I took the taxi home. When I got home I said to my husband, "I need to wash, it is *sulke tyd* [that time]." I washed and curled my hair and then I said to him, "We can now go back to town, to the hospital." Our neighbour took us. When we got to the hospital they had no beds – it was a very busy day. So I went straight to the labour room and they told me to lie on my side. Of course, I did not, because the pain was very bad. And then my water broke, and my husband ran out of the room screaming, "Nurse, nurse, *kom, daar het 'n pyp gebars!" Dit was nou snaaks'* ('Nurse, nurse, come, a pipe burst!' That was funny).

She now starts rinsing my hair.

'Water okay, *Mevrou*? But him and the neighbour left right after that. About an hour later, the nurse peeped around the door and asked whether I was okay. I said the baby was coming and she looked and said, "Yes, there is the head, the baby is coming." He was born an hour and a half after I arrived at the hospital. All six of my children came so easily. The nurse was nice, a *blanke vrou* [white woman]. I was pleased to be done before the night shift, because they were all coloured nurses and they were very busy. I saw them just walking past women who were screaming, just looking the other way. And there was a young girl who screamed so hard. She was in labour the whole night. I told her to breathe, to breathe, to breathe. No one was helping her. And in the end the nurse got the cleaning woman to hold up the girl's legs and she pushed them up and down like a pump so that the baby can come out. By that time, it was just the one nurse and the cleaning woman. That was terrible.'

She carefully folds a clean towel around my neck, gently pressing my shoulders.

My neck is stiff when I walk across the salon in my cloak of black plastic, my print-outs of papers about women and control and birth under my arm. '*Moet nou nie vergeet van die werk nie* [Don't forget now about the work], *Mevrou*,' says Marion. '*Ek kan enigiets doen* [I can do anything].'

I think of Marion who can do anything, and hair and food, and I think about Foucault and the agency of the seemingly powerless in the midst of social constraints. He says:

> Power is employed and exercised through a net-like organisation. And not only do individuals circulate between its threads; they are always in the position of simultaneously undergoing and exercising this power. They are not only its inert or consenting target; they are always the elements of its articulation. In other words, individuals are the vehicles of power, not its points of application.[11]

Marion is a powerful woman.

## Maids and madams

> We are aware of another gigantic wall being constructed in the Third World, to hide the reality of the poor majorities. A wall between the rich and the poor is being built, so that poverty does not annoy the powerful and the poor are obliged to die in the silence of history.
>
> — Pablo Richard, in Paul Farmer, *Pathologies of Power*

> I live on a periphery of an existence that I don't understand.
>
> There are superficial points of contact: a few words to the petrol pump attendant, good morning to the man who delivers the milk. And there is the black woman who works in my house.
>
> She is closer to me than a sister and she is more intimately acquainted with my private life than a sister ever could be.
>
> — Elsa Joubert, 'Agterplaas'

Young women in the valley learn about being locked into hierarchies at an early age.

We have a group session about careers and hopes and dreams with our thirteen-year-old schoolgirls. They are uncharacteristically subdued until they tell us about the dream of becoming a madam with a maid and playfully start to act out different versions of the maid-madam interaction.

Rodine starts by saying that her dream is to have her own house: 'Have my own house with a big garden at the back. Tennis court. Get up in the mornings. Say you get tired then you go: "Tring tring tring."'

Sandra chirps in: 'We will live like this. Then you just have to press a button for the woman, the woman who works in the house.' In a high-pitched voice, '"I want that and that." Nice life.'

Rodine is engrossed in her fantasy: 'Then you go "tring, tring", then the woman comes, then she says: "Yes, my lady?"'

The therapist, with agency and empowerment on her agenda, plays along with the fantasy, but tries to bring the girls back to reality. 'Okay, my lady, now tell me, tell me, how will this dream come about? How do I get there? How will you get there?'

Rodine understands the question: 'I am going to finish Grade 12. Then I'm going to, for me, become a chef and so. Then I'm going to . . .'

Sandra completes her sentence: 'Then you get money after all. "Yes, my lady." House. A car.'

Interrupting herself, Sandra becomes thoughtful and asks the group, 'What do you call someone who works in your house? . . . You don't want to call her by her name now?'

'Servant?' Rodine says.

Sandra, however, is adamant: 'Not servant. I will call her by her name.' She again speaks in a high-pitched voice, hand in the air, limp wrist. '"Carol? I quickly need you here."'

The therapist asks Sandra how the maid will feel if she is called 'servant'.

Sandra says: 'Bad!'

Rodine agrees: 'Bad, says she's a slave. Then she comes.' Now she acts out the maid. In a syrupy friendly voice, she says 'Yes, my lady.' And then immediately in a dark and down voice, 'Yes, my lady.'

Sandra imagines another possibility. 'I'll make her feel nice. Later make tea and so on. Then I'll say, "Sit, sit." Then I'll tell her she mustn't say, "Yes, my lady", she must say my name and then I'll tell her to sit and then I'll make her some tea because she must feel comfortable in the house and she must feel that we care about her, not that she must just go here, just go there, just go everywhere.'

The therapist inquires further. 'So Sandra, you want her to call you by your name and Rodine wants her to call you "my lady"?'

'Yes, my lady,' Rodine says.

The group does not blink at Rodine's ironic response to the therapist. They are seriously engaged.

The therapist wants to know more. 'How would you feel if I called you "my lady"?'

The girls are clear. 'I'll feel important,' says Rodine.

Wildene agrees: 'I feel good . . . when I think about it.'

'I feel excited,' adds Rodine. 'I want to be there now, I want to be there now.'

'Me too,' says Sandra.

'Oh, oh,' says Rodine, 'lifestyle dreams . . . a garden, a house, a swimming pool, dresses, a nice relationship with my family and every weekend to the sea. All the places . . .'

'Goudini,' says Wildene. 'It's nice there.'[12]

Spoilsport therapist once again interrupts the fantasy. 'Now, how far in the future do you think this dream is?'

'Wow, we still have four years of school. And it will take even longer.' This is Sandra.

'It's still long, yes.' Rodine.

'It's not nice,' says Sandra.

Rodine has the last word: 'If I think how long, it makes my *plak sak*' (it makes me feel really down).

The wall that has been erected and is maintained between rich and poor (in South Africa) is most permeable and most threatened when poor black people are employed by wealthy or middle-class white South Africans. In her book *Soos familie* (Like family), Ena Jansen writes: '*Sonder twyfel is swart huiswerkers die belangrikste kontakfigure in Suid-Afrika tussen wit en swart, stad en platteland, ryk en arm*' (Without a doubt black domestic workers are the most important contact figures in South Africa between white and black, cities and rural areas, rich and poor).[13] In this relationship, the privileged and underprivileged, the powerful and the seemingly powerless, the dominant and dominated are exposed to each other and can potentially obtain knowledge about each other. It has been pointed out, however, that 'the mutual knowing which occurs between the employer and servant is of a particular kind which involves as much – perhaps more – wilful ignorance as knowledge'.[14] Therefore, despite the fact that almost one million black women are employed as domestic workers in South Africa, this 'special form of servitude' continues 'to be largely invisible in our society, their needs ignored and their voices unheard'.[15]

In the valley, many of the women who work are in the service industry, with many of them working as domestic workers on farms and in the neigbouring towns.[16] Alicia is a domestic worker, earning a small wage every second week. She lives with her husband in a labourer's house on a farm in the valley. He also earns very little and is also paid every two weeks. She left school after Grade 8. She and her husband are active members of a church called the Sacred Heart Crusaders. When we interview her for a research project on motherhood, she is 26 and expecting her third child; she has two daughters aged ten and six. The interaction between the white female interviewer and interviewee is strained; the interviewer awkwardly and clumsily does her best to make Alicia comfortable.

The white student interviewer is acutely aware of the awkwardness of the interaction. 'The house was neat inside and looked like all the other small houses in which I've already been, a bit poky with a small table and four chairs around it,' she writes in her journal.

> There were quite a lot of flies in the small kitchen, probably just because the weather was so close to raining. I tried not to take notice of them, because she was also aware of the flies and I wanted to show her that it didn't bother me. I just wanted her to feel comfortable. Suddenly I was a bit more aware of what I was wearing, how I acted, what I said, how I said it. I wanted to fit in more, but she was a bit tense and I couldn't look past it.

In this rather stiff interview, Alicia says that motherhood and pregnancy are not difficult for her, her work is. 'Um, working conditions, yes, things at work. That make me feel discomfort, make me feel uncomfortable. But I don't express emotions. I just kept it inside the whole time . . . maybe – how can I now say? – I worked two, three days a week . . . and there are some things that she . . . now she isn't really nasty to you, but [with] some things she makes you feel as if it is your fault, maybe, like plates that are chipped or so, now she tells you, you must work carefully, then you know by yourself, but you're not the only one who works with those dishes. There are more people who – the children just chuck the plates down, things and then, then I feel rather *opstandig* [rebellious], but then I just keep it inside. One moment things are fine and then they are not.'

Much is revealed in this brief narrative about domestic work. For Alicia, her workplace is an uncomfortable space where she does not speak about her emotions, where she keeps things inside. She says that there is not direct abuse ('she isn't really nasty to you'), but Alicia is perpetually held responsible for things that go wrong. She is made to feel guilty and it is implied that she is careless. She feels resentful about being blamed for what goes wrong, thinking that the children of her employer are quite careless. While she relates feeling *opstandig* (rebellious) about all of this, she does not feel that she can voice this resentment. Her not feeling safe in the workplace is enhanced by the fact that the environment feels unpredictable – she feels that she has little control.

Her employer's critical attitude is not only limited to how she does her work. She is also criticised for how she lives and the life choices she makes. In this case, her employer is critical about the fact that she is pregnant again. 'Then she found out that I was pregnant. Then she asked, but how can I think about falling pregnant again because my first girl child had cancer, the second one got meningitis at one and a half years and she was left with a hearing problem because of it. Now, how can I think of falling pregnant again? I felt, see, us *bruin mense* [brown people], we don't interfere in them white people's lives, now why must she always . . . she is always busy with me . . . she cannot think, how you can . . . you can't provide for the one and then you fall pregnant again. I say our school fees aren't as expensive as their school fees and, look, as long as we don't lie in front of their doors for a piece of bread and so – not for food or so – and if I feel if I want to make another boy and that . . . then it is just . . . I'm the one who's going to struggle and not her. Struggle you just have to. If you plead for something from the Lord, then you must just believe, but our faiths aren't the same. I survived and every day I have with the Lord's help and power. Every day my daughter's hearing gets better and her use of language gets better and the eldest girl child, she was in Tygerberg [hospital] for eight months, she's healed from the cancer. And the one of six is still in the crèche, but hopefully she'll go to school next year. To an ordinary school, to see whether she'll progress there, but she talks everything. She is okay.'

Alicia is now indignant. 'Yes, to think that she tells me how I can fall pregnant – she has two girl children and they were also eager for a little boy, got a little boy, but now she is pregnant again with the fourth one, after lecturing me.'

Alicia is clear why she wanted another child. Already having two girls, she not only wants a boy, but also wants a small child to 'cuddle'. 'I think if your children's growing-up years and the best for you is just to, while they are still small and you can cuddle them and they do just as you want them to do, but when they are now this stage then they don't want to listen anymore.'

She experiences her employer as intrusive and inconsistent. Implicit is also her awareness of how she as a coloured worker will not 'interfere' with a white person's life, thus suggesting that she is frustrated by the arrogance (the critical opinionatedness) associated with power. For Alicia, pregnancy and motherhood are not problematic, work is. 'Yes, you just sometimes have to . . . or keep quiet about certain things to keep the peace. To be unhappy at work every day, it makes me mad. It's just not a nice face.'

Alicia's account of her life as domestic worker is not unique. In the literature, when domestic workers are interviewed, the talk is mostly about what has been called 'verbal and non-verbal bullying'.[17] The kind of belittlement and false accusations Alicia talks about are rife. The domestic worker is constructed, on the one hand, as an irresponsible child that should be looked after and reprimanded and, on the other hand, as a dangerous and threatening intruder. The employer's stance of both patronising and benevolent parent and strict authoritarian and disciplinarian is thought to be warranted.

Alicia is one of the few women we interview who herself explicitly brings up the issue of race. She is the only woman who insists on using her own name in the interview and is experienced as slightly withholding by her interviewer, a young white woman. In the interaction, much of what Alicia describes in the domestic worker relationship is repeated: the interviewer is asking questions that can be experienced as intrusive, Alicia is resisting the intrusions by refusing any intimacy. She feels suspicious, the interviewer feels guilty. The interviewer feels needy, Alicia seems uncomfortable and withholding. The very serious and perturbed interviewer writes about Alicia in her journal:

> [Alicia] wasn't very enthusiastic, and I wondered whether she really felt like doing the interview. I asked her again and she said that she wanted to do the interview . . . Her discomfort rather made me feel that I had to do it in as big a hurry as possible so that I wouldn't prolong the discomfort unnecessarily . . . She didn't get really excited during the interview . . . I felt rather guilty when I left because I would have wanted to do more for her. On the other hand, maybe I was just tired and I was the one who felt uncomfortable because according to me she didn't seem that enthusiastic.

After every interview, Alicia asks the interviewer how the interviews will be used. The interviewer is acutely aware of Alicia's presence and power. The relationship is fraught. Neither party seems to like what she has become in the interaction.

Elsa Joubert, award-winning author of the much-acclaimed *The Long Journey of Poppy Nongena*, an account of the life of a South African domestic worker in the years of apartheid, writes in her journal about the mutual antipathy that she felt when interviewing Poppie, who worked for her as a domestic worker:

> I have become aware of a strange antipathy. I have no more desire to proceed with the book.

I have become aware of an antipathy in her also. It is as if I must dig, bore, scratch out of her, details that I have no right to know.

We have evidently reached the point where I do not want to go closer and she does not want to expose more.

There is a wall not of incomprehension but of complete unwillingness to comprehend. For me there is something repulsive in what she must expose, for her in the breaking down of the walls that must stand between us.

Maybe I will gain a book, but will lose a servant.

But I think it is more than just a barrier or resistance on a human level.

The excitement of discovery, of spaces and realms of experience that were strange to me, is gone.

In the mass of material that lies before me there is a threat like that of a cancerous growth in the body.

Do I want to have this knowledge? My whole being rejects it.

It is unpleasant for me to work with it.

Contrary to what it would be if I described the life of a redskin or an eskimo. It is all the time a constant, constant gnawing at myself. Even my environment is being eaten away, like mice nibbling cheese from the inside.

Tonight, Klaas had to fix the key for her room, and the door was open and I went inside, which I do not like to do. I am not fond of the smell, of the strangeness, of, why does the word come to me, of the threat.

It disturbs me that the walls have been smoked black, by whom? I must get it painted. Tomorrow. Get another chair. A table. Why must the conditions that she tells me about be reproduced in my own back yard?[18]

Why indeed must the conditions of poor working women be reproduced in my own back yard? And in the back yard of my own academic and clinical work?

The walls that have been erected are smoked black, but they are still there.

What further complicates the relationship of the domestic worker with her employer is that while the worker is treated like an unruly child who is dependent on the employer not only for a living wage, but also (or so we tend to think) to live and behave in irresponsible ways, the employer is also hopelessly dependent on the worker. This dependence is complicated: the domestic worker is entrusted with the running and maintenance of the household and taking care of children, as well as with intimate knowledge about the household and its members. In the South African context, domestic workers are often described to be '*soos familie*' (like family), being closer to the employers than their sisters, mothers or friends.[19]

There thus is an extremely complicated intimate relationship of mutual dependence, characterised by a constant negotiation of power and vulnerability. Reading the literature about this relationship,[20] one is immediately struck by how the paradoxes, contradictions and ambiguities are always highlighted. Shireen Ally writes about how the institution of domestic work is fraught with contradictions, where humiliation and depreciation is bound up with intimacy and care, a 'dialectic of attachment and denigration'.[21] Service work, she says, can be brutalising and estranging, or affectionate and devoted. She cites Ann Stoler, who refers to tense and tender ties and states: 'In this zone of contact, that was so "forced and intimate", a contradictory cauldron of affect included distrust and fear as much as abiding forms of compassion and love.'[22] Jansen talks about *afstand* (distance) and *vertroudheid* (familiarity).[23] Tamara Shefer refers to love and humiliation, intimacy and estrangement, care and denigration.[24] Sarah Nuttall describes the relationship as an 'entanglement, a condition of being twisted together or entwined': 'it speaks of an intimacy gained, even if it was resisted, or ignored or uninvited . . . entanglement is a term which may gesture towards a relationship or a set of social relationships that is complicated, ensnaring, in a tangle, but which also implies a human foldedness.'[25]

With such a chaotic entanglement, splitting is very likely to happen.[26] The Other will either be romanticised and idealised, or denigrated and demonised, with defensive processes like projection and projective identification becoming inevitable.[27]

Shefer describes 'the painful but sweet comfort of nostalgia, confessions of shame and guilt' of white people when they talk about the domestic workers of their childhoods, confessions inspired by 'the imperatives of avoiding discomfort of a deeper confrontation of white investment in apartheid'.[28] The 'nanny' is idealised as the other mother: idealised, powerful and desirable.[29] In the words of Afrikaans rock musician Koos Kombuis:

> I remember her as yesterday
> Since I was this small, she was there
> With her eyes like kaffir beer she lets you think maybe the Mona
>     Lisa was brown
> Kytie Adams was the woman installed in our kitchen
> She could do dishes and wash clothes, look after children and
>     show us manners, show manners
> Kytie, Kytie, Kytie, you didn't live with us for twenty years for
>     no reason
> Kytie, Kytie, Kytie, you were not just a maid, but a mom to me.[30]

Like Alicia in the interviews, domestic workers themselves contest this idealisation of themselves as other mother (or sister), powerful and desirable. They insist, like Alicia on being seen as *die meid* (the maid):

> my auntie Katie was sixteen when she started
> working in service she just went to school until standard 5
> my grandmother auntie Katie's mom was also a domestic worker
> my auntie Katie was a very glamorous woman her
> hair always had blonde streaks in she only
> wore gold jewellery and went nowhere without her musky
> perfume and rouge lipstick
> except
> to work one must always do one's work with pride
> my grandmother told her but she couldn't she answered
> she wanted to look like
> she felt she said like the maid.[31]

The white man constructs the domestic worker as mother and Madonna, consistent, caring and *ordentlik* (decent, respectable). The coloured domestic worker is a glamorous person in her community, but insists on being the '*meid*' when she works as domestic worker – nothing glamorous about that. In remembering and reflecting, the white employer and researcher want to humanise; the domestic worker wants to insist on exposing the inevitable dehumanisation of being a domestic worker.

However, Alicia's description of her relationship with her employer suggests that in the household it is the domestic worker that wants to insist on her humanity, while the employer refuses to see it. Jansen cites Ntombi who writes: 'I tried to tell my madam my baby was hungry. But she wasn't listening to me. She wasn't thinking about me or Lindiwe. She didn't even look at us. She was thinking only of the supper I was cooking.'[32]

When writing about domestic workers, Antjie Krog quotes Drucilla Cornell: 'The nothing of the failure of representation itself becomes a form of listening.'[33] She then cites her domestic worker Victoria, in conversation with another domestic worker:

> The woman next door keeps her polony slices in our fridge, that's okay. is it your daughter that just got off? yes she's going to going to fetch that childs's grant yesterday morning another woman saw the dogs eating something in her yard then she saw it was a fetus the dogs were busy with the arms the eyes still moved like this but there was no more sound.[34]

Victoria instantaneously becomes a person. Someone with a fridge and a yard and dogs and death in her life.

South African psychologist Wahbie Long asserts that Karl Marx's notion of alienation is highly relevant when we consider the psychology of poverty in the South African context. He explains:

> For Marx, if human beings are not to lose themselves they must succeed in relating actively to others and to the world. The problem with the capitalist mode of production, however, is that it engineers a society in which that definitively human activity – work – is transformed into an endless exercise of mindless, joyless routines.[35]

I tell my friend, the philosopher, about the stories of the working women. She tells me to read Hannah Arendt. I read about Arendt's distinction between the human activities of labour, work and action. Psychologically speaking, it makes absolute sense to arrange labour, work and action in an ascending hierarchy of importance. For Arendt, labour is the activity that is related to biological processes and the necessities of human survival. As a result, labour is never-ending, repetitive and creates nothing permanent. Its products are quickly consumed and therefore it is a perpetual activity. Because it is a necessary activity, it is not an activity associated with freedom of choice. For Arendt, labour thus defined is contrary to freedom and to what is distinctively human – labour constitutes the basis of the institution of slavery.[36]

Someone said about domestic work, or domestic labour then, what is at stake is nothing less than what it means to be human.

The thirteen-year-old girls in the valley know the maid-madam script: it is a well-known and predictable story. It is seldom that something new is created in the relationship.

'The figure of the servant casts a long shadow.'[37]

## Bosses and labourers

And yet, as a path to happiness, work is not highly prized by men. They do not strive after it as they do after other possibilities of satisfaction. The great majority of people only work under the stress of necessity.

— Sigmund Freud, *The Freud Reader*

For working-class women there may be a different kind of settlement between motherhood and work, the projects understood as complementary in different ways: with motherhood providing motivation for work, breadwinning demonstrating maternal competence, or motherhood providing an attractive alternative to low-paid insecure work.

— Rachel Thomson et al., *Making Modern Mothers*

In the valley women who don't work as domestic workers or in the service industry typically work as seasonal farmworkers or in factories. We rarely hear from domestic workers that the work is intrinsically satisfying. It is relentless.

The women work to feed their children and they miss their children while working. Delize is a seasonal farmworker with a Grade 7 education.[38] 'We do the vineyard work,' she says. 'There are not so many vineyards now because they took out most. They want to make it a wine farm. They are going to plant other vineyards. They are actually busy getting the land and so ready. Trees that have been cut down and logs that they are busy taking out to get the land ready for vineyards. But at the moment we are cleaning bones. The vineyard's bones. That is the stick thing. That has to be cleaned, because they have wild shoots, shoots that do not carry grapes. They grow wild and make the vineyards ugly. Now we are cutting them off, breaking them off. As soon as the grapes grow more, one can say the growth is more in the wild shoots than in the grapes.'

When asked whether the work is difficult, she says, 'It is outside work and the whole day in the sun. I am used to it. When I was a child I started working. I started on a farm then and on a farm, I grew up. I was used to that work. I was probably about twelve years old. Twelve years and I still went to school, but at the end of the year it was harvest and I stopped going to school.'

A student brings me a song by the South African rap band Dookoom:

I'm fed up,
I'm fed up and I have had it up to here, fed up
My soul and my body, I feel crippled
All I say is fuck off I'll burn your farm down
Now you can work same as me.[39]

If Delize feels anger, she does not articulate it.

For her, as for most women, the most difficult thing about working is co-ordinating the work schedule with childcare. Just after giving birth, she had to leave her baby with her mother. Intergenerational childcare is common in the valley, but for Delize, as for many women, it is not ideal.[40] 'My mother is old now. She is not the person she used to be. Before, before, I could leave my kids with her. Now I buy a can of milk, the baby drinks that, then I go to work and then three times, like three times a day I come home to give her breast, not matter where I work. I have to make sure that I get here to give her breast. My mother can't do everything anymore. She can't pick her up, her arms get just too tired. My mother is 64 now. But she can't do many things. Many people of that age are still fit, but not her. I just leave her there and trust that things will be okay when I leave the house. I have to think, nothing will happen during the day.'

'But I worry. Sometimes I think, you know, she also is a *bloedlyer* [has high blood pressure]. She once had stroke. I thought last week I should ask my neighbour that *sy moet altyd so draaitjie maak* [she should come by every now and again]. But they will probably know quickly – my baby, when she cries, she has a very loud voice. They will hear her from afar. But still, I have to make sure that she has eaten, everything done, yes. And nappy, that she has a dry nappy. And in the mornings, before I walk to work, perhaps like ten minutes before, *dan bollie sy altyd klaar* [she does a pooh]. *Sy bollie altyd so eenmaal per dag* [She poohs always one time a day]. So I wait until she has made her pooh and then I change her nappy and *maak haar lekker skoon* [clean her properly]. Then it does not matter if she walks with nappy until twelve. Then I change it again.'

I ask her about lunch.

'We go home for lunch, yes. It's half an hour. It's funny.' She laughs. 'We don't actually really have food for us. We coloureds, our men are so spoilt. Nowadays they also want to eat well. I don't know what we ate when we grew up. When we go home lunchtime and there is leftover food from the evening, especially Mondays, afternoons, then there is just no food left over from Sunday. I always keep every . . . evenings when I cook, then I keep some of the food for my husband for the afternoon. But me, if I eat a piece of food at eleven o'clock, I'm not hungry. Then I maybe take a slice or two of bread to work. For if I get hungry around three, four o'clock, then I'll quickly eat it during work time. Four o'clock we get a small break of about fifteen minutes. Then we have to work again until five o'clock.'

As the baby gets older, Delize cannot leave her with her mother anymore. The schedule is still tight. 'But she must also eat every morning before I take her to the carer. She must have finished eating in the mornings and we drop in for work at eight o'clock, half-past eight. But I mean when the husband comes to eat breakfast at eight o'clock, everything must be done. The house must be clean, the child must be clean and ready. I must be ready. Our foods, we just always take a piece of bread along for eleven o'clock, or some of the evening's leftover food, then I dish up a little bit. Here around eleven o'clock or so, one gets hungry. Yes, if you get some rest here at eleven o'clock. But now after that time, after eleven o'clock one always feels tired, then I feel sleepy. Then I can feel now I'm getting tired and in those fifteen minutes – we only get fifteen minutes free – in that time then, if I just put my head down then, even if I just doze off a little bit, when I wake up there, then I'm ready for the day again, to carry on working. Just *so klein slapie* [such a little nap].' She laughs. 'When I wake up there, then I'm now ready again. Then my body feels ready to continue again. Until tonight, ten o'clock, eleven o'clock, before going to sleep.'

Seventeen-year-old Blondie, abandoned by the father of her child and forced to go back to work as a cleaner at a guest house, explains her decision to go to work, rather than to go back to school. 'I'm just happy I now at least have a job and things are going much better and so I feel fine.' She hesitates and speaks softly. 'And further, it's just . . .' Her voice becomes even softer. 'I just miss her so much when I work.'

She laughs shyly and is silent. She is asked more about the job. 'It feels okay,' she says. 'Now I can help my mom and I can buy for my child what she needs and so. I'm a *bietjie* [little bit] sorry that I don't have much breastmilk because she now mostly just drinks . . .'

On cue, the baby on her lap makes a protesting sound, a long 'Uhhhhh'.

Blondie and her therapist laugh. 'Ja,' says Blondie, 'she now drinks bottle milk. I buy it at Shoprite. It actually is cheap, say R15 for a *boksie* [little box]. When I went to charge her father, the woman at the court said I should go to school. But I thought, and I could not go back to school. I will now have to care for her. I know my mother will care for her, but the money is too little, the money that my mother earns. *Om vir haar kos te . . . sy eet mos nou eintlik een kant* [To give her food . . . she eats actually on one side]. *En sy makeer mos nou pap en sy makeer mos nou melk en sy makeer mos nou miskien diapers* [And she needs porridge and she needs milk and she needs perhaps diapers]. And who will now buy it for her? Her father *hoeka* [already] does not worry. And the woman wrote on the letter to her father that I am going back to school. Okay. So I accepted that, but I said to myself, "I am not going back to school." I need to work where I worked last year. Even if I don't earn the same. I am back to acceptance and determination. And my mother said, "It is your decision, my child." And I said, "*Mammie, Mammie* can't buy everything for the baby that she needs." And what is she has to . . . for my school and my sister's school, where will *Mammie* get the money? So I said to her, "No, *Mammie*, I am going back to work." And my work people are pleased that I am coming back. They thought I will stay home with the child. I will have my break at ten and then again half-past two.'

Her voice becomes listless, she seems to be losing her drift. 'And then it's clean and then we go for lunch again, then we come again at half-past two, then and in that time, I do such a lot of things. I have a quick look, then I go to her and say hello and maybe bring her a biscuit, or a sweet or so. And then I must now hurry again to get to work. But fortunately it's at least not taxi money or so. It's quite close to the house.'

Nineteen-year-old Millicent, beautiful but very sad, is a quality manager in the cold rooms of a factory. 'I work with fruit and the quality of fruit, that's all,' she says. Despite being the main breadwinner of the household, she stopped working when six months pregnant after she almost had a miscarriage. She explains, 'I actually work in a factory and it's very cold there and I have to work nightshift sometimes and it's now one week nightshift and one week dayshift. If we work dayshift in the morning, then it is five o'clock that I need to get up in the mornings. Then some mornings I walk and then I must walk in the rain to where the bus picks me up. That also had an effect on the miscarriage, the almost miscarriage that I then also went through.'

Millicent is ambitious and very ambivalent about her baby. She says she will not have a baby again in the next ten years and that she wants to do a computer course, so that she can become a secretary. She is one of the few non-working women who misses being at work. 'I am bored some days,' she says, 'then I wish I could still have worked, but not now. Probably next year I'll be able to go and work again.'

## Masters and slaves

What is the meaning of a handshake between somebody with an empty stomach and somebody who gets off on snow-covered peaks?

— Marlene van Niekerk, 'Labour'

It goes without saying that the history of South Africa is a history of masters and slaves.

— Wahbie Long, 'Shame, Envy, Impasse and Hope'

I want to see the valley after hours and go wine tasting with my friend the anthropologist.[41] We go to one of the very wealthy farms in the valley, a farm that markets itself as progressive and politically astute. We meet our host for the evening, Monique. She greets us cheerily, 'Welcome to XX farm.' Monique is a plump 21-year-old, but looks older, wiser.

'I am sorry – I forgot the most important thing, to introduce myself. I have just completed a hospitality course. Good afternoon. My name is Monique.' In perfect English, she explains the wines to us while she pours us generous glasses. Monique grew up on XX farm, but now lives in Pniel with her boyfriend, Martin. Martin is a security guard on XX farm. It is a good job. Everyone is treated well, she says. 'Craig [the farm owner] stops at the gate every day and chats to Martin.'

Only twice during the wine tasting she forgets the hospitality and reverts to Afrikaans. '*Nou is julle twee getroud?*' (Now, are you two married?)

'No.'

'*Nou weet Mevrou se man dat jy hier wyn drink saam met hom?*' (So does *Mevrou*'s husband know that you are drinking wine with him here?). Concerned.

And then she suddenly starts, vigorously, to scratch herself and then discloses earnestly: '*Ek jeuk. Ek jeuk altyd as ek hier op hierdie presiese grassie staan*' (I itch. I always itch when I stand on this exact little patch of grass).

With the afternoon becoming cooler, the shadows longer, the face and voice of hospitality seem to retreat even further. Monique becomes more confiding. When pouring the red bubbly, she giggles as if inhaling the bubbles and tells us that this is her favourite wine. 'You can drink it from the bottle. It is like grape juice. When I feel down, this is what I drink. And don't worry about the low alcohol. It really hits you. Three, four glasses and then I am gone. But otherwise I am not really a wine drinker.' She giggles and starts to hum. 'You know what I am humming?' In a clear voice, she sings 'Put your arms around me' and explains how she sometimes has to put her arm over someone when serving them and then she sings this song to herself. 'Yes,' she muses, 'I thought I was going to be a singer and actress and now look at where I am.' Her people, she says, still live on the farm. 'We were not happy when we were sold to Craig. Because no one told us. We did not know. We were invited to this party and then we were told we have been sold. We were not happy.'

Martin comes to fetch her and she has to leave. 'He comes and gets me early, because his shift starts at five. Otherwise I have to take the taxi.' Before she locks the doors, she pours us each another generous glass of her favourite bubbly and leaves us at an outside table overlooking the farm. We become aware of the birds in the vineyards and down at the river; they seem noisier now. It is suddenly cold. There is a full moon rising. When we drive away there is a change of the security guards at the gate. Martin is on duty.

I wonder if tonight is a night for bubbly in Martin's little house in the valley.

We drive away from the farm. The fields are luminously green and the mountains even more formidable than usual, with chilly caps of snow.

Our next stop is the shebeen in Kylemore.

The shebeen is in one of the poorest streets in Kylemore. The houses on this street are small, like dolls' houses, with the people seeming big in comparison, almost grotesque and slightly awkward. In all the back yards, there are other structures: Wendy houses, shacks or even more brick houses . . . and always those lean, hungry-looking dogs.

Tonight, fires are glowing in most front yards, with people huddling around them. The shebeen is an ordinary brick house behind the highest wall on the street. One enters through a small opening in a big security gate. There are seven people in the sandy front yard of the house, four men, two women and a baby. The Castle beer is sold by a stern-looking older man at R9 for a one-litre bottle. Everyone has brought their own glasses.

The woman sitting on the bench is Melody. She is holding the baby. The other woman is her daughter and it is her six-month-old baby Shandre that Melody is holding. Shandre is wrapped in two blankets. His eyes are alert, staring then at the neon light above, then at his grandmother, who tells us how she struggles to survive on R60 a day. I take Shandre from the grandmother. His mouth grabs my hand and sucks on it hungrily. He stares at me intently. The mother tells me that she is a security guard at Woudenmeer, a luxurious security village outside Paarl. She works in shifts, three days on, three days off. This is the end of such a three-day shift. She slurs. It might be the beer, it might be the fact that her front teeth are missing. She takes the baby from me, stumbles once, finds her balance and starts to light a cigarette. She laughs with a wide mouth, fumbling when lighting the cigarette with the baby on her shoulder. '*Maak toe die baba se voetjies*' (Cover the baby's feet), she says. One of the men takes the baby from the mother. '*Moenie my kind leer tik nie*' (Don't teach my baby to *tik* [use methamphetamine]), says the mother. The grandmother accidentally kicks over a half-empty bottle of beer, precariously positioned on a cement block. She puts down her glass and declares, 'I am going home. I know when to stop.' The beer fizzes on the concrete.

The moon is full and brilliant when we leave.

# Hunger

*'. . . some mother's milk (sometimes not) . . .'* *

And then on every table in the world, salt.
> — Pablo Neruda, *The Book of Questions*

If you had a difficult childhood, you sleep more so that there are fewer hours in the day. My uncle can sleep the whole day. When my mother asked him once why he sleeps like that, he said: 'I am damn hungry, if I sleep I dream about how I enjoy eating, then you come and wake me up. I had not even finished eating . . .'. Being hungry brings out the poet in you and it can make you crazy.
> — Nathan Trantraal, *Wit issie 'n colour nie*[1]

As long as the woman from Rijksmuseum
in painted silence and concentration
day after day pours milk
from the jug to the bowl,
the World does not deserve
the end of the world.
> — Wisława Szymborska, *Poems: New and Collected, 1957–1997*

'What does it mean to be hungry?' the anthropology student asks her focus group of three women, all of them mothers of infants she met in

---

\* The quote in the subtitle of this chapter – '. . . some mother's milk (sometimes not) . . .' is from Sen, 2005: xi.

the line at the local soup kitchen. It is midday, but the sun is feeble and it is still cold outside. It is August. The group is sitting in the community hall where the weekly soup kitchen is held. They have finished serving food and, having tidied up, they are having a picnic of sorts. The ensuing conversation is disturbing.

> Jessica said that hunger was 'not having something to eat'. Yes, sometimes, she experienced it. Veronica said she did, too, especially when her father's construction work had ended without notice. 'You just go to sleep,' she said. 'You just sleep, and you wait.' Jessica said: 'One gets headaches from hunger. It's something everyone in our community has experienced.'
>
> A little later, after the last shreds of cheese had been nibbled and Jessica had cut and shared slices of cake, we began to talk about food diaries. I had planned to request that the women keep food diaries (see Zimmerman and Wieder 1977) in order to detail their daily food intake and the sources of food. I handed out the diaries, and began to explain about the columns to fill in daily. The women started trying to recall what they had eaten, wondering out loud. Lydia's silence rang like a siren. She had been unusually quiet throughout. I asked her if she was ok? She looked at the small book, and the other two women making entries under what they ate yesterday (Tuesday). Lydia? Her voice cracked and with her double stream of tears came the words: '*Ek het Saterdag laas geëet*' (I last ate on Saturday). In the fraught pause that followed I calculated how many days that was – three. We were all in shock. Lydia was sobbing. I moved to comfort her. The others commiserated, expressing their shock and anger at Lydia's family. The hunger that had been spoken of in past tense and general terms came to the present. It was painful.[2]

The anthropologist wanted data. She got the soft crying of a hungry woman.

## Madness and hunger

'I am hungry. My child is hungry.' Dreaded words for a psychologist to hear. But much more dreadful words to speak. Psychologists do not know what to do with hungry people.[3] Social scientists refer to hunger as 'food insecurity'.[4] The food security literature seems to be far removed from what we experience in the valley.

Hunger 'was a base and vulgar instinct from which science had averted its gaze' the anthropologist Nancy Scheper-Hughes writes in her book *Death without Weeping*.[5] She has written extensively about what she calls 'the madness of hunger' (*delirio dé fome*) or 'hunger neuroses'.[6] She describes the psychological symptoms accompanying the physical changes associated with hunger:

> [Initial] depression followed by faintness, lightheadedness, silliness, giddiness, brilliant flashes of insight, bravado, often accompanied by irritability. These are often followed by uncontrolled weeping; fierce crazy anger; and the lashing out even at those who may be of assistance. Alternating with the rage are passivity and indifference, as if one were absorbed by some distant or interior reality.[7]

As David Orr, a social work researcher studying the narratives of carers in southern Peru states: 'Food . . . is also often central to explanatory models of how the madness arose in the first place.'[8]

The word '*honger*' in Afrikaans, 'hunger', evokes powerful reactions in people. When we think of hunger, we might see an open mouth, lips, teeth, tongue. A naked bony body with bones, an anorexic girl, kwashiorkor or an obese man. We associate hunger with discomfort, pain and distress (caused by lack of food or nurturance or love), but always, implicit in hunger is also desire (the desire to eat, to be loved, to be nurtured).[9]

Over the years we have realised that many of the women we interview or do psychotherapy with are hungry when they speak to us. Often, they have hungry children at home. According to Stephen Devereux and Keetie Roelen: 'In South Africa, where a constitutional right to "sufficient food" exists, 20–25% of children are undernourished. This has been identified as a "national scandal" and a source of shame for the wider society that allows the persistence of "hunger and malnutrition in a food-secure nation".'[10]

Another day in the valley. It is the first day of the third school term. It is cold. The students are running psychotherapy groups with thirteen-year-old boys and girls at the high school. Today's topic is 'difficult emotions'. The therapists want the children to think about thoughts, feelings and behaviours that they feel they must keep secret or hidden from others. To facilitate discussion, the children are asked to make masks.

The instructions are read:

> There are parts of ourselves that we feel more comfortable sharing than others. We all wear a mask sometimes. Take the paper plate, cut out some eyes, like this. Then on the front of your piece of face-plate, draw a picture or write about the face that you show to the world outside. On the back of the face-plate draw a picture or write about the face that you keep hidden from others. Everyone gets a chance to share their mask with the group. You only have to share your hidden face if you feel comfortable doing so.

We do this exercise every year. On this freezing August day, the kids seem impossible and the therapists struggle. 'My first group was very restless, and I struggled to go through the activities with them. I tried to bring order by reminding them of the values which they chose for our group. This helped a bit, but after a few minutes they were busy with their own things,' one therapist writes in her journal. She continues:

> Some of the boys told me that they are restless because the food scheme at school did not provide food today . . . it seems as if it is a common thing for the food scheme to not provide on the first day of school and also on some other days as well, without warning.

Another therapist is perturbed to see the emotional impact of hunger:

> Many of the boys reported feeling 'sad', 'powerless' and 'empty' on the emotion wheel. Upon further inquiry, it emerged that

the food scheme was closed on this day, and these emotions were connected to their experience of hunger. Their attention deteriorated towards the end and they told me how difficult it was to focus when hungry.

The therapist is painfully aware of how the children try to alleviate the pain. 'They seemed to use humour as a defence as they joked about who was the hungriest and what they were going to eat when they got home.' She is also aware of her own defences. 'It was difficult to hold this. So foreign. So awful. But it seems being listened to helps – although that's probably just a fantasy which makes it a bit more bearable (for me).'

Another therapist, who usually has funny stories about his energetic (often quite unruly) boys' groups, writes a subdued journal:

At school today, things were more out of control than usual. The children were hungry because the food scheme wasn't open. The discipline in both my groups was poor and at times I felt like a headmaster as I had to command order – especially with the boys. I feel guilty, because I try to create a safe and a free space, but if I don't intervene things get out of hand.

He clearly struggles to write about his experience: 'For some reason I struggle to reflect on yesterday – is it because I switched off as a therapist when I went into headmaster mode? Maybe I'm tired – didn't sleep much.'

After this session, the students cancel their supervision session. Or was it I who cancelled, after reading the reports?

When I eventually see the students they are despondent, almost listless. I know the feeling. We talk about how one cannot think about emotions when you are hungry. How can one think about anything when hungry? Maths, grammar, science? We decide that we have to give the children something to eat when we see them, even if only as a token that we have heard them. One of my long-term private patients, a graduate student in engineering, studies the bruising of apples. This means that he gets apples by the truckload for his experiments. He brings me apples in black bags, which the students take to their next therapy sessions. We carefully take out the bruised ones and eat them ourselves. My engineering student, himself in pain in different ways, is pleased that he can help and that the apples are useful.

The student therapists are surprised by the impact of the apples. 'My first group was a lot less restless than last week,' one writes in his journal. He continues:

> I do believe that it is because they have had a week to settle in at school, however, I do feel that it is greatly due to them having had the apples to eat. Both groups and other children passing by asked if they could have one more apple and I felt bad in having to say that I have just enough for my two groups. It was very insightful to see how big a change in behaviour there was once they had something to eat.

Another one writes: 'Yesterday was a better day in Kylemore than last week. The children were not as hungry. The apples really helped.'

I don't know who the apples are more useful for – the children, the therapists or me.

One of the therapists immediately extended the apple strategy to another patient that he is seeing in the valley, a sad and hungry twenty-year-old man who came back to school to finish matric. Orphaned at a very young age, he is sleeping on the floor of an older brother's shack. The therapist is clear that his patient benefits from the therapy, but also, definitely from the Monday apple. 'Of course, I gave him an apple this week . . . he eats once a day . . . there was no doubt that I would offer the apple.' He adds: 'But he wants someone with whom he can share stories, and talk to. He also says he is ashamed but grateful for the apple that he received. He is starving.'

Ashamed and grateful.

## Shame and care

Our Father in heaven,
hallowed be your name,

your kingdom come,
your will be done,
on earth as it is in heaven.

Give us today our daily bread.
And forgive us our debts,
as we also have forgiven our debtors.

And lead us not into temptation,
but deliver us from the evil one.[11]

Evil. Temptation. Debts. Guilt. Forgiveness. Bread. All in the prayer of the Lord, recited before food is handed out at the valley soup kitchen. Bread and guilt are clearly related, as is pointed out in the stern little sermon that precedes the prayer at the soup kitchen. The forlorn-looking people standing in a line, children in their arms or hanging onto their legs, listen politely to the sermon, mumble the Lord's prayer with bent heads.

Carina Truyts, an anthropologist, describes a typical morning at the soup kitchen. As part of her fieldwork, she works at the soup kitchen:

The soup was ordinarily distributed with a set of conditions. Everyone had to line up with their own containers. When the pots were ready at the tables there would be a sermon or speech. This was premised on moral sentiments including appeals to leave drugs, alcohol and abuse; work harder and better; stand together as a community; and remember God and the church always. Then the Lord's prayer would be recited.[12]

Trained as a chef, she helps making the soup.

It was 2:30pm, on a cold winter day. The queue of people waiting for food at the soup kitchen exceeded the length of the hall. Our work had begun around 9:00am, when the food usually arrived. The food was delivered regularly (twice a week), although the content was inconsistent. Most weeks the major food items were starch (maize and samp) and bags of chopped, mixed frozen vegetables, sometimes containing raw beans. Routinely, the cooking process began between nine and ten in the morning. A large pot was placed on the stovetop to which was added the frozen vegetables and enough water to cover. Other foodstuffs (which varied according to the delivery and stock) were then added. On one occasion this was an enormous bone with some meat on, on another day it might be mince, or fresh vegetables when the nearby school garden project provided some. In a second pot the women would cook up starch. The beans in the vegetable packs were not pre-soaked, or cooked. By the time the queue started to form (around 1pm) the beans would still be hard, the vegetables uniformly soft.

On this particular day we were running later than usual. Two extra bags of donated foods had arrived from an NGO [non-governmental organisation] in nearby Stellenbosch. The first bag contained freezer-burnt pizzas, chicken nuggets, giblets, and fish fingers, loose from their boxes. Following the usual procedure, this collection was added to the water and vegetables in the pot. The pizza was torn into chunks and added to the soup pot along with the now-defrosted vegetables. The pizza floated to the top, dough-side up. The gizzards sank. The fish fingers bobbed around with the chicken nuggets.

The second bag contained bread, cakes and pastries in various state of freshness and decay. The mould from white bread rolls contaminated fresher loaves, mixing with a crush of red velvet and chocolate icing. Three women took the bags to tables and began to sort the goods, without a sound. I watched their hands at work trying to keep the oozing sugar away from doughnuts away from the loaves away from the rolls sprouting the blue/green wreath of mould. I broke a long silence, asking, 'Why couldn't they just separate this?'

There was a long pause before Aunt Sara responded, 'No man. I know we have to be grateful. But they can also treat us right. It's not nice. It's not nice. People are hungry but they are *still people!*'[13]

The anthropologist/chef, perhaps in protest against the ghastliness of the fish finger stew/soup, decides to make a peach cobbler:

> Just then, a donation from a local culinary school arrived. Having trained as a chef, it was my habit to try and fashion such donations into some sort of edible dish. Form and quantity always posed a problem (what to do with three bags of left-over chocolate glaze and a bagful of custard? How to distribute it fairly between an indeterminate number of people?) There was an assortment of pastry, and some icing delivered that day. There was a large stock of cans in the larder. The cans had no labels or expiry dates. The prior omission was source of amusement because you never knew if it would be peas or peaches upon opening. And so we took bets. (At a later date I ate from one such can and got ill). I had a peach tart in mind, and was lucky to hit on a shelf of exclusively peaches on my first attempt. I used a wine bottle to roll out the base, and flour from Aunt Sara's own kitchen to dust it with. I cobbled the base together from short crust, nut, and puff pastry offcuts, arranged the peaches, glazed with over-mixed icing (we gave that culinary student an internal rating of 2/10). I dotted them with frozen berries that arrived, luckily still packaged, in the same bag as the freezer-burnt pizzas, chicken nuggets, giblets, and fish fingers. As the queue lengthened I took two large sheets of trays from the oven. The golden brown pastry, uneven as it was, generously covered in yellow peaches and speckled with purple berries, looked and smelled delicious.
>
> I suggested that we cut them into small pieces and distribute them amongst the attending adults. A decisive chorus of 'NO!' shunned my proposal. I was sternly told we would distribute tarts to children only.
>
> As the food neared readiness, the waiting line was divided into two – one for the adults to get their jugfuls of soup, and another for the children to receive the (unwieldy) tarts, which had been portioned into disposable cups.
>
> The dishing up began, I refused (again) the offer to ladle up soup, but could not really justify hiding in the kitchen. So

I stood near the table with the cups of tarts, where the children were collecting a cup each. One young boy took one cup, then reached for another. A woman who was dishing up soup noticed this, lurched in his direction and confiscated both the paper cups. 'Out!' she shouted at him 'get out!' and proceeded to discipline him. The people in the queue quietened and turned to watch the commotion. The boy quickly dropped his shoulder, face cast down, and retreated outside. His mother re-entered the double-door she had just exited, realising what had happened. 'Where is my child?' she asked, softly, looking at his back as he walked away. She looked on the verge of reproach but instead mirrored his bodily reaction. They left with only her recycled margarine tub of fish finger stew.[14]

The anthropologist remarks: 'Food can be simultaneously nourishing and frightening.'[15] She is interested in food and the restoration of dignity, she encounters shame.

Stephen Devereaux, who also works on shame and hunger, writes about the many ways in which hungry women are shamed. He says:

Public policies such as social protection programmes are intended to alleviate poverty, but being dependent on 'handouts' from the state can be a source of shame in itself . . . In South Africa, women who receive social grants feel shame on three levels: firstly because they are poor ('poverty is seen as undignified and shameful'); secondly because they are dependent on support ('poverty forces them into degrading and embarrassing dependence on others'); and thirdly because they are stigmatised for collecting social grants ('those who don't have the grant look down on those who get the grant, they are saying like they are lazy, they don't want to work').[16]

He quotes from the film *The Grand Seduction*:

It's been years since the fishing dried up here – years. And we line up every month and collect welfare cheques. Did you ever collect welfare, Paul? Well you collect more than your money, let me tell you that much. You collect shame. You collect a good deal of shame. The money only lasts 15 days but you get enough shame to last the whole month.[17]

I wonder again about shame and anger and how the anger is projected at those who shame us. Or how the anger is introjected.

When hunger is talked about, shame often seems to surface, not only for the one who is hungry or has been hungry, but also for the one who is confronted with the hunger and is helpless to do something about it. In the cases cited above, the students' shame when they hear about hunger (a hunger they feel helpless to do anything about) is perhaps of a similar kind to that which women feel when their children are hungry – even if it cannot match the intensity. For the women, shame is often pertinent when they experience or think or talk about hunger. They are ashamed that they are not able to provide for the basic needs of their children, or afraid that their children might be taken away from them if they acknowledge their incapacity to care for them. Erica Burman, a prominent critical developmental psychologist, writes about 'the hungry child as signifier of need' and the moral imperative to care for the child that implies 'an interpellation of a singular adult addressee', typically the mother.[18] The neo-liberal discourse of privatised responsibility that maintains that citizens should accept and assume individual responsibility for their own well-being is gendered: women are typically held responsible for taking care of children.[19] In particular, women are expected to feed children, an expectation held not least by the children and felt by the mothers themselves.[20]

Many of the depressed women we encounter talk about the demands of their children and how hungry children are implicated in their emotional distress.[21]

Leila, who has been diagnosed with depression, describes the relentless demands of a hungry child on a mother: 'Only for the fact that the child goes to no one else . . . only comes to me: "Mommy, there is no sugar today, Mommy there is nothing of this" and Mommy just has to provide . . . "I cannot buy you food, I have . . ." What I have I must use so sparingly now.'

Another mother diagnosed with depression, Sterretjie, play-acts to show us what her children are like: 'You come to me, you must eat. You come to me, "Mommy, is there bread?" "Mommy, is there sugar?" "Mommy, is there coffee?"'

Gendered neo-liberal discourses clearly inform the narratives of the women in this community, specifically when they discuss notions of ideal motherhood. Implicit in the narratives of the women is the ideal of the all-providing, ever-giving, self-sacrificing mother, an ideal that the women cannot live up to, given their context. In this community, a 'good' mother is clearly equated with one that can nurture her child.[22]

The women of the valley consistently articulate this ideal. Jenna is only sixteen years old, but knows what she has to do as a mother. 'As I said before, [a good mother is] a mother who cares for [her] child, that looks well after [her] child, who always keeps him clean and . . . always gives him his food, feeding [him] fat.'

Conversely, a bad mother is one that, among other things, fails to feed her child. 'A bad mother,' she says, 'is someone who does not look after her children, who does not care, who drinks and goes wild, who allows her child to go hungry, and things like that.'

Sam, another young mother, contends that if you don't feed your child, you cannot even be called a mother: 'She should look after her baby first. She must look after the child first. The child should not be wet and dirty and without giving food to the child and with bathing him. No, that's not a mother.'

The tension between low-income women's constructions of ideal motherhood and their inability to meet these ideals because of poverty-related constraints means that children's inexorable and continuous demands are experienced as unbearable rebukes of women's failures as mothers.[23] This means that they inevitably feel that they have failed as mothers.

Angry Dora says, 'This makes me feel so useless. I am not worthy of the word "mother", I cannot provide for them.'[24]

Many women, like Dora, say that they feel it is their responsibility to feed children and they feel guilty and ashamed when faced with their children's hunger.[25] Florrie, a 40-year-old woman with two children, who is employed part-time, speaks of feeling guilty: 'It almost feels as if,

I feel now, I feel guilty. I cannot give it. I really want to help the children, but there is nothing; I cannot give to them because I don't really have it – financially, I don't have enough.'

Leila, also overwhelmed by the relentless demands of her children, talks about how her mother tries to convince her that she is not a bad mother. 'Your mother comes to tell you today you are not a bad mother. Take it from your thoughts that you have been a bad mother, perhaps, or a bad wife. You were never. She said, "I can watch you and wonder at you today. You are a single mother."'

It is clear that for the women of the valley, feeding children is their responsibility.[26] Despite appealing to others, they are ultimately alone in this responsibility.

Sterretjie is a 54-year-old woman with four children, who is also employed part-time. She talks about a sense of responsibility, juxtaposed with a clear sense of helplessness. 'It does, yes [make me feel worried] . . . because everything has to come from me. I must make sure that there is bread, that there is food to eat. Let the children have all the food. It is not always easy to do that . . . It is, yes [a lot of pressure] . . . It makes me feel uneasy. How am I going to get it, where am I going to get it? I think about the day of tomorrow as well . . . [what] am I going to do if the children don't have milk? . . . And it is not [easy] to always ask people . . . for things . . . And then the, [I] went to the doctor, I did not know it was depression . . . And then the doctor said, but my whole body . . . my whole . . . body . . . was stressed.'[27]

Often women talk about feeling frustrated and angry when talking about hungry children. Leila, who struggles to provide for her children with her salary as a part-time factory worker, talks about being angry about the demands of her children: 'And these are things I cannot handle, I become flipping angry so to speak. Only for the fact, the child does not go to anybody else . . . comes to me.'

Their anger and frustration are often directed at the hungry children themselves. Women report feeling resentful about what is experienced as an insatiable hunger. Sterretjie speaks about her son who makes coffee all the time: 'And this stresses me because it's sugar and such stuff is expensive. And now his friends also sit there and he makes [coffee] for them. I then just hit him with a stick – in front of his friends. And I take the coffee and I pour it down the sink. See, everything is frustration that comes inside of me . . . I just take the things. I will take the bread, then I just throw it for the dog . . . He, he already ate. Don't take again and eat, ask me . . . And he eats . . . that child eats continuously! I must lock everything.'[28]

Some mothers talk about feeling as if they are competing with children for food. Delize tells us about how food is shared in her house: 'I just eat most of the food which I actually use in the house. Potatoes and rice. I make sure that if I make porridge for her, then I also make a little bit of porridge for myself, so that I eat porridge and milk. Then I take some of that to work. So, at about eleven o'clock I eat my porridge and piece of bread with butter. If there was a piece of meat the [previous] evening I would *skelmpies* [secretly] put away a piece of it for myself. If one breastfeeds a child, then you get very hungry.'[29]

Delize, a mother of three children, hides food away for herself, even if at the expense of her children. Scheper-Hughes, in her study of impoverished mothers in Brasilia, found that it was common practice for heads of households to take a disproportionate share of available food, 'so as to be able to work'.[30] This practice of 'parents first' is also described by Trevor Lubbe in his account of a workshop with South African HIV-positive parents and their children, where 'parents and councillors pushed past the children and jostled for places at the tables while piling their plates up high'.[31] He interprets this as a matter of survival, stating: 'What if a mother's health and intactness should be placed first because she must survive in order to continue to be a mother and produce the next generation?'[32]

I think of myself, also a therapist of middle-class patients: 'Remember the instructions when flying: to always put the oxygen mask on yourself, before putting it in on your infant.' I say this to convince mothers to look after themselves. The relevance of this is even more obvious in the valley.

Women feel despondent about their unbearable circumstances, especially about their children's hunger.[33] Leila describes her stuckness: 'And these are things that I cannot handle . . . but unfortunately, I am just a human being, and I can't carry everybody's things.' She starts to sob. 'I sometimes don't know what to, I don't know what to do anymore . . . With my situation, my circumstances.'

Guy Standing's description of the anomie of the precariat comes to mind: 'Anomie is a feeling of passivity born of despair . . . Anomie comes from a listlessness associated with sustained defeat, compounded by the condemnation lobbed at many in the precariat . . . castigating them as lazy, directionless, undeserving, socially irresponsible and worse.'[34]

We (the student psychologists and I), mostly middle-class women of different races, have often felt alarmed and sometimes even (unfairly) judgemental about the apparent lack of agency of the women we encounter. Similarly, anthropologist Elysée Nouvet recounts her ambivalent response to a despondent impoverished mother:

> At the front of my mind was one thought, illuminated like on a neon sign, predictable and moralistic: The kids! There are kids! I wanted to yell at Juana: Isn't it better to get something to eat, however little? Isn't it better to try? But another thought was wrapped around my throat. Is there a difference between carrying on or staying in bed in a context of acute structural violence? Is one action more productive than the other? Of what? On what basis?[35]

These accounts of middle-class alarm and judgement in the face of the anomie of poor women seem to be in line with what is described in the literature and are tied to larger societal discourses concerned with individual responsibility.[36] Also, too often, poor people, and specifically poor women, are so easily stereotyped as anomic, lazy, directionless, undeserving, socially irresponsible.[37] The point here is that hungry children can lead to anomie in certain women at specific times, not that anomie is an inevitable consequence of having hungry children. The important question is: why or in what circumstances do hungry children lead to anxious, angry and anomic mothers?

It is clear that food insecurity, and in particular, children's hunger, should be investigated as a key dimension in the link between poverty and mental health where women are concerned. As Orr states: 'Food and hunger are integral themes in how *campesinos* [peasant farmers] conceptualize madness and that formal mental health services are largely unaware of this significance.'[38] Hunger, Ivy Pike and Crystal

Patil conclude, 'may serve as the most potent physical and psychological stressor for women across the globe'.[39]

The failure of psychiatry and psychology to engage with the problem of hunger seems to be related to the powerful gender and neo-liberal discourses within which mothers are interpellated to care for children, and more specifically, to ensure that children are not hungry. If mothers fail at doing this, they are thought to be failing to fulfil their responsibility. Given these expectations, women's emotional responses to children's hunger are complex and range from sadness and pain to anxiety, anger, anomie and alienation.

Impoverished women are kept captive in complex and vicious cycles of hungry children, sadness and anxiety, shame, anger and anomie, aggression and withdrawal, negative judgement, and more shame. The unbearable rebukes of hungry children can be thought of as evoking a kind of 'madness' in low-income mothers.[40]

## Greed and love

> You must remember that sometimes bread is just bread . . . But hunger is also a metaphor.
> — Michael Jackson, *Life within Limits*[41]

> Food moves about all the time. It constantly shifts registers: from the sacred to the everyday, from metaphor to materiality, it is the most common and elusive of matters.
> — Bernard Lyman, *A Psychology of Food*[42]

How then to think about hunger in my world of want and my world of excess?

Trained psychodynamically, the word 'hunger' is one that I often use, also in my private practice. Sigmund Freud wrote about hunger, linking hunger (a so-called ego-instinct) and emotional well-being, citing the poet-philosopher Friedrich Schiller, who said that 'hunger and love are what moves the world', hunger and love thus being 'the most powerful motive forces.[43] This link between hunger and love was taken even further by object relations theorists, with their emphasis on the oral developmental stage, with Melanie Klein (perhaps infamously) linking the depressive stage with the infant's longing for the lost good breast of the mother. It is not the milk, Klein said, it is the breast, or then the relationship with the mother that motivates:

> The object which is being mourned is the mother's breast and all that the breast and milk have come to stand for in the infant's mind: namely, love, goodness and security. All these are felt by the baby to be lost, and lost as a result of his uncontrollable greedy and destructive phantasies and impulses against his mother's breasts.[44]

In my middle-class practice I inevitably use the word 'hunger' metaphorically. Here, I also see starving women and girls, but these are women and girls who starve themselves. I also see women who binge and purge. When I say at a dinner party that I yet have to meet a woman who does not have an issue with food, a friend of mine, a very tiny and extremely well-preserved chef, says, 'Well, you are meeting the first one then. I don't have an issue with food. If I have eaten too much, I just don't eat anything for a few days.'[45]

The dinner party laughs. 'I rest my case,' I say.

I am invited to speak about eating disorders at a local school (a prestigious, wealthy girls' high school in Stellenbosch). I speak to a hall packed with high school girls with names like Jana and Cara and Mia and Nina. Most of them are blonde and straight-haired, their ponytails too quirky, seemingly confident and scarily in control. I show them video clips and poems and photographs. I start with Dr Seuss: 'Oh the places you'll go. You have brains in your head. You have feet in your shoes. You can steer yourself. Any direction you choose. You're on your own. And you know what you know. And you are the [girl] who'll decide where to go.'[46]

I tell them that in our culture eating has become a way of talking for women. We sometimes stop eating because we are angry at ourselves or at others. We eat more than we need to eat because we are scared. We are obsessive about what we eat because everything else feels out of control. We eat and vomit, eat and vomit because we don't think our bodies deserve good food. We over-exercise because we want to punish ourselves. We use eating as a language because we have learned not to speak about the difficult emotions. We have learned that it is unacceptable to have emotions like neediness and fear and sadness and being out of control and hopelessness. We are expected to conceal these emotions, but of course they surface, in this culture, often in the ways we treat our bodies, and in the ways we eat or don't eat.

I end the talk with the poem *Love after Love* by Derek Walcott:

The time will come
when, with elation,
you will greet yourself arriving
at your own door, in your own mirror,
and each will smile at the other's welcome,

and say, sit here. Eat.
You will love again the stranger who was yourself.
Give wine. Give bread. Give back your heart
to itself, to the stranger who has loved you

all your life, whom you ignored
for another, who knows you by heart.
Take down the love letters from the bookshelf,

the photographs, the desperate notes,
peel your own image from the mirror.
Sit. Feast on your life.[47]

They listen politely and quietly, almost too quietly, to my little sermon. In question time, the first question is asked by a (too thin?) sixteen-year-old: 'Is it true that it is your parents' fault if you have problems with eating?'

I am a parent of a daughter myself, so defensively, I immediately say, 'Well, maybe we as parents are implicated, but you know, you yourselves are doing a good job to police yourselves and your eating; you are the agents of this culture.'

But standing on the stage, microphone in my hand, an enormous arrangement of proteas on my left, the South African flag on my right,

Klein and her notion of greed in my head, I think: what are these children greedy for and what are they self-defensively denying themselves?

Klein writes about the infant as a needy, helpless creature, abjectly dependent on the mother's breast for nourishment, safety and pleasure. Understanding that the mother (the nurturer) is all plentiful and powerful, the infant becomes suspicious, suspecting the mother of enjoying the power, refusing to give the infant continual and total access to nourishment. In reaction, the infant wants to possess and control, not to destroy. But, says Klein, greed can become ruthless in its acquisitiveness.[48]

We can be greedy for food, literally, but we can also be greedy for love or control or meaning. Different people are hungry for different things.

> In understanding what it means to be well we must therefore take into account not only what we need as a bare minimum to survive but what we need for our lives to be worthwhile – for we do not live by bread alone, and well-being is never simply the satisfaction of biological needs, the possession of primary goods, or the attainment of personal fulfilment and happiness. Nor is it a matter of adaptation, since getting what we want invariably leads us to conceive of new wants, as if satisfaction is always a matter of possessing more than we have, even when we appear to have everything we could possibly wish for . . . Amartya Sen's view that impoverishment is never simply a lack of income but a deprivation of opportunity to exercise one's ability 'to achieve various valuable functionings as a part of living' is a valuable corrective to those who would reduce well-being to material circumstances or see it as a mainly clinical question of physical or mental health.[49]

When I think about this kind of hunger, I am not only thinking about the too-skinny, blonde, straight-haired girls, I am thinking about the desolate women standing in line for the unpalatable mix-up in the soup kitchen, the school kids who are hungry on Mondays, the many young women who crave a baby, Wilmien Wilders who wants a job,[50] the Wolf

Man who dreams of being mouthless,[51] and Dora whose hungry children make her crazy.[52]

And I think of Anna.

Anna is a 41-year-old white woman who is single and unemployed. She has been in psychotherapy for fourteen years, sometimes once a week, sometimes every second week. She was diagnosed with bipolar disorder.[53] If she is not on medication or in therapy, she really suffers. Once she stopped coming for therapy and was hospitalised for three months. Another time she booked herself into an addiction centre for an addiction to food. After three months, she left the treatment centre with four new addictions diagnosed (alcohol, anxiolytics, shopping and sex) and came back for therapy.

As always, Anna is on time for her session. She starts talking as she walks into the office. 'Your money is on my lips and in this bag,' she says.

She puffs up the pillows on the couch as she always does and takes off her shoes. 'I hope there is no smell,' she says. 'The shoes are old.'

She crosses her legs into a yoga pose and sighs. 'Russian Red,' she says and touches her lips. Broad smile. 'The lipstick that I bought with the money that I withdrew to pay you.'

'And look here.'

Long interlude about the three pairs of socks paid for with the other half of the money for the session. Socks she could not resist.

'Feel how soft. I will pay you next time for two sessions.'

'And look what I found in my doctor's waiting room.' She takes out a magazine. 'Don't worry, I will take it back once I have read the whole thing.'

'*Cleo*, wonderful, wonderful magazine,' she says. '*Cosmopolitan* is simply too terrible, below the belt. Maybe I should subscribe to *Cleo*. But I am not allowed to. My budget.'

'Look at this article. "Dickipedia". Sex tips for all kinds of penises.'

'That's why I took the magazine. Just for in case. One never knows.'

Anna has been single for ten years. It is a sore point.

'Okay. So here are the kinds. Carrot (thick). Asparagus (thin). Baby marrow (long). Mushroom (short). Eggplant (turns down). Banana (turns up). And you must see what one can do with these vegetables. Oh, how I miss a man in my life.'

'But wait. I have an agenda for today.'

'I made soup. You can call this the soup-making episode. So, let's start with the soup. How much time do we have left?'

'First the bad part. I gained six kilograms in the last two months. So, I know what I have to do. I have to eat right. That means real homemade soup. Not the Woolies shit. But I wanted to do it right. Real roast chicken stock and real vegetable stock. So, I was going to make chicken, leek and potato soup and cauliflower soup and broccoli soup.'

'It was terrible. Six pots.'

She counts with her fingers.

'The roast chicken. The chicken stock. The vegetable stock. The potato soup. The broccoli soup. The cauliflower soup. Two recipe books. Three big bags of vegetables from Vegetable City.'

'Now I can say the soup operation was relatively successful. The cauliflower soup was fantastic. Cauliflower and fine almonds, a cup of almonds. Roasted almonds. And then the soup is so creamy you can't believe it. Like meringue or something. You should try it.'

'But. It took me two days to make the soups. And in the end, I only had ten servings in Tupperware.'

'And the broccoli soup I will have to say was a disaster. I forgot that it was hot and I was in a rush and so I put it in the smoothie maker and then it exploded. Basically. Over the whole kitchen. Over the new toaster. In the cutlery drawer, between the knives and forks. The ceiling. The floor. Everywhere. Green. But I was so determined that I did it again. And then it happened again. Explosion. Everything covered in green again. So then my mother chased me out of the kitchen.'

'So that was the soup-making episode.'

'So next on the agenda is the dinner party.'

She tells me about how she had finally met her neighbours, two pleasant-looking bachelors, while walking her dog, Fred. She now wants to invite them for dinner. Detailed descriptions of the neighbours, Fred and the interaction.

'I told them Fred sleeps with me on the bed and I don't know whether his backside or his front side smells worse. I think they were a bit disgusted.'

'Now the dinner. So much to do. How much time do we have left? I thought I will invite them today for Friday night. Then I have two days to do everything. I must choose a beautiful outfit. That will take time. At least a day. I have to make soup. Two soups. Potato and leek soup. Mussel soup. Then a playlist. Then I must get the house ready. But everything is going to take long.'

I ask her what I will say about this plan.

She interrupts me. A long question about how I think the invitations should work. She does not wait for my answer.

'To get the place ready, I have to make pillows. And new curtains. Then I have to hang the curtains. Plant out my succulents. Lanterns in the trees.'

'I am just thinking this *Cleo* magazine, much better than *Cosmopolitan*, definitely, says that single women should not have any pillows or fluffy toys on their beds. It scares men off.'

I ask again, 'What am I going to say?'

She sighs.

'So, you are going to say I can't do it all. So, I can't get the place ready. Maybe my old pillows are fine. And maybe I can't hang the curtains, only make them.'

She laughs a deep laugh.

'And if I don't have time for lanterns in the trees, I can hang the fluffy toys from my bed in the trees.'

'And I have to talk less and listen more.'

Another big sigh.

'I struggle to dress myself. I look so terribly dreary and sad. Even though I have so much colour in my head. I think I look sad.'

I look at her. Her eyes are bright, her cheeks pink and smooth. Her big wide mouth is still red, Russian Red. She wears a pink jersey. She is beautiful. There is nothing sad about her at this moment, although I know that the pain is always close.

'I just must not drink too much. Before the party I should not drink too much.'

'Last night I had the best time ever with Fanny in Durbanville. We spent the night in our pyjamas. She bought Chinese takeaways. Deep-fried prawns. Clouds of dough that melt in your mouth with the prawns bursting in your mouth, like grapes. After this spring rolls, sushi, ice cream, malva pudding, doughnuts. We ate it all.'

'I don't know which soup to make for dinner. I have to call Liesl about her blasphemy soup. It is called blasphemy soup because when people eat it, they say: "Oh Jesus, it's three cheeses."'

'There is something else I need to tell you. This afternoon on my way here I was in the wrong lane and I should have turned left and I am confused and while I am confused I think I am going to miss our appointment and suddenly I am happy and it is not a personal thing and I would not have said it if I thought it was and I know you would not think it is . . . But it is just so exhausting to come and the thought of not having to go to school today.'

'On my way here, I think about what I am going to tell you and then I think about what I am going to say about what I am going to tell you and how I think about what I am going to tell and then it is mirror upon mirror upon mirror and then I say, "Anna, you are driving. Concentrate."'

'But that is how it is. I think too fast and too much. I don't want to be like this. I realise if someone watches me in Canal Walk, they are going to see how anxious I am. They may not say, "Oh fuck, move away from her", but they will know I am worried. And I don't want that.'

'But actually, I don't have time for this dinner party.'

'I have to go now and invite the people.'

She puts on her shoes.

I say, 'Anna, we still have time left.'

She sighs. 'Sorry.'

'I have people to invite. Vegetables to buy. Bye.'

# Distress

*'. . . a bit of play (amid pestilence and panic) . . .'*\*

Tell me: Is the rose naked or is that her only dress?
— Pablo Neruda, *The Book of Questions*

Illness is the night-side of life, a more onerous citizenship. Everyone who is born holds dual citizenship, in the kingdom of the well and in the kingdom of the sick. Although we all prefer to use only the good passport, sooner or later each of us is obliged at least for a spell, to identify ourselves as citizens of that other place.
— Susan Sontag, *Illness as Metaphor*

And so often, when you get to know a patient, they lose their diagnosis, you know.
— Elvin Semrad, in *Semrad: The Heart of a Therapist*

I interview Dora in the back yard of her parents' property, just outside the wooden hut she calls home. We are each sitting on an upturned wooden crate. Dora has been referred to me because she has been diagnosed with depression.[1] Her small-boned body makes her seem young, but her eyes are old and tired. She is chewing bubblegum. Dora's youngest child, a two-year-old boy, sits on her lap. Her other son is ten years old and visually disabled. He is clumsily kicking a ball around in

---

\* The quote in the subtitle of this chapter – '. . . a bit of play (amid pestilence and panic) . . .' – is from Sen, 2005: xi.

the dusty back yard. Dora also has a sixteen-year-old daughter who is nowhere to be seen. The two-year-old is fidgety, constantly trying to get his mother's attention. Early in the session, while still answering the basic demographic questions, Dora starts crying when she talks about her husband's work.

'He works on the road.' The boy on her lap says something to her. 'But if it rains, they don't work. Stellenbosch municipality.' The boy puts his arms around her neck and asks her something. 'They sweep the streets.'

The child places his hands on Dora's cheeks and forces her to look at him.

'My parents get old-age pension.'

The child whimpers. Dora blows a big bubble with her bubblegum, takes it from her mouth and puts it in the child's mouth.

'To be honest, at this moment, it is only his money,' she gestures to her disabled son, 'and then the baby gets Mandela money [a grant]. That is the only proper income. And if my husband works, then he gets R90 a day. If he works a full week, then it is R450, but if it rains – it depends, sometimes he works one day, then it's R90 income. Just that for the whole week. And sometimes he works two days, sometimes he does not work at all, then there is not an income. It is very, very difficult.'

'So, there is not really money, there is not really food in the house.'

She starts crying.

'Now, last night we again went to bed without food. It was the third night in a row.'

Loud sobs.

'Or what stresses me out a lot. Ashlyn [her daughter] goes to school without bread and if she comes back from school . . . I believe that there must be a small piece of bread for her because in the end it breaks her down because she goes to school without bread and if she comes home from school, there is nothing for her to eat . . . for me, it is not . . . it is not right . . . And this is not nice for me. Because everyone asks me for little piece of bread and then I don't have it for them. And my mother and them don't always have to give me, you know. My brother is also without food.'

Still crying, she cracks her finger joints.

'And I then went to see if I can't carry the thing because it is difficult for me. Because I talk to no one. And there's no one really that helps me with my situation.'

She looks at me. 'I sometimes do not know what to do. With my situation, with my circumstances. And my oldest one says that she is going to kill herself, or my husband says he is going to kill himself. Then I have to try to give everyone courage, I have to be the strong one, but unfortunately, I am just a person and I can't carry everyone's stuff. It feels as if there is a mountain on my shoulders.'

Three nights without food. Everyone asks me for a piece of bread. A mountain on my shoulders.

The boy on her lap is not satisfied with the bubblegum. Dora takes out her breast and starts feeding him.

Dora only attended school until Grade 5, but is very articulate about the intricacies of her emotional suffering. In tears throughout the rest of the interview, she relates feeling sad, feeling stuck, feeling lonely, feeling anxious, struggling with sleep, but also talks about being able to cope and to laugh. Diagnosable depression. But there is more.[2]

Dora says that because she feels it is her responsibility to feed her children, she feels guilty and ashamed when faced with her children's hunger. She clearly blames herself and speaks about the overwhelming shame she feels. The boy on her lap is now asleep, seemingly content. She gently rocks him while telling her story.

I tell Dora that she has been sent to me because she was diagnosed with depression. Does she know what that means? She clenches her hand into a fist. 'For the anger that I have inside me. The, the, the, the . . . I am almost . . . There's not a day that goes by without me feeling frustrated, irritated . . . There's not – really. There. Is. Not. A. Day. In. My. Life. You do not even have food to eat . . . I have more anger inside me than, than, than anything else.'

When asked to explain her depression, how it feels and what causes it, Dora says, 'Yes. Like . . . I, I . . . The whole situation, the whole problem, I take on me. Because I think if things were perhaps different, if I perhaps could work and all the things then . . . Then we wouldn't have stayed in such a place, then it would not have been so hard for my children and they would not be hungry.' Her head moves slowly as she speaks.

She talks about the shack that they live in. 'It's a *gangetjie* [corridor], it is too small for all of us. It is not right for the children. We have no bathroom, we wash in a *kom* [plastic tub].'

She tells me about her resentment at what she experiences as her children's insatiable hunger. At this point the two-year old wakes up and says, '*Mammie, Mammie*.' Dora does not look at the child and continues talking.

'They moan at me . . . Then, probably, everything becomes too much for me, because everyone moans around me. Ashlyn says she's hungry. Now this one [she indicates child on her lap] asks me, looking in my eyes, "*Mammie*, what I eat now?" Because I say, I told my husband yesterday, my longing is to have enough food in the house. I said last week – I perhaps shouldn't say that – but I am more than one day sorry I got him.' She gestures in the direction of the child playing in the yard.

'Last week I, then I said, um . . . Sometimes I feel sorry I have him as well.' Now she lifts up the child on her lap. The child stretches out his arms to be hugged.

'You are going to get a *klap* [slap], you hear? *Jy is lekker onbeskof* [You are really rude],' she says to the child. She wipes her eyes and looks me straight in the eye. 'Because he also has to suffer through all these things.'

'All these things,' she says, 'all these things I think about during the night.'

She is angry with her husband, but also with her children. But mostly she is angry with herself. 'So I blame myself . . . Most of the time I blame myself for my circumstances, my situation. It makes me feel very, very inferior. It makes me feel as if I am a zero. A zero, I don't exist . . . A zero . . . I am a nothing, yes. This makes me feel very, very inferior. This makes me feel so useless. I am not worthy of the word "mother", I cannot provide for them.'

She talks about her 'crazy' fantasies of setting fire to the shack.

'Yes, because I, I, I will do something, really. I will do something. I said to my mother just the other day, I will set fire to everybody in my house and not feel anything, just for the, the . . . how they [treat] me. I'm always crazy, I'm always stupid. So, I said, "*Mammie*, if something happens to me one day in this house, not even the [dogs] should attend my funeral." That is how I feel sometimes. Then I say to him [her husband]: "I will kill all of you. I will think nothing of it."'

'Will you really do it?' I ask her. I have to check how violent she really is.

Dora answers my question by talking about a recent incident where she realised that her daughter was skipping school. 'I freaked out and I scolded her, and I swore. I said, "How the bloody hell?"'

She makes a fist.

'I beat her terribly. I punched her like a man would punch another man with a fist. Then I grabbed her hair, I slammed her face here in front of my family.'

She punches down with her right hand. She grabs her own hair and punches the air three times.

'I hit her. With the fist. And, um, but I was still not satisfied, but it, because it was still not enough for me. It was as if I couldn't fully express my emotions. And I went – she went around the house and I followed her – and I took my belt and I beat her with it.'

She hits her own leg.

'Then my sister came and said no, she thinks I have done enough.'

She punches the air again, now talking very loudly.

'I freaked out. I'm always crazy, I'm always stupid. And I say to myself, "Dora, you can't want to do this." But now he [her husband] says, and my daughter as well, *Mammie* is full of stress". Then I say, "Yes, I am full of stress because no one carries what I carry in this house."'

Talking even more loudly, she says that she realises that her behaviour is out of line. The child on her lap is now whimpering softly. She raises her voice and says to the child, 'I am going to hit you.'

Still talking loudly, she continues, 'I am used to saying . . . I am crazy.' She taps the side of her head. 'I see my family look at me as if I am crazy. Then he asked me: "Are you crazy?" Now is, is, is, is, is . . . It breaks your self-esteem down, but I am so used to it that I don't . . . I don't pay attention to it. Now I have the attitude that I say to everyone: [pointing to herself], "This Crazy Dora – I am Crazy Dora, according to you – I am so crazy."'

She sighs, sits back, sobs quietly. She puts the child down, gets up, looks for tissues, she finds some, but they all look used. Irritated, she throws them down on the ground. She gets a roll of toilet paper and sits down again. She continues talking about her hungry children, about feelings of despondency and hopelessness.

'Sometimes I don't know what to, I don't know what to do anymore. With my situation, my circumstances. Yes . . . The feelings that I have, because, because, because . . . The feeling that there is no way out for me.'

Dora puts the tips of the fingers of her two hands together in front of her face. 'I am caught. I feel like a spider that is caught in a web.'

The child on the floor watches her intently.

On my way home, I think of the spider caught in her own web. I remember Louise Bourgeois's giant mother spider at the Guggenheim in Bilbao. I wish I were in Bilbao.

## Diagnosis and its discontents

There is, thank goodness, an obdurate grain of humanness in all patients that resists diagnostic pigeonholing. Most experienced psychiatrists learn to struggle to translate diagnostic categories into human terms so that they do not dehumanize their patients or themselves.

— Arthur Kleinman, *Rethinking Psychiatry*

Dora is depressed. She has all the emotions typically associated with depression: dysphoria, sadness, guilt and shame,[3] but as is the case with many women in the valley, she also speaks of anxiety, anger, frustration, resentment and anomie.

Formally Dora has the same clinical diagnosis as most of the women whose stories I am trying to tell in this book. Anxious Wendy. Frowning Eve. Traumatised Karesha. Despondent Delize. Weeping Wilmien. Ashamed Lettie.[4] All of them have been diagnosed with major depressive disorder by a health professional (a psychiatrist, a doctor, a nurse or a psychologist).[5]

I also diagnose the Wolf Man with major depressive disorder. I have been seeing the Wolf Man, a 41-year-old, single, white male, in psychotherapy for a year.[6] He is a private patient. I see him in my office at my home in Stellenbosch. He is a tall, thin man who wears a heavy black coat, even in summer. He has beautiful long fingers, hairy fingers. A professor in theoretical physics, the Wolf Man reads voraciously. His face is sombre and he never makes eye contact. Every few weeks he takes to the mountains for a few days, wanders around on his own, drinks only water and eats nothing. Unlike Sigmund Freud's Wolf Man, he has never related seeing his parents having intercourse nor does he dream of white wolves. Apart from his perpetual sadness and rage, specifically with women (but never acted on), he has a recurring nightmare in which he does not have a mouth. The Wolf Man and I talk about the meaning of his dream. He thinks his mouthlessness in dreams has to do with a fear of not being able to talk (something he does very well). I wonder if it does not have to do with the fear of being hungry, the fear of needing others (something that he is petrified of). I tell him to write the history of his mouth so that we can get behind this dream. He writes 21 pages in his small, dense handwriting, starting with the fact that he 'refused' to be breastfed and ending with how he sometimes roams the streets of cities, amazed that people do not run away from him, that they do not notice that he actually is a wolf and can devour them.

If I were to work with standard psychiatric diagnostic systems, I would have focused on Dora and the Wolf Man's and all the others' symptoms and signs, how those symptoms and signs cluster together and how they develop over time.[7] With this information, I would have made a psychiatric diagnosis and chosen an appropriate treatment plan.

However, this is not how I work. Like many other clinical psychologists in South Africa and elsewhere, I am criticised for my seemingly obstinate resistance to adhere to what is called the biomedical model.[8]

Why is it that clinicians like myself resist manualised treatment based on psychiatric diagnosis?[9]

I would argue that clinical and counselling psychologists' apparent resistance to ubiquitous psychological knowledge and treatment, informed by such universal models, has to do with clinicians' intimate knowledge of the subtleties and nuances of people's pain and the large range of emotional needs that people divulge to them behind the thin walls of sparsely furnished community clinic consulting rooms, but also behind the closed doors of our comfortable private practice rooms.[10]

Clinicians working in the field of mental health have been questioning the relevance of diagnostic categories such as depression for decades,[11] particularly when applied to marginalised people in developing countries.[12] On the one hand, it has been questioned whether the diagnostic criteria for diagnoses such as depression aptly capture or describe the emotional distress of individuals with very different histories, situated in very different contexts. On the other hand, the fact that individual diagnoses can serve to obscure adverse socio-economic and political conditions has also been highlighted.[13]

What then lies beyond a diagnosis of depression?

When I diagnose a person with depression or when another health-care worker tells me a patient is depressed, I know that the patient is feeling low and perhaps sad, she may cry a lot, she has no energy, she has little hope, her sex drive, her sleeping, her eating are all compromised ('neuro-vegetative symptoms', we call it). She is probably struggling to function in the world. She may find it difficult to work and to have relationships. Work and love, Freud said, are the big ones.[14]

These 'symptoms' may or may not be what trouble the so-called depressed patient the most.

They, or those close to them, may have problems with living. With finding a home or being at home, with falling pregnant or being pregnant, with giving birth, with being loved or not, with working or studying, with eating and drinking, with illness and death, as described in the chapters of this book.

But even those 'co-morbid conditions' may not be what cause the most distress.

Patients may actually be most concerned about their relationships. Our patients are mothers and fathers, lovers and spouses, neighbours and friends, but always also the children of their parents and grandparents.

As described in the other chapters of this book, these problems of living may manifest as emotional issues. Patients typically oscillate between hope and dread. There may be a longing for home (belonging) and a fear of homelessness. Patients may need containment and holding. They may struggle with boundaries and intrusions. Identity and obscurity may be issues. In their lives, patients typically are confronted with the abject and desire, care and cruelty, pain and pleasure, intimacy and violence, parenthood and childhood, guilt and shame, tenderness and brutality. We sometimes see the compulsion to repeat, sometimes desperate attempts to separate and to do things differently. Sometimes life is experienced as meaningful, sometimes as meaningless. Many times there is the longing to be recognised, attended to, loved, but often people want to be left alone and need space. Some people struggle to survive. They may be hungry and greedy in different ways. They may want to nurture and be nurtured, but they often are poisoned instead, or become toxic themselves. All human beings suffer loss and may be in mourning or collapse into melancholia. We are acutely aware of patients always oscillating between agency and disempowerment.

The emotional sequelae of these issues include fear, sorrow, grief, misery, melancholy, anger, rage, shame, guilt and pleasure.

The patient may defend herself against these painful emotions by using a range of defensive strategies: enactments, repression, projection, projective identification, denial, splitting.[15]

Most practising psychologists are acutely aware of all these complex layers of patients' functioning and will therefore typically question using diagnosis as the only basis for psychological treatment.[16] In most cases I contest the use of manualised treatments for all people with the same diagnosis. Rather, I insist on paying attention to the complexity of each individual. This need for the acknowledgement of complexity is perhaps even more pertinent in low-resource settings.

## On assessment: Beyond diagnosis

Such indeed is the condition of things . . . I do know that however long I did so, I would not get anywhere near to the bottom of it. Nor have I ever gotten anywhere near the bottom of anything I have ever written about. Cultural analysis is intrinsically incomplete. And, worse than that, the more deeply it goes, the less complete it is. It is a strange science whose most telling assertions are its most tremulously based, in which to get somewhere with the matter at hand is to intensify the suspicion, both your own and that of others, that you are not getting it quite right . . . There is an Indian story – at least I heard it as an Indian story – about an Englishman who, having been told that the world rested on a platform which rested on the back of an elephant which rested in turn on the back of a turtle, asked (perhaps he was an ethnographer; it is the way they behave), what did the turtle rest on? Another turtle. And that turtle? 'Ah, Sahib, after that it is turtles all the way down.'

— Clifford Geertz, *The Interpretation of Cultures*

What then do we as clinicians look for when we meet a patient, when we try to understand her distress, what she needs emotionally, how we can perhaps help or support? We do what we call 'clinical assessment'.[17]

### Lived experience

What brings you here? And: Tell me more?

These are the only sentences my students have to know when they start doing therapy.

As a psychologist I am interested firstly in how a patient subjectively experiences her world. I want to know what worries or distresses her and how she feels about it. I want to try to answer the question, 'Why did this particular person, given his or her particular personality, current life circumstances, and personal and family history, develop this specific psychological problem or issue at this particular point in time?'[18] My focus is on 'how a particular patient differs from other patients as a result of a life story like no other'.[19] The particular is what is important. Psychological practice therefore 'embodies an attitude of inquiry, deliberation, and discovery. It eschews rules, but loves questions – questions about what is wise to do with this persona, at this time, for this reason.'[20]

When I try to establish who the person is and what she needs, I look at her subjective experience of her emotional distress, how she feels at this moment, what she is thinking, how she copes with or how she defends against painful or unacceptable feelings, thoughts and memories, how she relates to me and others, her history, her specific context, her body and how her own beliefs about herself and the world's impact on her experience of psychological distress.

I am interested in the complex inner world of the patient: feelings, feelings about feelings, fantasies, dreams, fears, hope, impulses, wishes, self-images, perceptions of others.[21] The patient herself is the only one who can accompany me into her inner world, even if she is not an expert on illness or disorders.[22] Patients may not consciously know everything about themselves, no one does, but we also cannot get into their inner worlds without them.

Every single word the patient says about herself is important to the clinician, even if the patient is not always aware of all her feelings and thoughts, or may not have the words to name them. The patient may also feel embarrassed or ashamed about her feelings. She may feel ambivalent about talking about them. I, as clinician, therefore do not only pay attention to what is said and explicitly communicated, I am also focused on and acutely aware of what is implicitly communicated about the inner world of the patient. I pay attention to body language, the location of emotional intensity and/or emotional discomfort, the pace and style of talking. I can learn much from how a patient interacts with me and how I subsequently feel about her. The negotiation of power is also of crucial importance. What is not said is sometimes as important as what is said.

### Feelings: 'Affect'

The most important source of resistance in the treatment process is the therapist's resistance to what the patient feels.

— Paul Russell, 'The Role of Paradox in the Repetition Compulsion'

Many contemporary psychotherapists agree that it is crucial to understand the patient's feelings in the moment, what is called their affective world.[23] When I sit with a person, I want to know what she hopes for and dreads, her longings and her fears, her desires and the anxieties that accompany them. If we think of affect as any inner experience characterised by intense mental activity and a certain degree of pleasure or displeasure, one needs to look out for the following innate or hardwired affects: interest-excitement, joy, surprise-startle, fear-terror, distress-anguish, anger-rage, contempt, disgust and shame-humiliation. But there are also other feeling states that must not be ignored: love, lust, hate, envy, gratitude, boredom, spite, resentment, guilt, pride, despair, exasperation, tenderness, vindictiveness, pity, scorn, the feeling of being moved or touched, loneliness, resignation, hopelessness, powerlessness, energy.[24]

I want to explore all affect. Does the patient act on the feeling? How does the patient feel about the feeling? The patient's shame about feeling angry is often worse than the feeling of anger. Frequently, the anxiety about anxiety is most debilitating for an anxious person. The clinician also has to determine whether the feeling disclosed by the patient is perhaps a defence against another feeling.[25]

I first encourage my patient to feel the feeling in the room and to be with it. This is called mindfulness.[26] However, in initial sessions people will often first talk about a feeling before they feel safe enough to experience it. When a feeling is felt or talked about, I want to further explore the feeling with the patient, helping them to name it and to think about it. This is called reflective functioning, or mentalisation.[27] I want to think with the patient about what caused the feeling. Are there other feelings? Working with the patient, I try to understand what can be done to make the feeling less overwhelming and how to manage it. This capacity for linking feelings to what has happened before and what happens after (putting feelings on a timeline) is crucial in the therapeutic process, but also in general. A capacity for reflective functioning, or mentalising, frees us from being caught up or embedded, not only in our internal world, but also in a daunting external reality. If we feel embedded or caught up in our internal world or in external reality, we are more likely to become defensive and to act in destructive or self-destructive ways.[28]

Some people become paralysed because they stay caught in the feeling. They are so sad or anxious that they cannot act, or they are so angry that they act in destructive ways. Other people keep the feelings at bay by overthinking. Overthinking the anxiety or sadness also can mean that they cannot act in effective ways.

Dora is not simply a 'depressed' woman. In the initial stages of the first session she is still giving basic demographic information about her income and employment, when she is overwhelmed by sadness. She cries when she talks about feeling powerless and needy. Without any prompting, she links the sadness to her children's emotional pain, their hunger and their disobedience. Speaking about this, she becomes more animated: she speaks loudly and fast, her tone is urgent, she gesticulates and sits upright. She snaps at the child on her lap and threatens him with a slap.

I am the therapist. I feel myself withdrawing in aversion and maybe even fear. Talking about her own sense of responsibility at the end of the session, Dora is in tears again, ashamed about what she has told and showed me, but also probably ashamed about what she imagines I may have heard and seen.

Dora's subjective experience of the world oscillates between feelings of sadness, anxiety, anger, anomie, shame, guilt, hopelessness, madness, strength, feistiness, energy. My job is to understand with her what triggers which feeling, why she feels the way she does and how she can manage the feelings. I have to take all feelings seriously. Her most important problem at this stage is not her 'traditional' depressive symptoms, but her rage and her violent behaviours. I understand that her rage is an extreme defence against feeling vulnerable, anxious, hopeless and ashamed. My biggest concern is that she acts out the rage against her children. Even though I can understand her anger and identify with it, I have to think with Dora how to manage her anger in less destructive ways.

It is clear that the therapy has begun, even in the first moments of the initial session.

### The relationship: 'The intersubjective space'

While we listen to the patient's words and respond with words of our own, we need to pay as much, if not more attention to the emotional, relational, and visceral/somatic undercurrents that shape the verbal exchange. The words, in their own right, may or may not convey significant meaning. The implicit, nonverbal subtext almost always does. It is the feeling of what happens here – the sense of what is actually going on in the therapeutic relationship – that can lead us to what is most immediately salient both in the patient's experience and in the interactions, we co-create.

— David J. Wallin, *Attachment and Psychotherapy*

I pay attention to the feelings or affect the patients bring into the room, but much about what I get to know about a person has to do with how she is with me: how she feels about me and how I end up feeling about her. The interaction between the patient and the therapist provides psychologists with crucial information. We refer to it as the 'intersubjective space', created when patient and therapist meet, aware that both patient and therapist, each with their own unique history, in the specific context of their meeting, are contributing to this space. I know that I have to take my feelings about my patients (countertransference) and their feelings about me (transference) seriously. My feelings may have to do with my own history and what is evoked with regard to that history in a session. However, it is also possible that my patient's feelings or words evoke in me what the patient unconsciously wants me to feel.[29]

In the case of Dora, I feel how an intersubjective space of 'mutuality and recognition' waxes and wanes and gives me even more information about Dora.[30] In this, I am sometimes drawn in by Dora and sometimes repelled by her. At moments I am 'overwhelmed by aversive affects and . . . unable to think'.[31] In my fluctuating feelings about Dora, I perhaps get information about Dora's ambivalent feelings about herself, but also about how other people and society in general may respond to a poor woman who feels hopeless and despondent, but also enraged. Dora lacks agency, but people are also scared of her because of her powerful rage and her violent acts.

In these moments of fluctuating feelings, both my patient and I are 'subject not only to a dynamic unconscious, but also to social discourse' (when I use the word 'discourse', my friends roll their eyes, but I do find it an important concept, despite the rolling eyes).[32] I am aware that my feelings about Dora have to do with societal expectations of mothers.[33] 'Good' women, 'good' mothers, should not experience, much less express, anger. And, certainly, we don't expect them to act on it. Easier for me are moments when I feel drawn in, able to hear and digest what seems like the toxicity of a life, able to process the painful feelings and with Dora, make plans to do something about them.

## Coping with difficult feelings: 'Defences'

People's defensive styles are almost as individual as their voice or their fingerprints. Some people use sadness as a defense against anger, while others get angry to defend against sadness. Some defend against a pervasive underlying shame; others seek not to feel guilt. Some have an extensive repertoire of defenses, while others perseverate with one or two tried-and-true mechanisms, no matter what the circumstances. In order to help a person, we need to appreciate the particular way in which he or she is using thoughts, feelings and actions to relieve upsetting internal states.

— Nancy McWilliams, *Psychoanalytic Case Formulation*

Psychodynamic psychotherapists start with the subjective experience of the patient, but there is always the assumption that in any person's experience of herself some salient aspects will be missing, whether the person is aware of it or not.[34] Wilfred Bion refers to these unacknowledged feelings as 'the nameless dread', while Donald Winnicott speaks of 'unthinkable anxiety'.[35] Because it is often these unconscious (not thought about, not named) feelings that cause the psychological distress, it means that the therapist has to get to what is not there by paying exquisite attention to what is there.[36]

People protect themselves against painful or unacceptable feelings in very distinct ways. In psychodynamic language we talk about their defensive styles; we can also talk about their coping mechanisms. Defences can be cognitive, getting relief from painful feelings by thinking about things in particular ways (rationalisation, intellectualisation). An emotional defence is when someone copes with distress by developing an emotion that will obscure the more painful one (reaction formation). People also defend themselves against painful feelings by how they behave, thus escaping painful feelings by forgetting (suppression, repression, denial, dissociation) or by external enactments (acting out).

Dora's defensive style is different from many of the other women that I write about.[37] She defends against her sadness by being very angry (emotional defence) and against both her sadness and anger by violent acts against her children (behavioural defence of acting out). As her therapist, I may initially focus on Dora's violent enactments, but I will have to take into account that Dora already feels deeply ashamed and guilty about her behaviour.

If I could see her in more long-term therapy, I would focus on the sadness and pain that she is so desperately defending herself against.

### The larger world in which we find ourselves: 'Context'

Our embodied and personal worlds of experience are both nested within and continually emergent from the larger worlds in which we find ourselves.

— Donna Orange, 'Kohut Memorial Lecture'

I take note: a wooden shack, the icy breeze, the stench of an outside latrine, a scolding mother in the house next door (not too steady on her feet), a nine-year-old boy, who cannot see, happily humming to himself while playing with a ball in the back yard, men's laughter in the yard next door, a girl's screams in the distance, dust everywhere, a despondent dog somewhere. The shack is in a back yard, the back yard is in a street, the street is in a town, the town is in a valley, the valley is in a country that still reels from the aftermath of apartheid and persistent inequality.[38]

'How what is outside becomes the inside.'[39]

A psychiatric diagnosis of depression does not tell us anything about the context or life circumstances within which the emotional distress is experienced.[40] As a therapist I need to understand the life circumstances of a patient.[41] I have to understand how a person like Dora internalises her context.[42] The individual does not exist, and cannot be understood, separately from her relationships, her community and her culture. This is true whether the patient lives in a shack or in a mansion, whether she is in an abusive or supportive relationship, whether she lives in small South African town or in Vienna.

When psychological distress is addressed in this context, it is important to understand how inequality and domination are ingrained onto the psyche and body and life of Dora, who passes the mansions and vineyards and Mercedes Benzes of millionaires when she goes in an overcrowded taxi to collect her son's disability grant.

I think of Dora's answer to my question about how depression feels to her. 'For the anger that I have inside me. The, the, the, the . . . I am almost . . . There's not a day that goes by without me feeling frustrated, irritated . . . There's not – really. There. Is. Not. A. Day. In. My. Life. You do not even have food to eat . . . I have more anger inside me than, than, than anything else.'

And then her explanation for why she is feeling this way? 'Yes. Like . . . I, I . . . The whole situation, the whole problem I take on me. Because I think if things were perhaps different, if I perhaps could work and all the things then . . . Then we wouldn't have stayed in such a place, then it would not have been so hard for my children and they would not be hungry.'

Dora is clear. She is more angry than depressed. And she is angry about what she calls, 'the whole situation', which 'I take upon myself'.

### Parents and partners: 'Developmental and relationship history'

> If you really want to hear about it, the first thing you'll probably want
> to know is where I was born, and what my lousy childhood was like,
> and how my parents were occupied and all before they had me, and all
> of that kind of Copperfield kind of crap, but I don't feel like it.
> — J.D. Salinger, *The Catcher in the Rye*

When people talk about themselves and their pain, they almost inevitably talk about their histories.

'How will I ask a patient about her parents? How do I bring it up?' my students often ask. I can reply quite confidently, 'Don't worry, they will sooner or later bring them up themselves.' Those infamous culprits, mothers and fathers. This makes me think of Philip Larkin's poem, 'The Verse':

> They fuck you up, your mum and dad.
>    They may not mean to, but they do.
> They fill you with the faults they had
>    And add some extra, just for you.
>
> But they were fucked up in their turn
>    By fools in old-style hats and coats,
> Who half the time were soppy-stern
>    And half at one another's throats.
>
> Man hands on misery to man.
>    It deepens like a coastal shelf.
> Get out as early as you can,
>    And don't have any kids yourself.[43]

At some point in the first session Dora shows me a scar that she got when her mother threw a fork at her. She says: 'Oh, so unhappy, I could have killed that woman – really, truly . . . How can a mother hurt her child like that?' She continues, 'And I always said, one day if the Lord gives me children, I will never, ever treat my children the way my mother treated me and raise them in the circumstances that we were raised in.'

Dora describes her father as a 'quiet man', who was very strict. According to Dora, her father hit her more than he hit her siblings. 'For me, my head is very sensitive, and I was hit on my head many times.' Dora left school at fifteen when she was in Grade 5 and then worked at a clothing manufacturing company, a job she held until her second child was born. She had to give most of her wages to her parents, while her father's abuse of her continued. He once broke her nose. She ended up in hospital. The hidings she got with the sjambok were so bad at times that she had to cover her body when she went to work: 'It doesn't matter if you, if I got a smack, or if I was hit, I must wake up at 5 a.m. I must go to work. I must put on long-armed clothing, so that they can't see at work.'

What is relevant here are not only early relationships, but also current ones.

Dora's parents are still present in her life, as she lives in their yard, but their mental representations of her are perhaps even more powerful. After all these years, she is still Crazy Dora – to her parents and sister, and now also her husband. And when Dora's eldest daughter also seems to disrespect her, Dora gets enraged and violently attacks her.

I pay attention to the unique history of each patient.[44] While most psychological theories posit the importance of the developmental history, the familial history and the relationship history in the development of psychological problems, they differ in profound ways as to which events and relationships are crucial and how exactly they impact on the psyche of a person. If psychotherapy is seen as an opportunity to rework previously thwarted processes of development,[45] therapy is thought to give the patient a corrective emotional experience.

In Dora's stories, I hear how she hates her mother, fears her father, resents her husband's inability to change her circumstances for the better, feels disappointed by her children. She violently re-enacts this hate and fear. When she feels the dread, the horrendous repetition comes to consciousness.[46] However, still repressed, maybe, is her longing for her mother, a mother. A dreadful longing.

There is an Audre Lorde poem that reads in part:

My mother had two faces
and a broken pot
where she hid out a perfect daughter
who was not me
I am the sun and moon and forever hungry
for her eyes.[47]

A hunger for her eyes.

## Our bodies, ourselves: 'Embodiment'

The body keeps the score.

— Bessel van der Kolk, *The Body Keeps the Score*

The body speaks.[48] Look at Dora shivering in the iciness of a winter's day, the tired eyes, the baby's snot rubbed off on her face, her own snot later, the missing teeth that become visible when she chews her bubblegum, the scrawny breast, a scar on the cheek, a broken nose, tears, tears, tears and an angry fist.[49]

We experience our psychological distress in our bodies. People use their bodies to speak and experience distress.[50] Our bodies also cause us distress. Bodies are therefore important to us as psychologists.

In the therapy process I have to pay acute attention to the concrete details of the body that I am  encountering. Is the body healthy? Is the body disabled? Is the body hungry? Is the body overweight? Is the body fit? Is the body well looked after? Some of it we can see, some of it we have to ask.

## The rules and requirements: 'Discourse'

While I always start with the stories of my patients, wanting to pay attention to the details, I am also very aware that these stories are shaped and informed by larger societal narratives. In these larger narratives ideals and standards are set, rules and practices are determined. Every individual story is always also political. In their own telling of themselves, individual women compare who they are and what they do with cultural expectations of women and mothers. This often is what causes them the most distress.

These (sometimes explicit, but often implicit) rules and requirements (in academia we call them 'dominant discourses' and immediately lose our readers) are also present in the stories of Dora.[51]

These ideals are implicit in Dora's stories.

There is the ideal of the all-providing, ever-giving and self-sacrificing mother, an ideal that many women in the valley cannot live up to, given the context within which they are mothering.[52] The tension between low-income women's ideas about good motherhood and their inability to achieve this because of poverty creates feelings of disappointment, inadequacy, psychological distress and desperation.

Mothers such as Dora are ashamed for not being able to live up to this ideal.

There also is the Calvinist idea that suffering is virtuous, that a greater good is obtained through suffering.[53]

The neo-liberal notion of individual responsibility is also subtly present in all Dora's narratives.[54]

The personal is indeed political. Dora's distress is linked to and maintained within a particular socio-political context and through certain dominant discourses. Dora is grappling with several social expectations: mothers are always caring and nurturing, women do not get angry, the individual should take responsibility. Ashamed about not being able to live up to such expectations, Dora becomes enraged and directs this rage at her children.

But shame is fundamentally a social emotion, often reflecting comparison with cultural or idealised norms. Yongmie Jo describes it as emanating from the scorn and contempt of others, real or imaginary, imposing feelings of denigration of the entire self and instilling a sense of failure or inferiority.[55] Paul Gilbert describes it as 'an inner experience of oneself as an unattractive social agent'.[56] Feeling shame is therefore inseparable from being shamed; it involves a sense of powerlessness, of being judged by others, 'who consider or are deemed to consider themselves to be socially and/or morally superior to the person sensing shame'.[57]

Any intervention with Dora should inevitably also include some political dimensions, where the rules and regulations that determine the 'standards' against which individuals in all contexts are measuring themselves should be challenged.

### What we believe about ourselves: 'Emotional convictions'

Man is an animal suspended in webs of significance he himself has spun.

— Clifford Geertz, *The Interpretation of Cultures*

When I see a person in therapy, I am not interested only in how she feels about the world, others and herself, I am also interested in how she thinks about all of this. In contemporary psychoanalytic literature such beliefs are called emotional convictions/truths or organising principles (some call them pathogenic beliefs). They are the 'emotional conclusions a person has drawn from a lifelong experience of her emotional environment'.[58] Such organising principles are powerful because they are both thought and felt. They are typically held rigidly, with absolute certainty. Emotional convictions are formed through individuals' relationship experiences within their original family contexts and are typically then confirmed in later relationships. Inevitably, such convictions are also shaped by larger societal narratives or discourses. They can be understood as an individual's core convictions that operate either consciously or unconsciously and have relational consequences, subsequently compelling individuals to assume particular relational positions.[59] Sometimes the belief itself may be conscious, but the interpersonal processes that created such ideas may be obscured.[60]

Dora has different sets of core convictions.[61] There are convictions that are compatible with a traditional diagnosis of depression, a 'Depressed Dora': I am alone, no one cares about me, I am worthless, my life is meaningless, I do bad things. She says things like: 'I feel worthless. I feel that I mean nothing for them in the house; I am just there because I must be there, but further than that I mean nothing for them . . . I struggle, but on my own . . . nobody, but nobody really knows what I'm going through.' These convictions seem to be related to her sense of not living up to ideals of motherhood, but also perhaps because of her sense that her own mother was not the ideal mother.

She also has convictions that are more compatible with her notion of herself as 'Crazy Dora': the world is unfair, the world (including my family) is treating me badly, my children should not disappoint me, I am enraged and rightfully so, my rage is crazy. While Dora feels rage and acts on it, she can articulate why she considers it to be mad. Good women do not get angry and good women do not show how they feel.

Dora has a third set of convictions related to her sense of responsibility and her shame for not living up to expectations. This is 'Disappointing Dora': 'Everyone asks me. If only I could . . . I have to . . .'. Implicit here is not only the discourse of idealised motherhood, but also the neoliberal discourse of individual responsibility.

On the one hand, Dora expects something from the outside world and is angry; on the other hand, she feels she needs to do something herself and feels ashamed. These emotional convictions inform her shame and anger in complicated ways. She is ashamed about not living up to expectations and is angry about feeling ashamed. She is angry about others not living up to her expectations, but her anger makes her ashamed.

### Responsibility and agency: 'Self'

Women as passive dupes, rather than active agents who continuously make sense of and interpret the social sphere, and their own bodily experiences.

— Jane Ussher, 'Are we Medicalizing Women's Misery?'

In my interactions with patients there are at least two different ways in which the self, and feelings about the self, become important. First, I am interested in how a person feels about herself, her self-esteem or her healthy narcissism: 'How secure is her self-esteem? On what is it based? What undermines it? How is it restored when it is injured? How realistic are the aspirations on which it depends?'[62]

But I am also interested in the extent to which a patient locates power in herself or in the external world. Does the patient have a felt sense of agency and empowerment or does she feel disempowered? Is her locus of control internal or external?[63]

Dora feels hopelessly lost in the world, but also shamefully responsible for everything that has happened to her. In our work together she has to figure out what she can and cannot do.

### How we talk about it all: 'Language'

But we have speech, to chill the angry day,
And speech, to dull the rose's cruel scent.
We spell away the overhanging night,
We spell away the soldiers and the fright.

There's a cool web of language winds us in,
Retreat from too much joy or too much fear.

— Robert Graves, *The Cool Web*

I listen to a person. I do not only listen for content. I listen carefully for how they talk: 'The method consists in recording not only what the patient said, but also how he gave the information.'[64] I listen for how much she talks, or how little. I take note of the kind of language she uses. I listen for stories and metaphors.

People use language to understand themselves and their worlds.[65] Mikhail Bakhtin says:

> [Language] is not an abstract system of normative forms but rather a concrete heteroglot conception of the world. All words have the 'taste' of a profession, a genre, a tendency, a party, a particular work, a particular person, a generation, an age group, the day and hour. Each word tastes of the context and contexts in which it has lived its socially charged life.[66]

People create themselves and their worlds through talking and through the stories that they tell.[67] They tell stories to make sense of themselves and their worlds, to create order and meaning.[68] 'Narrative is,' Julia Kristeva says, 'in sum, the most elaborate kind of attempt, on the part of the speaking subject, after syntactic competence, to situate his or her self among his or her desires and their taboos.'[69]

As a therapist I listen to the narratives not only as representations of patients' worlds, I listen to how they are used to make meaning. If the self is a telling,[70] the work of the therapist is to determine how that telling came into being, what functions it serves and what it conceals.[71]

Conversely, it is also interesting if there are no narratives or if there are many and if they are conflicting. Donna Orange asks, 'Why do some patients become mute, some speak compulsively and repetitively in ways that feel dead and deadening, some just scream, and others keep searching for words and expression?'[72]

Much has been written about the breakdown of narrative in the face of vulnerability, especially embodied vulnerability. Elaine Scarry, in her book *The Body in Pain*, talks about pain as the shattering of language.[73] She describes how physical pain does not only resist language, but actively destroys it, bringing about an immediate reversion to a state anterior to language, to the sounds and cries a human makes before language is learned.[74] Sometimes people are surprised that they walk into a therapist's office and simply cry. Their pain seems unspeakable.[75]

In the psychotherapeutic hour metaphor also assumes central importance. Orange writes about how 'the shared search for the more and more adequate metaphor becomes the search for emotional truth'.[76] She says that patients use metaphor to share something of their lifelong-developing experiential world. The metaphor is used to imply that there is something yet to be grasped.[77]

Dora's metaphors reveal much about her experience, more than she can probably articulate in explicit explanations. Her words 'I feel like a spider caught in a web' suggest, in quite a profound way, the victimhood of the predator, how she feels trapped in her own predatory web. When she states at the end of the first session that it is 'almost like a tap that is turned open', she is suggesting a lack of agency, but she also conveys her felt sense of being vulnerable and overwhelmed by an uncontrollable stream of emotions.

In the first sessions Dora tells many stories about herself and her world. What can I do with her narratives? If we had had time for a long in-depth therapy, I would have explored the different narratives in detail. Given that Dora will not be in therapy for long, I will point out the different narratives to her, think with her how each narrative in different ways informs her actions and rather pragmatically talk to her about what her next steps will be, taking all these stories into account.

As psychologists we have to take language seriously, investigating how realities and selves are constructed in words: 'Language both expresses the symbolism of the unconscious and is the means for unravelling it. It therefore embodies subjective experience but also provides a route to the source of that experience – the construction of the subject itself.'[78]

Human beings are complex, multifaceted, situated, in process, under construction. What does this say about what psychotherapists do in psychotherapy?

It means that we need to pay attention.

## On care:  On becoming human

> The old Mediterranean norm – that a wise person needs to acquire and treasure an *amicus mortis*, one who tells you the bitter truth and stays with you to the inexorable end – calls for revival. And I see no compelling reason why one who practises medicine could not also be a friend – even today.
>
> — Ivan Illich, 'Death Undefeated'

If we are to think that we need to highlight the uniqueness of each person and the specificity of each case, how are we to think about treatment?[79]

### The therapeutic stance:  Curiosity and attentiveness

> I have always felt that a human being could only be saved by another human being. I am aware that we do not save each other very often. But I am also aware that we save each other some of the time.
>
> — James Baldwin, *Nothing Personal*[80]

Edmund White, in his somewhat sceptical essay titled 'Me and my Shrinks', considers all his many psychotherapies and muses about the meaning of it all: 'Psychoanalysis did leave me with a few beliefs,' he says, 'including that everyone is worthy of years and years of intense scrutiny.' 'That scrutiny is better left to writers,' he adds. 'To Proust, the supreme psychologist in fiction; to Nabokov for his respect to details, the sensuous surface of experience – preferable to the reductiveness and aridity of a Freud.'[81]

Larry Beutler, perhaps the scientist/practitioner who has done the most traditional research on what he calls the science of psychotherapy, writes about the importance of scrutiny:

I believe there will always be a place for people who can listen and who can provide, through whatever means they can, the experience of help to other people. There will always be a place for that. I don't think that we will continue to support it through health care indefinitely, because we will have to accept the fact that it is not health care – it is life care . . . Within the narrow view that we use psychotherapy to treat psychopathology we're going to have all kinds of medical, biological, chemical treatments to do away with symptoms. What we won't be able to do is change a lot, through this chemical interjection, some of the basic angst that people experience in not being connected to other people, not being heard, not feeling relevant. Having another person, someone who is trained to do something that is helpful and optimal, who will listen and care for them, is going to continue to be very important.[82]

Not surprisingly, Beutler's research findings correspond to what prominent psychoanalysts have discovered in their practice rooms and have documented in different ways, often in the form of case studies. Freud considered psychoanalysis to be the cure of love, love demonstrated through 'the evenly-suspended attention'.[83] He states that the analyst must 'turn his own unconscious like a receptive organ towards the unconscious of the patient'.[84] While psychoanalytic theory has assumed different forms across continents and over time,[85] most psychoanalytic theorists and clinicians do assume the 'complexity of the mind, the importance of unconscious mental processes and the value of sustained inquiry into subjective experience'.[86] In other words, while psychoanalytic theories can be said to 'radiate in different directions', they do so 'from a common, core commitment to a sustained, collaborative inquiry into the complex inner textures of human experience, established in the complex interplay between past and present, actuality and fantasy, self and other, internal and external, conscious and unconscious'.[87]

Wilfred Bion describes the therapeutic stance as one of curiosity, evenly suspended attention (focusing on the client without memory or desire) and speaking from the heart and mind.[88] This 'psychological state of receptivity', Thomas Ogden says, involves a 'to-and-fro of experiencing and reflecting, of listening and introspection, of reverie and interpretation'.[89] He cites the novelist Henry James: 'Experience is never limited, and it is never complete; it is an immense sensibility, a kind of huge spider-web of the finest silken threads suspended in the chamber of consciousness, and catching every air-borne particle in its tissue.'[90] For Ogden, our receptivity must be

> for  the stuff of ordinary life – the day-to-day concerns that accrue in the process of being alive as a human being . . . the lives and the world that the lives inhabit . . . [they are about] people: people working, thinking about things, falling in love, taking naps . . . [about] the habit of the world, its strange ordinariness, its ordinary strangeness . . . our ruminations, daydreams, fantasies, bodily sensations, fleeting perceptions, images emerging from states of half-sleep, tunes and phrases that run through our minds, and so on.[91]

If we are really to pay attention to the uniqueness of each person, no two treatments will be the same. Ogden highlights the fact that mothers and fathers learn '(with a combination of shock and delight) that each new infant seems to be only a distant relative of his/her older sibling(s)'.[92] He says that a mother and father must reinvent what it is to be a mother and a father with each child and must continue to do so in each phase of the life of the child and the family. Similarly, he says, the analyst must learn anew how to be an analyst with each patient in each session.

The contention is that the empathic immersion in the subjective experience of the patient and the attempts to understand her are more important than applying a technique. Understanding a person's unique personal subjectivity should be the basis for determining the best treatment approach. What helps one person can damage another.[93]

The work of the therapist is to be compassionate, to have the relentless desire to accompany and to understand, a capacity to share the experience and the suffering of the other.[94] This kind of compassion is more than simply witnessing, but it is also not pity, condescension, or mindless and inauthentic 'making nice'. This therapeutic stance can 'gradually restore to the shattered, alien-feeling, frozen, lost, dehumanized other a sense of belonging to the human community'.[95]

This, of course, means that training as a therapist is not about technique, but about a certain way of being.[96] A therapist should thus be connected to herself, be able to be appropriately open, show herself as a kind and caring expert, be able to put the illness in perspective, show knowledge, deal with doubt and be able to instil hope.[97]

No easy task.

## On theory

> Experience is messy . . . When human behaviour is the data, a tolerance for ambiguity, multiplicity, contradiction, and instability is essential. When we at last sit down at a clean desk in a quiet study and begin to assemble the vivid images and cryptic notes, searching for a coherency, we must constantly remind ourselves that life is 'unstable, complex and disorderly' everywhere . . . our job is not simply to pass on the disorderly complexity of culture, but also to try to hypothesize about apparent consistencies, to lay out our best guesses, without hiding the contradictions and the instability.
>
> — Margery Wolf, *A Thrice-Told Tale*

If the therapist focuses on what is unique, specific or particular, the patient becomes a person, rather than a diagnosis. If we are to think of each case as unique, the care or treatment will emerge in the relationship (psychologists call this the 'dyadic process'). What is healing will not be determined by psychological theory (which typically posits universal motives, stages of development and curative interventions), but will be discovered during the therapy process and in the specifics of the relationship (in psychological jargon it is called 'dyadic specificity'). As a responsible therapist, I will not only be receptive to the needs of the patient, but also simultaneously to any theory that may illuminate my understanding of and responsiveness to those needs.[98]

This means that the therapist must be determined to name the distress, to think about it with the patient and to thus transform it into metabolised and non-toxic feelings.[99] This is where theory becomes important.

When I teach theory, I tell my students that we hold on to theory lightly and with each new case anticipate that the theories we know might not be applicable, may have to be altered or even discarded.[100]

Theories are there simply to guide us lightly in our explorations; they can never determine what we find. In psychotherapy, theory should raise questions, not answer them.

Theory can be too prominent and can become problematic,[101] but not applying our powerful theoretical tools to people (especially to those on the margins) can be perceived as patronising and actually uncaring.[102] Inadvertently, while both therapists and patient overtly and authentically share desires for experiences that reveal new relational possibilities, 'potent forces that invite repetition' may already be at work.[103]

Any case that we are confronted with allows us to build theory, refine theory, contest theory. Every case is an opportunity to find out more and understand more about being human. For instance, in the case of Dora, we slowly start to construct a theory that we think might explain the dynamics of violent motherhood: a demanding and disobedient child creates an anxious and sad mother, who in turn is ashamed because she feels that a good mother should be able to feed and control her child. Ashamed, she becomes angry and her anger (in contexts where it is impossible to feel and name and manage anger) leads to acts of aggression and anomie. And even more shame. And so the cycle is repeated.[104]

### On writing

> If there is nothing written there in the margins, it is as if those stories were never written . . . There is nothing less important than the lives of poor people. If poor people die, they leave nothing behind, no trace of them exists. For me, my writing is history as told by the losers.
>
> — Nathan Trantraal, in Murray la Vita,
> 'En ôs stuck innie mirrel'[105]

> In understanding and writing up our cases in more complex ways, we are documenting lives that are otherwise invisible; important interactions that can serve to illuminate something about human minds, human interactions, human processes . . . [Case notes] are accounts, stories and a way of being accountable to a process that often defies description, a counting – of bodies and breaths and heartbeats.
>
> — Sally Swartz, 'The Third Voice'

Writing up cases is part of the therapeutic process.

Poignantly Dora speaks about her longing to have her story heard: 'And I wish I could do something about my situation. And so I wrote a letter. And I got it typed up and printed, and then I faxed it to *Huisgenoot*, but they haven't responded yet. And I also want to email it to *Touching Lives*.'

I am very sure she has neither email or fax; maybe she simply has a fantasy of sending her message to the world, of talking to the world? I think she has no way to get anything about her life out there. But there is the fantasy.

I ask about the TV programme *Touching Lives*. She says, '*Touching Lives* is on SABC. In Afrikaans. It sends people to come and see where I live and then they show it on TV . . . unfortunately I don't have those kinds of facilities, but I do try and reach out to improve my situation because I feel I can't live like this for the rest of my life. I am at home. I must try reach out. I've got to do something about it.'

As Paul Farmer says: 'The poor are not only more likely to suffer; they are also less likely to have their suffering noticed.'[106]

## The curative factor

And two people may be talking to each other, at any moment, in a civilized way about something trivial, or something even complex and delicate. And inside each of them there runs a dark river of unconnected thoughts, of secret fear, or violence, or bliss, hoped-for or lost, which keeps pace with the flow of talk and is neither seen nor heard. And at times, one or both of the two will catch sight or sound of the movement, in himself, or herself, or more rarely in the other. And it is like a quick slip of waterfall into a pool, like a drop into darkness. The pace changes, the weight of the air, though the talk may run smoothly onwards without a ripple or a quiver.

— A.S. Byatt, *The Matisse Stories*

What is it then that cures? Perhaps Heinz Kohut's notion of twinship, of 'being human amongst humans' and thus giving the patient an experience of being human amongst humans, is useful.[107] While treatment of each patient will be different, the therapist's stance will always have to be the same: one of curiosity and loving attentiveness.[108] This is true when we listen to the patient, when we apply theory and when we write up our cases.

When saying that patients benefit from this kind of attention, how exactly does it help? Again, the answer will be different for different people and different for the same people at different times.[109]

In her last session Dora talks about therapy. She touches her heart and says, 'I feel I can get comfort. I get rid of my feelings. It makes me feel better than when I react with bottled-up feelings in my house. After we were done, I felt much better . . . What does not help me is to go on and to react. That does not help me because I don't get my way. To swear and to scold, it brings me nothing. It does not give me peace of mind . . . I am just looking for help so that I can be a better person, someone to lift me up . . . I will say psychological help is . . . I think it is the best. Really, because you get someone that you can talk with. It is that one does not always want to express your feelings to anyone. Now you come specifically and yes, really, then you get rid of it, almost like a tap that is turned open that lets the water out for the first time.'

I ask how she feels now, at this moment? 'Again, a little better,' she says. 'Again more. Not a hundred per cent, but a little better. I am actually thankful you came on my path.'

The melancholic Wolf Man and I will argue about the meaning of his mouth for some time still. Like Freud's Wolf Man, this Wolf Man does not feel cured by me, not if 'cured' means the absence of all symptoms of depression. Like Freud's Wolf Man, he may never be 'cured' by psychotherapy. He will stay at least a little sad and a little angry. However, I know that he is always pleased to see me and that he likes to make me laugh. Every now and again, ever so rarely, he will look me straight in the eye and I will see the slightest of smiles on the face of the mouthless man. For a moment, only a moment, he has the mouth of a man and is living with his hunger. When I asked the melancholic Wolf Man whether some of his case material can be used for this book, I also asked him why he is still in therapy. 'You don't seem to be less melancholic than a year ago,' I say.

'You keep me sober and you keep me alive,' he says, without hesitation.

I ask hungry Anna about writing up her session, referring to the red lipstick session.[110] She immediately starts talking, 'Red lipstick should not be worn on a first date because in Egyptian mythology lips painted red represented the labia majora or the labia minora.' She does not know which, so her uncle Awie suggested that, to avoid this association if one wants to insist on wearing red lipstick on a first date, one should put the red lipstick on one lip only. She laughs boisterously. 'Can you imagine?'

Anna becomes very quiet when I ask her why she is still in therapy. I am moved, remembering again how she has suffered over the years, bravely so. She says that maybe she can't answer because it is beyond words. Then she thinks more. 'All I know,' she says, 'I know that when I started therapy I knew I was not alone anymore. And I am not the only one. I still feel that,' she says.

A human amongst humans.[111]

# Death

*'. . . and then things end (without a rumble)'**

Why does the earth grieve
When violets appear?
   — Pablo Neruda, *The Book of Questions*

I want to give thanks . . .
. . . For Frances Haslam, who begged her children's pardon
For dying so slowly,
For the minutes that precede sleep,
For sleep and death,
Those two hidden treasures.
   — Jorge Luis Borges, *Jorge Luis Borges: Conversations*

Lettie, sick with AIDS, is referred to me by the clinic nurse. My clinical notes start with the poem 'Report from the Hospital' by Wisława Szymborska:

We used matches to draw lots: who would visit him
And I lost. I got up from our table.
Visiting hours were just about to start.
When I said hello he didn't say a word.
I tried to take his hand – he pulled it back

---

* The quote in the subtitle of this chapter – '. . . and then things end (without a rumble)' – is from Sen, 2005: xi.

Like a hungry dog that won't give up its bone
He seemed embarrassed about dying.
What do you say to someone like that?
Our eyes never met, like in a faked photograph.
He didn't care if I stayed or left.
He didn't ask about anyone from our table.
Not you, Barry. Or you, Larry. Or you, Harry.
My head started aching. Who's dying on whom?
I went on about modern medicine and three violets in a jar.
I talked about the sun and faded out.
It's a good thing they have stairs to run down.
It's a good thing they have gates to let you out.
It's a good thing you're all waiting at our table.
The hospital smell makes me sick.[1]

Lettie is 42 years old. She carries her head low, mouth slightly open, white tongue, body visibly shivering, big jacket, slippers, small, bare, brown ankles, sweatpants that are too short and too red and too bright for everything else. I ask her why she is here. She says that she is cold and tired. She cannot eat, has not been able to keep food down for almost a month. I say to her that she looks sick. Is she sick? 'I came with a lift. I stay in Factory Street.' Is she is in bed all the time? 'I get up a little. If the sun shines, I get up. Then I sit in the front room. The lying down works on my sides.'

She does not look at me. Her head stays low. I open her file. The last inscription in her files reads:

Make appointment with Lou-Marié.

1. Prepare client for death.
2. Talk to her about gratitude. She has a supportive family.
3. Repentance about promiscuous life.

Before that the list of most recent physical symptoms:

Complaint of bad cough. Vomiting. Productive cough. Yellow bile. No appetite. Temperature: 39.4°C. Weight: 50kg. Respiration: bilateral crepitasis. Candidas in mouth. Referred to hospital with pneumonia. Admitted Emergency Unit.

I ask to be excused and go next door to find the sister. I tell her that the client referred to me seems very ill, too ill to do a session with me. 'Oh yes, Lettie,' she says. 'Her count is 92, too low for treatment. It went down overnight. Such a pity. She comes from such a good family. There is always a *vrot kolletjie* [rotten spot]. I will come and look at her; we probably will have to hospitalise her again.' Behind the nurse's desk, beneath a poster advertising female condoms, a handmade poster with a picture of a nurse's cap and a stethoscope: 'Save one life, you're a hero, save a 100 lives, you're a nurse.'

I go back to Lettie. '*Vrot kolletjie*'. I put one of the clinic blankets around her shoulders. I wait for the nurse. In the meantime, I do what I usually do – I ask questions. History. Her father was a builder and her mother a housewife. She is the youngest of nine children, seven brothers and one sister. It is the sister she is staying with in Factory Street. Her own children are 25, 12 and 8. The younger two live with their father in Worcester. The oldest son is a cabinet maker and 'my girl works at Kekkel en Kraai. They take care of me, the children.'

She struggles to talk, I struggle to listen. I watch the movements of her white tongue. She says she got divorced four years ago. Her ex-husband initiated the divorce. 'And Lettie, do you have someone new?'

'I now have a boy, Koos Swart. He is also positive'. Her sentences are short. She is not interested in the conversation.

*Three violets in a jar.*

She is still trembling. 'I am just tired and I can't get warm.'

So much for the history.

'To get a history is to get the longitudinal information,' I teach my university psychology students. 'The mental status exam is the cross-sectional picture. Both kinds of information inform the diagnosis and the formulation, and ultimately the treatment plan.' I think about what I will write down for Lettie's mental status exam:

Affect: Blunted (disturbance in affect manifested by severe reduction in the intensity of externalised feeling tone).
Motor behaviour: Anergia.
Disturbances in speech: Poverty of speech (restriction in the amount of speech used; replies may be monosyllabic). Non-

spontaneous speech (verbal responses given only when asked or spoken to directly, no self-initiation of speech).

Levels of memory: Immediate, recent and remote intact. Cruelly so, it seems.

Insight (ability to understand the true cause and meaning of a situation – such as a set of symptoms): Impaired.

*Who is dying on whom?*

There will be no diagnosis. No formulation. And certainly, no treatment plan. I tell her that she seems very sick and that the sister will examine her, but she will most probably be hospitalised. Her face changes for the first time during the session: 'The last time I went to the hospital, I sat there, waiting, for six hours. Later, I was lying in the corridor, crying. It was so cold. I don't want to go.'

*It's a good thing they have gates to let you out.*

I do not know what happened to Lettie. I never saw her again.

In writing about my failure to help, I realised that when I left Lettie I was filled with shame. I was ashamed to be a psychotherapist, ashamed that I could do nothing, ashamed that I was looking forward to leaving the clinic for my warm house, two blocks away from the hospital where Lettie would probably lie shivering in the corridors. Lettie, sitting with me, might have felt, in Szymborska's words, 'embarrassed about dying' in this way.[2] Ashamed. I don't know. She was perhaps in too much physical agony to feel anything. The nursing file reads like a litany of shame.

I do think, however, that our metaphors helped us in the session, whether intended or not. In her few sentences about the hospital, Lettie succeeded in telling me about how very cold and stark and lonely the world had become for her, how very cold her future seemed. How she did not 'want to go'. I believe this allowed me to understand something about her emotional world, without her saying anything directly.

I also realise that the only useful thing I did in the session was to call the nurse, to put the thin clinic blanket around Lettie's shoulders and to sit with her, waiting. In turn, I used metaphors to say to her: I hear you are cold. I can do almost nothing. I will sit with you. I am sorry.

My enactment provided me access 'to highly significant, as-yet-unrecognized facets of the client, the therapist, and the relationship they share'.[3]

## Loss and melancholia

In mourning it is the world which has become poor and empty; in melancholia it is the ego itself.

— Sigmund Freud, *The Freud Reader*

An object-choice, an attachment of the libido to a particular person, had at one time existed; then, owing to a real slight or disappointment coming from this loved person, the object-relationship was shattered. The result was not the normal one of a withdrawal of the libido from this object and a displacement of it on to a new one, but something different . . . an identification of the ego with the abandoned object . . . object-loss was transformed into ego-loss

— Sigmund Freud, *The Freud Reader*

In Jonny Steinberg's *A Man of Good Hope*, he recalls asking his protagonist, Assad, why he is unable to read the book, the story of his life:

'What is it that upsets you when you read it?' I ask.
'It is two things,' he says crisply. 'The one is the loss, loss, loss . . . Everywhere it is loss, loss, loss.'[4]

Nathan Trantraal, in an interview, describes how poverty means that people almost become accustomed to death and loss.

Because poverty and struggle necessarily mean that people process things at a hyper-accelerated speed. I know of a family where the whole family, except one sister, died in one year, I know of brothers who all were shot within a year or a few months. The people who stay behind move on, accept it as a normal part of a painful life, not acknowledging that it mostly is a painful existence. It is like fantasy and reality that, with time, melt into each other.[5]

In my work as a therapist I am confronted with loss every day. Sometimes it is death. Thirteen-year-old Rodine has had three serious suicide attempts. She explains what made her want to end her life. 'That afternoon my mom's little baby died. It was born dead. That's a lot of dying in our family. First my granny, then my uncle, then another uncle, now my granny, aunt . . . my granny, then my uncle Piet, then uncle Boetatjie and uncle Andy. I wonder why, why do these people have to die? People are so needed.'

Sometimes it is not an actual death that leads to distress, but the loss of relationship or even the loss of a longed-for or hoped-for relationship.

In our work in the valley it seems that women often specifically relate their psychological distress to the pain and disappointments associated with the mother-child relationship. They are disappointed and distressed about not being able to be the mothers they wanted to be, but they are also disappointed and distressed that their children are not living up to their expectations, not fulfilling the hopes and dreams they, as mothers, had for them. Ideal mothers and ideal children seemed to be implicit in all the narratives.

A different kind of loss to be mourned. A loss that renders mothers melancholic, in the Freudian sense of the word. The mothers longed for grateful and satisfied children, but instead they are faced with demanding children whose needs they cannot fulfil. This loss of the idealised object also leads to a loss of the ideal self, the sense of being an all-giving, nurturing mother.[6]

Sterretjie explains, 'It makes me stress because I do not have money. Then they [the children] come, "There isn't bread". But now I say, "Gosh, ask your father for a change!"' Shaking her head, she says, 'I become, oh, I become very angry and become, become emotionally worked up.' She waves her hand to illustrate. 'I think it's because I stress.' Now she makes her hand in a fist. 'Now, I can't handle everything and then I become, and then I shout at everyone. He [her son] will, one evening while we were sitting he, then we were talking and then he told me my kitchen's ceiling board has fallen off, but every time he tells me I must buy a board and I say, "I don't have money now!"' She shows her empty hands. 'I say they all come running to me and they all say "*Mammie* do this. *Mammie* do that."'

Dora also ascribes her distress to not being able to meet the demands of her children. 'Or Lydia [her daughter] moans, she wants food. Tasha [another daughter] moans, she wants food. Jerome [her son] moans, he wants food. "Mama, I am hungry." And then he looks irritated. And everyone comes to me, everyone asks me. They moan at me . . . Then, probably, everything becomes too much for me, because everyone moans around me. Ashlyn [another daughter] says she's hungry. Now Tasha asks me, looking in my eyes, "*Mammie*, what I eat now?" Because I say, I told my husband yesterday, my longing is to have enough food in the house.'

The tension between low-income women's constructions of ideal motherhood and their inability to meet these ideals as a result of poverty-related constraints leads to feelings of disappointment, inadequacy, psychological distress and desperation. Children's relentless and continuous demands thus may be experienced as unbearable rebukes for their failures as mothers.[7] In the words of Dora, 'It leaves me feeling so useless. I am not worth the word "Ma", I can't provide for them.'

Apart from wanting to feel nurturing and giving, many so-called depressed mothers also expressed a distinct need to be nurtured and supported themselves.[8] However, instead of being attended to, supported and nurtured as caregivers, mothers in the valley are often lone mothers (even if they have partners or husbands), receiving little or no support from others. Those with partners are often in abusive relationships. When their own needs are not being met (partly because of the demands of their children), the mothers are put in 'the untenable position of giving what [they feel they] should be getting'.[9] Maria, also diagnosed with depression, says, 'Sometimes I feel that they [her children and husband] must also help me to do something.' She pauses and shakes her head. 'Then they don't want to, um, then they say, especially my husband says, "It is a woman's plight, her plight", but sometimes I also feel they must do something for me and so.'

Sterretjie also complains about a lack of support. 'Look, I am actually the man in the house. Because my husband, he, he, he is not worried at all about what goes wrong in the house. I must make sure that everything is right in the house.'

Mothers were particularly enraged when even their children do not help or support them. Leila, speaking about her depression says, '"Make me a fucking cup of tea! And you see I came from work, but you won't even make me a cup of tea!"'

Twela, speaking about her depression and the aggression that she associates with it, also talks about her fantasy that her child will help her and support her. 'I don't want to lift my head up to do a thing. I just call my son, Ashley, must do things for me. And I just just get aggressive.'

The longing was for a considerate and supportive child, but it is loss again when the child turns out not be that child.

The distress experienced by participants when they were not cared for, helped and supported happens in a context where there often has been a history of neglect and a continuous denial of needs.[10] When the women turn to their children and, yet again, their needs are not met, they are very likely to re-experience past ruptures and unprocessed painful experiences. The neediness, frustration and sense of abandonment they subsequently feel manifests as a deep melancholia, a sense of self-doubt and self-denigration.

Furthermore, cultural discourses of femininity portray the 'good mother' as someone whose activities are oriented toward relationship and family caregiving and as someone who has no needs except for those that are functional for her children.[11] When women put their needs first or make self-care a priority, they are at risk of being seen as selfish,[12] something 'a good woman' must strive to avoid. Their own need for care and support may thus further add to women's distress. Not only do they lose the caring child, they also lose the sense of themselves as the selfless and all-giving mother.

Mothers do not only long for respectful, helping children, they also want children who are disciplined and in control. Depressed Leila says, 'I will laugh with a child, I will play with a child, but there is a certain point where you must not make me angry. If I told you, "But it must be like this", then you must not tell me you will just do it tomorrow quickly. If I tell Lucinda [her daughter] to put water on for Mom, then you leave what you are busy with, because Mom spoke, Mom gave me a task.'

Sterretjie also speaks about the importance of discipline. 'Yes, and I have told them [her children]: "If the school is out, I am at work, you arrive at home. You see that Gladys [her neighbour] can't look after you, because she has two children on her name. You will finish that work for me. If I come through the kitchen door, I don't want to see, see a fork lying in the basin because it upsets me if I arrive at home and there is is lot of dirty dishes because I did not dirty them. Why must I clean them now?" Those are things that upset you. And they are big. "First, make your beds before you go through the door. Afternoons, when you come back, undress, hang you school clothes over that chair, put your bags on top of the cupboard."'

In the working-class context a caring, respectful, responsible and disciplined child is the idealised child that potentially can ensure a new life and a new identity for the mother.[13] An acting-out child confronts a mother with the possibility of losing her child and the fantasy of what the child may become. Mothers feel distressed when their children do not live up to this ideal and therefore do not allow them to feel good about themselves and their role as mothers.

Given their investment in responsible and disciplined children, mothers report severe distress when their children fail to conform to social rules and engage in illegal activities such as gangsterism and substance abuse. In the words of Leila, 'I said, now you [her daughter] want to tell me, "Mommy enjoys beer." I say, "I am an adult. Yes, you are a child. You are not a grown woman yet, and Devlin [her son] is not a grown man yet. That stuff will mess your lives up. You, who does not want to go to school." I say: "Today I am sorry, look where I have to work. On a farm with little money due to leaving school early." I say, "Do you want this future? You have big ideals; no one who wants to become an attorney does not go to school. No, you will have to get your butt into gear girl! You can't do it like this." But she insists. It's these types of things that work on me.'

Maria also talks about wanting to give her children the best. 'I feel that I always want to give my children the best, so that they do not grow up like I did, and so that they can have a future. And I must, I always watch them and so on. But sometimes when things become too much in the house and things then [pause] then I panic on my children or I panic on my husband, or I stress on them or something. But sometimes I think they don't understand me. I will always, never leave my children with what they are busy with I will always, always be hard on them because, because I don't want them to also . . . there in a house people lived in, or sometimes the environment outside is different. Children use *tik* [methamphetamine], children smoke, children use drugs and things.'

The mother of the acting-out child is also confronted with the possible loss of the longed-for maternal identity – she cannot think of herself as a good mother anymore. In other words, an acting-out child causes a mother to simultaneously experience the disappointment of not having the ideal child *and* she has to confront the reality that she is not the mother that she hoped to be – she is not the ideal mother. Women are generally very clear that mothers are typically blamed for the acting out of children.[14] Leila says, 'My son, I recently found out he is using marijuana, and these are things that work on me. And then I ask myself each time as mother, "Gosh, where did the problem come in? Where did I make a mistake? Is the problem with me or is it maybe because they are involved with the wrong friends?"'

## The anger of melancholia

While a deep sense of melancholia can be discerned in the disappointed mothers, the distress also often manifests as outbursts of anger and acts of aggression directed at their children. We encounter many angry women and women who are angry with their children.

In the valley, when asked about depression, women typically associate their psychological distress with anger.[15] Consistent with a larger feminist literature, the anger seems to be related to relational experiences and their disappointments within the context of relationships.[16] What is diagnosed as women's depression is actually better described as anger about relationship deficits, in that low relationship mutuality is associated with more anger suppression and/or less control over the experience and expression of anger.[17] While the relational difficulties of volatile, angry and demanding women are often attributed to internal instability (leading to a diagnosis of borderline personality disorder), women are often simply reacting to a disturbed and disturbing intersubjective field,[18] which is, in turn, situated in a very specific context.

Mothers seem to be uncomfortable with their anger and are often scared, even terrified, of it. They typically are especially ashamed if their anger manifests as violent behaviour against their children. For instance, implicit in Maria's rather self-critical description of how she disciplines her children is the notion that an ideal mother should not be so 'hard', but should be 'ever-patient'.[19]

Twela says, 'I don't want to be that person, that bad person, like swearing and whatever. And I don't want to be impatient. It isn't right to swear to express your feeling, to be impatient to express your feeling. It isn't right. Yes, and I don't want that angry. It's, it's frightening. I don't want that angry. I want to talk with a kind voice, but I don't want to shout back and ignore them or whatever, I don't want to do that. So I don't want to be that person. I want to be, um, calm, still and I want to be that person.'

Maria, crying when she talks about how she hits her children, says, 'But I always try to give my children the best, and, and, and, and, and, but the other thing is that I want to stop being so hard on them.'

Dora says that depression sometimes means that you become aggressive. 'You want to do things that you don't want to do. So the best is walk away. If you believe in God, you talk to God. I say to God, "I don't want to, I don't want to." My children can't suffer damage through this thing.'

We see that mothers who feel that they have lost the children they wanted to have also lose not only their sense of being good mothers, but they are also further distressed by their own reactions to the situation. A vicious cycle is created: loss, melancholia, anger, violence, shame and more melancholia. This is a cycle that is repeated from generation to generation.[20] In the words of Twela: 'That, that, that feeling what I had inside me, that, that, that bitterness and all that dark things that I had, um, how can I say? Um, that I can give them to him [her son].'

Many mothers talk about being hit as children themselves.[21] Cathy says, 'My mother was very strict. And I got hidings. If she called me, and I say, "Yes Mommy, I am coming", but I don't go immediately, then I get a hiding for that.'

Instead of becoming the ideal mother or having the ideal child,[22] in the words of Rozsika Parker:

The child has become her persecutor, and her love for the child and culture's expectation of maternal behaviour combine to accuse her of inadequacy. She slaps because she hates the child for behaviour that threatens her with the loss of an internal object called 'me-as-a-good-mother', for turning her into a monster, and for obscuring the love and concern that are obviously there.[23]

Children are experienced as demanding, inconsiderate and acting out and mothers are disappointed in their own abilities to live up to implicit ideals of motherhood. Women faced with these losses are not merely sad or in pain or even ambivalent, they are often and, perhaps, typically, also angry and outraged for very valid reasons. If such women are simply diagnosed with depression, their distress is medicalised and their anger is obscured.[24]

If we want to deal with women's distress, we should pay more attention to what mothers are angry about. Michelle Lafrance and Suzanne McKenzie-Mohr stress the importance of legitimising people's distress, but also of 'keeping visible the clear links between the social conditions of people's lives and their suffering'.[25] On the other hand, implicit gender discourses that determine women's idealised expectations of motherhood are also relevant, in that they lead to unrealistic expectations and fantasies about motherhood: 'At the root of women's depression are specific images of relationship – pleasing, self-sacrifice, self-silencing, compliance – that are culturally defined as feminine attachment behaviours.'[26] Such a notion of motherhood serves to obscure the possibility that motherhood simply may be a depressing and frustrating experience,[27] and seems to be part of 'a powerful web of discourses which position working-class women as inferior, irresponsible or even dangerous'.[28]

Interventions focused on individual women should be aimed at providing spaces where women can talk about their complex and ambivalent experiences of anger in safe ways: 'Feeling the anger, tolerating it, and judiciously putting it into words . . . is the essential task for the mother.'[29] Working within a psychoanalytic framework, Paul Trad discusses how feelings of ambivalence, regression and fear of separation and hostility are part and parcel of the mother's experience of pregnancy and child-rearing.[30] He argues that mothers need spaces to represent symbolically and discharge feelings aroused by these developmental crises, otherwise these feelings will be randomly discharged on themselves or their children.

## Anger turned inwards

The girls' group is grim. They are talking about how they deal with anger.

'Once there was a girl,' Sandra says, 'I cannot say her name. She was drunk when she got home. Now she can't, she was not allowed, she had to be at home at six. But she is in high school already. So she said, "I am mos not a *kleintjie* [little thing] that I have to be home at six. I will be home at nine," she said. So she got home at nine and her mother yelled at her. Her grandmother yelled at her. She was drunk. So there was this boy, a boy that she had sex with, but they were friends, friends with benefits. So he wanted to have sex with her, but she did not want to have sex. She said to him, "No, I don't want to give my virginity to you." And she was glad, she did not go because that evening, if she went, he would have had sex with her. And she would have done it because she was angry. She would have done anything at the moment. It would have made her feel better.'

Another girl explains: 'You want to forget. Say now your mother yelled at you. You want to go to a party, she says no. And they say to you, "Come to the party, come." And you go, you want to forget the yelling. They say to you, "Come, we have liquor. Pour yourself a drink." And so on. You will do that then – because you want to forget, forget about the argument. Just forget.'

The girls agree that forgetting is the best way to deal with difficult things like yelling parents. But Rodine says there are other options. 'You can just kill yourself. Because you are tired of life. You don't want to be yelled at by your parents all the time. Say your parents have a drinking problem and there is nothing to eat in the house and you are left alone at home. And you parents just keep on drinking and they don't worry about you, they don't care. Then you get tired of life. Like my friend, her mother and sister made her angry, they argued, so she cut her wrists. So she had to go to the hospital. They told if she does it again, she will die. The next time it was about a boy. And she cut her wrists again.'

Other girls in the group also know about suicide attempts. Wildene says, 'There's a girl, I won't mention names. She went to school and after school, it wasn't nice to get home, so she cut her wrists.'

The group feels subdued. They are more quiet than usual, their stories longer, the pace slower, no interruptions. Rodine says, 'I know a girl, she does not live here anymore, she moved at the end of last year. She had a boyfriend, he sold *tik* biscuits, so her aunt did not want her to go out with him anymore. She told me everything. And then she disappeared. And they went looking for her and they found her on the train tracks. Her wrists were cut. So her auntie whacked her with the broom. So she ran away again. Now there are pictures of her all over. She is still gone.'

The group listens quietly. 'I have also cut my wrists once,' Wildene says. 'My mother . . . it was on a Sunday, my mother and my sister went to town. My mother bought us these thin tops that I don't like. I told her not to buy it. My sister then got angry and said, "*Ek praat nie saam met jou nie*" [I won't talk to you]. Then she hit me. And then my mother also hit me. So I left. I walked down the road and they asked me why I am not in school. That was the day I cut my wrists.'

'And do you think your mother will think about you if something like that happens?' the therapist asks. 'Will she miss you?'

The girls look at each other. No one says anything.

On the way home the therapist takes a picture of the glass cabinet in the hallway of the school that displays the pictures of pupils who have committed suicide. On the opposite wall is the cabinet of the leaders and champions produced by the school.

## The ungrievable life

Who counts as human? Whose lives count as lives? And finally, what makes for a grievable life?

— Judith Butler, *Precarious Life*

The opposite of love is not hate, but indifference.

— Elie Wiesel, 'Insight'

I have seen death without weeping.
The destiny of the Northeast is death.
Cattle they kill,
But to the people they do something worse.

— Geraldo Vandre, 'Disparada', in
Nancy Scheper-Hughes, *Death without Weeping*

It was my first autopsy . . .

Then he took out the large and heavy heart, with its right side hypertrophied and documented its weight in grams.

I found myself strangely disappointed. There was nothing else to see. No hidden place, unexplored and unexplorable, no unpenetrable small black box, hidden in all these wiggly intestines. It was undeniable, Mr. Baker had completely disappeared. Autopsied, his body was nothing more than a suit of clothes lying disregarded in the corner . . . I did tuck away in the back of my mind the image of his body as a crumpled suit of clothes, abandoned in the corner of the white room.

— Victoria Sweet, *God's Hotel*

I am waiting for a patient. The waiting room smells like Dettol and sweat and Cup-a-Soup. There are twelve people waiting with me. Some people are watching the TV in the right-hand corner. Others are staring at the walls. The walls are covered in posters and notices. Recipes for *toe neus* (blocked nose) and *rehidrasie* (rehydration). Big, black, handmade signs with arrows indicate *Rehidrasiehoekie* (Rehydration corner). Against the wall a pine table with a plastic cloth and plastic flowers. Infant scale. Another table with three wooden boxes: *Kondome. Pos. Voorstelle* (Condoms. Mail. Suggestions). A white cardboard doctor's jacket, which serves as a brochure stand. The brochures are all about TB.

A man in the fourth row gets up slowly. He coughs violently and stumbles over the green plastic chair next to him. In the process he knocks over a few more chairs. He lands on the green melamine floor and lies still. The other patients watch him. The cardboard doctor's jacket does not move. The nurses laugh in the kitchen where they are having tea. The man stirs. I get up and fetch a nurse.

The nurse kneels at the man's side and feels his pulse. She puts her hand over her mouth. 'Dead,' she says. 'He just died.'

My patient never turns up.

It is spring in the valley.

# Epilogue

*'The world goes on as if nothing much has happened'*\*

If we had a keen vision and feeling of all ordinary human life, it would be like hearing the grass grow and the squirrel's heart beat, and we should die of that roar which lies on the other side of silence.

— George Eliot, *Middlemarch*

Is it really useless to complain? For my own amusement, perhaps, I ask the question out loud. The bamboo gives no answer. I hear only the faint sound of someone singing, a hoe striking the stony earth, a finch.

— Paul Farmer, *Pathologies of Power*

The space, at once empty and populated, of all those words without a language which allow the person who lends an ear to hear a muffled voice from below history, the stubborn murmuring of a language which seems to speak quite by itself, without a speaking subject and without an interlocutor, huddled in on itself, a lump in its throat, breaking down before it has achieved any formulation and lapsing back into the silence from which it was never separated.

— Michel Foucault, *Madness and Civilization*

In the valley our patients come to us in the way patients everywhere go to their therapists: with hope and with dread. And we, middle-

---

\* The quote in the subtitle of this chapter – 'The world goes on as if nothing much has happened' – is from Sen, 2005: xi.

class psychotherapists, approach our patients in the way that therapists everywhere approach their patients: with hope and with dread. These conflicting impulses mean that patients and their therapists everywhere sometimes activate a repeated relationship and sometimes the needed relationship: while there is inevitably the pull toward repetition in both patient and therapist, there are also desires for new relational possibilities.[1] This activation of both the desire for repetition and the desire for change are also evoked, in very profound ways, in the valley of hope and dread.

Dread is an uncomfortable feeling: it refers to anticipating something with great apprehension or fear. My students and I feel apprehensive about our sessions in the valley, worried and anxious that we will not be able to help, that we will be exposed as inefficient, incompetent or, worst of all, uncaring.

In his journal, one of my students reflects on the emotions he experienced while waiting in the reception area for his first patient at the community clinic in the valley:

> When I was told there was someone to see, I became instantly anxious. I hope this is not a hectic one, I thought. I envisioned the possible stress that may follow if the patient had a 'serious' problem. I became more anxious. Reluctant and irritated on the inside, I said cheerfully, 'Sure, can I see her now?'
>
> I desperately tried to scan her appearance, trying to convince myself that she was not going to burden my Monday afternoon. Don't have a hectic problem, don't have a hectic problem, I pleaded with her in my own private thought. 'What can I do for you?' I said in my now finely tuned professional tone. Don't be suicidal or abused. Don't be suicidal or abused, I thought, all the while displaying my serene therapist-like demeanour. Within minutes she was in tears, mostly about her lack of money and support, not knowing what to do.
>
> Shit! Poverty is real! I thought.

Our dread makes us feel distressed. We feel bad about our dread and our despair.

Our reactions of shame to our impoverished patients are not unusual.[2] Firstly, there is always potential for shame in the psychotherapeutic encounter.[3] There are many reasons for this: there is the risk of failure at his/her profession; the therapist (like the patient) risks exposure of painful vulnerabilities and personal shortcomings that may be felt as the shameful sense of being bad, disgusting or a failure as a human being; and emotional life itself is often felt to be shameful.[4] By making the therapist the expert authority who claims to know the patient better than the patient herself, a culture of shame is created.[5]

Apart from the fact that the therapeutic situation in itself is potentially shaming to the therapist, the potential for shame is even greater if there are class (or other) differences between therapist and patient. Rafael Javier and William Herron write about how analysts may respond to a patient's impoverished status:

> The psychology of most analysts that has developed long before they met their first disenfranchised patient, and that may well have been reinforced by the homeless panhandler or other encounters on the way to the office, tends to solidify a class dichotomy related to a mode of anxiety regulations commonly used by members of the dominant group . . . The resulting schism, often reflected in just enough distance to still appear politically correct by hiding overt discriminations, makes the development of true empathy and working alliances virtually impossible.[6]

Often my students write about what I would consider to be unverbalisable shame.[7] They also describe a seemingly common reaction to the uncomfortable feelings associated with shame: wanting to 'leave it behind' and the 'desire to run away'. Sometimes our flight is literal: going home early on particular days or leaving community work altogether. Often, we flee emotionally, using all kinds of sophisticated defence mechanisms. Shame, if not verbalised and acknowledged, can potentially lead to enactment in the shape of abandonment.

I myself often feel like fleeing, and I always do, inevitably, flee.[8]

This book, in a certain sense, is about arriving and leaving, about engaging and disengaging, connecting and disconnecting, love and abandonment.[9]

I end this book not knowing what I know and what I do not know.

In the words of Wendy Hollway: 'One consequence of Bion's emphasis on emergence and living in uncertainty is traceable in the way I have written this book, the shape it has (uncertainly) taken and the way I try to deal with the residual bits at this final stage.'[10]

Hope and dread.

And the feelings are always mutual, the enactments inevitable on both sides.

## The boy with the shiny shoes: The inevitability of re-enactment

> Constable N stepped away from the car, into the darkness where Darren could not see where his gun was pointing and fired two rounds into the air. The gunshots cracked the roof of the night sky and echoed back at us. My first thought was that they could be heard all over Toekomsrus; I wondered how many imaginations had in that instant conjured a different story to explain the gunshots; a record of all those stories, I found myself thinking, would probably document every fear this place has of itself and its young men.
>
> — Jonny Steinberg, *Thin Blue*

Trevor Tindall, a seventeen-year-old Grade 12 pupil, is referred to us by the valley's high school principal who says that the teachers are so scared of Trevor that they don't want him in their classrooms. He recently became involved in gang activities and got into trouble at school for fighting and carrying a knife.

He is interviewed by a young, white, female therapist in training. She is scared of him and his knife.

As is typical, the therapy session starts with the question 'What brought you here?' His 'presenting complaint', as we say as psychologists, is insightful. He does not talk about violence and anger or gangs. He immediately talks about his mother. He says that the school principal told him that he should talk to someone, a psychologist. 'And this is a problem that I have,' he says, 'I stress a lot. My mother, she drinks. She drinks every weekend – badly. And my father died when I was three and then my mother just gave me away. She says I am a mistake in life. Now I ask myself: Why are you saying such things to me? She is the one that brought me into this life. I did not ask to be here. Every day I say to her that I did not ask to be here.'

Then, with his head bowed, avoiding the eyes of the therapist, seemingly shrinking in his seat, he says, 'And then in 2007, then I got involved with a gang.'

The supervision videotape of the session shows an intense, sad, young man, tall and thin, but soft-spoken. His whole physical presentation seems to be one of shame: head bowed, avoidance of eye contact, shrinking of the body.[11] On the videotape the therapist seems terrified. At times she looks as if she is going to flee the room.

Trevor continues to talk about being enraged with his mother. She was drunk and recently had sex on the street with a random man. Trevor and his friends and everyone else who happened to be around witnessed this sexual encounter. He talks about how utterly humiliated he was. As he is talking, he bends down to his bag, fumbling around to find something. The therapist watches in horror and surreptitiously glances at the door, measuring the distance. She is waiting for the knife.

Trevor fumbles and fumbles in the bag and takes out a shoe brush. Continuing to talk, he starts polishing his shoes. Determinedly. Carefully. While he is polishing, he talks more about his childhood and his mother. 'I don't now want to think about her like that, that she does things like that. I told my grandmother this, probably the Sunday after it happened, that I can't continue like this. Yes, I always speak to my grandmother. Just before my father died, my mother gave me away. I remember that. I can remember it. I was three years old. Then my mother gave me away. And then my grandmother went to fetch me. And then my grandmother said to the people who took me from my mother, "You can't take him!" My mother and father took me just like that and packed my clothes and gave me to the people and said, "We don't want him." And my grandmother came and wrapped me in a towel. She has only one eye and she can't see that well. But she brought me up, not my mother. And my father actually also left my mother before he died.'

Trevor relates being a 'mistake' in his mother's eyes, abandoned by her as a baby. From the beginning she treated him with disrespect and contempt, she shames him when she says that he should not have been alive. She did not teach him to love himself. If shame is a deficiency of self-love, Trevor has been shamed since the beginning.

James Gilligan writes that it seems 'difficult if not impossible for a child to gain the capacity for selflove without first having been loved by at least one parent, or parent-substitute. And when the self is not loved, by itself or by another, it dies, just as surely as the body dies without oxygen.'[12] Trevor was not taught to love himself by either of his parents, he was not mirrored. But also, he was not able to idealise and admire them, and his mother still shames him by behaving badly in public.[13]

If we understand that Trevor is not merely a knife-carrying gang member, but also a young man feeling helpless and dependent, longing for love and fearing abandonment, we may relate to him differently.[14]

The therapist, however, does not see the fear and the longing. She wrote in her journal how scared she was to get this referral and how petrified she was throughout the session:

> I tried really hard during the session to hide my anxiety, and just really listen to what he has to say . . . I kept telling myself to not let the anxiety show on my face . . . I felt quite bewildered throughout the session and kept thinking that this must be my most horrible performance as a wannabe therapist to date.

Trevor is shamed once again.[15] He must have sensed the therapist's fear in the session: he is someone who terrifies white women – and again as a person he is rejected and treated with disrespect. In this sense, the session, which he must have approached with some hope, becomes a dreaded repetition. For him as patient there may be the experience Silvan Tomkins writes about: 'If I wish to be close to you, but you move away, I am ashamed.'[16] In her journal, the therapist admitted that she was 'quite ashamed' that she 'came across as so cold and detached'. Although she was deeply ashamed of her fear and her wish to flee,[17] she is enacting something for the patient, and her experience offers information about his experiential world as a young black man in South Africa, interacting with a white woman.[18]

Donna Orange's description of shame in a psychotherapy session seems to describe exactly what happens in the session with Trevor: 'Both [therapist and patient] begin innocently and with the best of intentions. Before long they are tied up together in an impasse that results from mutual shaming. The shame belongs [to neither]; it becomes like the oxygen in the room when they are together, all-pervasive.'[19]

Andrew Morrison also writes about the pervasive quality of shame: 'Shame settles in like a dense fog, obscuring everything else, imposing only its shapeless, substanceless impressions. It becomes impossible to establish bearings or to orient oneself in relation to the broader landscape.'[20] In his article 'History Repeats Itself in Transference-Countertransference', Neil Altman describes how history on the large-group social level and history on the individual, dyadic or small-group level may reflect each other.[21] Part of what is reflected in this psychotherapy session seems to be the vein of shame that endures for contemporary South Africans, even as we are all so desperately trying to close the door on our nation's shameful past.[22] Both patients and therapists feel deeply ashamed in these encounters.

In this situation it is possible that there might have been violent enactments in the therapy room. The therapist might have fled the room, both patient and therapist might simply have withdrawn, violently rejecting each other.[23] If Trevor were a different person, he might have taken out his knife (and one might actually have understood why).

Shame, however, does not always and inevitably produce violence.[24] Trevor first continues to talk about feeling guilty about joining a gang and carrying a knife, of losing his temper and acting out.

But then he does something remarkable.

While the pair is caught up in this terrible interaction, he starts polishing his shoes. His act is one of pride and self-respect. As he polishes and polishes, his shoes becoming shinier and shinier, another self emerges. Only in polishing his shoes can he move the conversation from his mother to his grandmother: his mother called him a 'mistake' and gave him away, his one-eyed grandmother wrapped him in a towel and took him home. Despite all the levels of shame, he uses the therapeutic space to connect to the other side of himself: he acts out pride and self-respect. At the same time, a discourse of shame and rage is replaced by a discourse of tenderness and gratitude. The therapist, in turn, is forced to be witness to these other sides of the knife-carrying young gang member.[25] In his enactment of the old and the new, the 'repeated relationship' and the 'needed relationship' are reflected in very subtle ways.[26]

Trevor is in no way a young man doomed to a life of violence. He had a person whom he could idealise and love from an early age, a person who also respected him and taught him to love himself, someone who even now takes him seriously and attends to him. He is aware of the fact that his joining the gang is not only part of a longing to belong, but also part of wanting to be respected and wanting to be with people that he can respect. Because he has loved and been loved, he has, somewhere along the line, developed the capacity for remorse and guilt. At this stage Trevor is aware of other (non-violent) ways of saving and restoring his self-image: he still goes to school, he still talks to his loving grandmother, he has friends. He even agrees to see a therapist on his caring principal's insistence.

Trevor's shoe polishing becomes a metaphor for hope.

## The girl with the sweaty hands: 'A feast of brief hopes'

So what kind of prophet am I?

. . .

Flawed and aware of it. Desiring greatness.
Able to recognize greatness wherever it is,

. . .

I knew what was left for smaller men like me:
a feast of brief hopes.

— Czesław Miłosz, *Selected and Last Poems, 1931–2004*

You put together two people who have not been put together before. Sometimes it is like that first attempt to harness a hydrogen balloon to a fire balloon: do you prefer crash and burn, or burn and crash? But sometimes it works, and something new is made, and the world is changed. Then, at some point, sooner or later, for this reason or that, one of them is taken away and what is taken away is greater than the sum of what was there. This may not be mathematically possible; but it is emotionally possible.

— Julian Barnes, *Levels of Life*

I see Wendy Winters for individual psychotherapy for about ten sessions.[27] While she was sad and anxious in our initial meeting, she was also almost immediately confiding and ferociously focused on wanting to get better. At only seventeen, she has somehow understood that she is entitled to have things better than they are. And she is clear that she needs help with this.

Her symptoms seem to be directly related to her stepfather's drunken rages. He drinks regularly on weekends and then becomes violent. Wendy becomes terrified. The terror manifests as an ongoing mild anxiety, sometimes culminating in panic attacks. We talk about how things can change, how the household can change, how she can change. I ask if she can send her stepfather to see me. I have two sessions with Moos, an exhausted man with a heavy presence and a reluctant smile. He is angry, yes. His family does not take him seriously. He can never watch the TV that he wants to. Another shamed man. But he does drink: '*vat 'n biertjie of twee met vriende*' (take a beer or two with friends). I see him again. His smile is easier. He is trying to drink less.

Wendy likes to work with the idea that her stepfather's fury is like an animal that he comes home with and wants others to look after. 'Don't take it on,' I say. 'Close your door. Go away. Refuse to take it on.'

'It works,' she says. 'I don't take on the animal. I stare it down. I run away.'

Her anxiety becomes less. The panic attacks disappear.

Wendy is more upbeat every week, bringing me photographs of netball matches and modelling competitions. She is still highly strung and excitable, but mostly happy – always focused on getting ahead and getting rid of all obstacles in the way.

Soon after this she decides that she does not need to see me anymore, she is fine. '*Ek deal nou met daai dier*' (I now deal with that animal). She puts her hands on the table between us, palms up. 'Feel, my hands are not wet anymore. I am not scared anymore.'

For a brief moment I cover her hands with mine. Her palms are white and dry.

I am taken aback, not clear that I have done anything for her. Her symptoms might be gone, but I feel that her life has changed very little. As a therapist, I feel ashamed again. Fraud in the valley.

For the first few months after we end therapy she drops by regularly when she sees my car at the clinic, with a photograph of an event or news about her latest achievements at school. Over time the visits taper off and I only get text messages: 'Hallo Auntie Lou-Marié, I am on the students' council.' 'Hallo Auntie Lou-Marié, *ek is af van die till af by* Meatrite. *Ek is nou die* manager' (I am not working on the till at Meatrite anymore. I am now the manager). I note that I have become 'Auntie' Lou-Marié. At some point in the year, I get a 'Please call me' from an unknown number. It is Wendy. 'Hallo Auntie Lou-Marié. I have decided that Auntie Lou-Marié has to drive me to my matric dance on the 1st of November.' I am not asked. I am told. Being a conscientious psychotherapist, I think: the frame, the frame, the frame. But because November is still far away, I decide not to worry.

I hear nothing from her for months. I assume it is off, but in the middle of October she calls to confirm arrangements. I have to pick up her boyfriend, Clinton, outside Lanquedoc and he will direct me to her house. '*Hy sal vir Auntie Lou-Marié wag in 'n wit pak by die ingang van Lanquedoc. Net oorkant die skool. Kwart oor ses*' (He will wait for Auntie Lou-Marié in a white suit at the entrance of Lanquedoc. Across the road from the school. Quarter past six).

Not knowing what to do, I disregard my concerns about the frame and I find myself and my daughter, Mia, waiting in the oak lane for Clinton. Mia has never been to Lanquedoc. I point out the mountains, the old oak lane, the one-lane bridge and the Herbert Baker cottages. We take many pictures. It is a spectacular early summer evening, the mountains, as always, looming large.

Clinton is eventually dropped off by a battered light blue Datsun with a Paarl registration. He has soft, toffee-coloured eyes and he wears mostly white: white suit, black shirt with white embroidery, white shoes. His fringe is in dreadlocks. In his hands is a red plastic flower, still in its plastic wrapping, price, bar code and all.

In the car I try to make small talk. Clinton is polite in trying to answer my questions, but his focus clearly is on his brief to direct us to Wendy's house. He seems to switch seamlessly and effortlessly between Paarl, where he first met Wendy and Lanquedoc, where he is taking us.

'Wendy and I met in the Paarl. She was with her cousin. She stood there on Main Street eating an ice cream cone.

Right here.

And I saw her and I checked her out.

Left.

And then she saw me and then I saw that she saw me. And then I walked on.

Left again.

Then they kind of followed me.

Up the hill. Keep going, straight.

So I saw that they are following me. I then asked her cousin for her number and then I messaged her and now we have been together since June. It was the last day of school.

Here we are. Turn left.'

We stop in a dirt road in front of a typical Lanquedoc house. 'Cute,' says Mia. It is a small, square house with pink trimmings and a miniature garden with pink shrubs – quaint to the middle-class eye so eager to romanticise simplicity. There is a large group of people outside the house, all of them clearly waiting for something to happen.

Shrieks when we enter the little house. Another small crowd. Wendy comes forward, hugs me. 'Wow, Auntie Lou-Marié, you look just like me.' I am also wearing black clothes, but I don't look like her at all. She is eighteen and beautiful. Knowing her, I can see the anxiety in her tight, bare shoulders, hear it in the shrillness of her voice. Also present is the very familiar deliberateness of her gaze.

It is obviously photo time inside the house. Clinton is hardly greeted before he is placed, next to Wendy, behind a table with a crocheted tablecloth and snacks of all sorts. Little chicken pies and samoosas, rows of potato chips and peanuts, two bottles of sweet sparkling wine. Behind the couple, against the wall in a silver frame, Jesus is benevolently and piously watching the proceedings, a golden halo above his head, fat sheep in his arms.

It is a long photo session. Pictures are taken of everyone, including me and Wendy. 'She is, after all, my godmother,' Wendy explains to the crowd.

Wendy heads for the door. 'Now for me and my car.' Outside the crowd, which has doubled while we were inside, welcomes the couple with cheers. 'Three minutes of fame,' Wendy says and waves. She poses next to the Mini, on top of the Mini, inside the Mini. The family is clicking away. The children in the crowd are mirroring themselves in the chrome bumper of the Mini.

When we get to the City Hall, where the dance is to be held, the pavements are packed with people. We are circling the block at ten kilometres an hour, with revving Hummers, Mercedes, BMWs. 'Ooh, we are getting closer,' says Wendy. 'My three minutes of fame.' She switches on the interior light.

'What are you doing?' says Clinton. '*Ag* no, man, Wendy!'

'They have to see me. If the light is off, they can't see me,' she says.

Inside the car we are now all brightly lit. The cars are bumper to bumper, facing the biggest crowd of the evening. I see several patients in the crowd. They wave. I wave back.

Auntie Lou-Marié, I think, what are you doing?[28]

We drive stop-start. Stop-start. Stop-start. We are in the parking lot of the City Hall. A stern-looking woman indicates that we should wait. We are approaching the drop-off point. Go, she finally shows.

Giggling on the back seat.

I drive the last ten metres and stop the car. The crowd forms a corridor. Clinton opens the front door and gets out. Wendy shrieks. She hugs me with dry hands and steps out of the car. The crowd cheers and cheers and cheers. Three minutes of fame indeed. Wendy takes Clinton's arm, tightens her shoulders in the way that I know and walks through the crowd, waving as she walks, her black skirt swaying. She does not look back.

I rev the Mini Cooper. My daughter rolls her eyes and reprimands me, '*Mamma.*' I steer the car through the crowds. We will have supper in town.

# Appendix

*Some Notes on Method and Ethics*

> I think anyone trying to create something, in the spirit that I'm trying
> to create something, wants it to not pass for life exactly but be as close
> as possible to what might be felt as true to anybody.
> — Rachel Cusk, in Alexandra Schwartz, 'I Don't Think
> Character Exists Anymore'

The original idea for this book was for it to be based on a single, rather
conventional qualitative research project, the Maternal Mental Health
Project (see below). This was a study conducted over four years and
involved graduate students interviewing low-income, pregnant women.
When I started writing up the data in book form, I realised that I could
not dare try to write about the lives of others if I had not encountered
their worlds myself. I realised that if I was going to write about the
lives of these women, I had to immerse myself in their lives in more
substantial ways. The book project was abandoned and I embarked
on a meandering, haphazard and rather strange journey in an effort to
understand the lifeworlds of the women I was trying to write about.[1] In
this effort I came to understand that I am not writing about the women,
I am writing about a specific encounter in a specific place between
specific people.[2] I attempt to explain this complicated and unfinished
journey in the *Prologue* and to explain how this book should be read as
the unfinished and incomplete notes of a psycho-ethnographer.

In this brief reflection on method and ethics I attempt to describe
in more conventional academic ways how all of this can be constructed
as social science research. I describe how the 'data' on which this book is

based was collected. I also discuss how I dealt with some of the ethical dilemmas I faced, how some of these dilemmas remain unresolved and how complicated such dilemmas are.[3]

In this book I refer to data that was generated in very different ways – clinical cases, ethnographic encounters and interviews conducted in conventional research studies. What these research strategies have in common is 'thick description', the kind of description that one can only find in so-called case studies.[4] Clifford Geertz's concept of 'thick description' perhaps best describes the value of a case study. The most important issue is not simply the facts themselves, but how the facts are framed. The case study involves an in-depth, intensive and focused exploration of 'natural occurrences with definable boundaries' over a period of time.[5]

## Ethnography

Ethnography is variously defined by different people. Geertz says that there are three characteristics of ethnographic description: 'It is interpretive; what it is interpretive of is the flow of social discourse; and the interpreting involved consists in trying to rescue the "said" of such discourse for its perishing occasions and fixing it in perusable terms.'[6]

In the *Prologue* I emphasise how individual biography has to be read against the background of larger social and political processes. Anthropologist João Biehl articulates this projects as follows:

> Our lives are part and parcel of small- and large-scale milieus and historical shifts colouring our every experience . . . As ethnographers, we are challenged to attend at once to the political, economic, and material transience of worlds and truths and to the journeys people take through milieus in transit while pursuing needs, desires, and curiosities or simply trying to find room to breathe beneath intolerable constraints.[7]

While my work is very much influenced by psychoanalysis (with its emphasis on the importance of unconscious processes) and discourse analysis (arguing for the importance of how lives are 'overdetermined by regimes of power and knowledge') ethnography has forced me from 'the sway of crude universals to attend more closely to the specificity and the world-historical significance of people's everyday experience'.[8] Ethnography has compelled me to ask some crucial questions, articulated beautifully by Biehl:

> How can we ethnographically apprehend these worldly fabrications and the lives therein, constituted as they are by that which is unresolved, and bring this unfinishedness into our storytelling? How are long-standing theoretical approaches able to illuminate these political/economic/affective realities on the ground? How can the lives of our informants and collaborators, and the counter knowledges that they fashion, become alternative figures of thought that might animate comparative work, political critique, and anthropology to come?[9]

Biehl then answers his own questions as follows:

> Through ethnographic rendering, people's own theorizing of their conditions may leak into, animate, and challenge present-day regimes of veridiction, including philosophical universals and anthropological subjugation to philosophy ... This sense of ethnography in the way of (instead of to) theory – like art – aims at keeping interrelatedness, precariousness, uncertainty, and curiosity in focus. In resisting synthetic ends and making openings rather than absolute truths, ethnographic practice allows for an emancipatory reflexivity and for a more empowering critique of the rationalities, interventions, and moral issues of our times.[10]

Ethnography helps to explain why we are to hold on to theory lightly, whether it is psychoanalytic theory or discourse analysis.[11] Or for that matter, any theory. We have to attend to the leakages, the animations and the challenges presented by everyday lives and interrogate our theories. In the *Prologue* I stress the importance of recognising the tentativeness of any academic project, the humility with which we should approach our findings or conclusions. Ethnography is crucial in making us more humble and open in our academic endeavours:

Epistemological breakthroughs do not belong only to experts and analysts. Simply engaging with the complexity of people's lives and desires – their constraints, subjectivities, projects – in ever-changing social, economic, and technological worlds constantly necessitates rethinking. So, what would it mean for our research methodologies and ways of writing to consistently embrace unfinishedness, seeking ways to analyse the general, the structural, and the processual while maintaining an acute awareness of the tentativeness of our reflective efforts? As anthropologists, we can strive to do more than simply mobilize real world messiness to complicate – or serve – ordered philosophy, reductive medical diagnostics, and statistics-centered policy approaches. Both the evidentiary force and theoretical contribution of our discipline are intimately linked to attunement to the relations and improvised landscapes through which lives unfold and to trying to give form to people's arts of living. At stake is finding creative ways of not letting the ethnographic die in our accounts of actuality. And attending to life as it is lived and adjudicated by people in their realities produces a multiplicity of approaches, critical moves and countermoves, an array of interpretive angles as various as the individuals drawn to practice anthropology.[12]

## Clinical work

Writing about clinical cases is notoriously difficult and controversial, but also necessary and important.[13] The writing up of clinical case studies contribute to what John Gabbay and Andrée le May have called 'practice-based evidence for healthcare' – 'gathering good quality data from routine practice'.[14] When writing up clinical cases, one aims at making tentative conclusions about a case, opening those up for scrutiny by a community of clinicians and researchers, and using the knowledge thus attained cautiously and reflectively and critically.

While it is generally agreed that the writing up of clinical cases is extremely important, practitioners disagree about how to do it, particularly about how to do it while also protecting the patient.[15] Generally, two approaches to this ethical dilemma are considered.

First, one can get informed consent from a patient in the same way that one would get informed consent in a research study. If informed consent is to be obtained, timing becomes crucial. Asking for permission at the beginning of therapy may have an impact on the therapeutic alliance and on the therapy itself. Getting permission in the termination phase of therapy means that the therapy itself is not interfered with, but the request can be discussed in the therapeutic space and the discussion can actually become part of the treatment process. However, as is true in all processes of informed consent, the person giving it is often not clear about what exactly it is that they are consenting to. A patient may give a clinician permission to write about her, but will end up feeling betrayed by how and what the clinician writes.

Second, many clinicians who write about their cases disguise their patients, so as to make them unrecognisable, even to the patients themselves. The disadvantage of this is that some of the facts of a life that are obscured may have been vital to the dynamics of the case.

Some would argue that a combination of both disguise and consent is necessary.

For this book I used various strategies. First, I believe I have disguised all research participants and patients by using pseudonyms, by changing identifying facts about their lives and by compiling facts from different cases to construct a case that is not recognisable, but still convincingly real. While I did change details, I did not change crucial facts such as age, race, gender and class. I have tried to ensure that no individual in this book is identifiable.

Second, I approached the question of informed consent case by case. I tell many of my patients that I write about my clinical work, so many of them know that I do this when they start with therapy. More specifically, when I started to do clinical work in the valley, I knew I was going to use the clinical material in my writing and told patients at the beginning of therapy that I would possibly write about their stories. When asked for permission to do this, they invariably said yes, possibly not knowing exactly what they were consenting to. Some of the cases written about in this book were retrospective write-ups and are the cases of people I have no contact with anymore and whose permission I thus cannot get.

Third, I have made extensive use of my own and students' journals – case notes. Sally Swartz argues for the importance of writing case notes. She highlights that even if they are often clumsy, they expose important, underlying subtleties:

Knowledge that truth is not 'fact', that our clumsy attempts to make language represent reality in some transparent way lets loose exactly what we hoped to capture in our web. The music, the shape of a word, its historical resonance, tells far more than any accounting column can. It argues that regardless of the therapeutic orientation of the practitioner, private musings, written outside the boundaries of professional surveillance, give access to subliminal, submerged, sometimes fleeting or hard-to-grasp aspects of therapeutic encounters.[16]

## Research studies

A lot of the data used in this book was generated in rather conventional qualitative research studies. The designs of these studies were quite different from one another, but all were broadly informed by a social constructionist feminist approach.

### Maternal Mental Health Project

The largest of these studies, the Maternal Mental Health Project, was conducted over a period of four years. All pregnant women reporting to the local primary health clinic were approached to participate in the study. Those that agreed to participate were interviewed at four different points by the same interviewer: after their first prenatal visit to the clinic, a week after giving birth, three months after giving birth and six months after giving birth. In the end a total of 93 women participated in the study (one-third of the 276 women who were on the clinic records as giving birth during this period). A total of 310 interviews were conducted: for various reasons not all participants were interviewed four times. These interviews covered a wide variety of topics (current symptomatology, personal and family history, coping mechanisms, violence, substance use, reproductive health issues, sexuality), but focused more specifically on women's experiences of pregnancy, termination of pregnancy, birth and early motherhood. The interview questions were aimed at exploring how the women themselves interpret and make sense of their experiences. In keeping with the assumptions of qualitative research, as researchers we used the emerging analysis to direct the data collection: interview questions therefore developed during the course of the study, as researchers acquire a more sophisticated knowledge of the subject area.[17]

Apart from the in-depth interviews, quantitative data was also collected. Several standardised psychological measures (Beck Depression Inventory, General Health Questionnaire and Edinburgh Postnatal Depression Screen) were also used, although it is very clear that any measures developed in other cultures have to be used with caution.

Interviewers (graduate students in psychology) were expected to keep a detailed journal of their interviews, with the understanding that journals would become part of the data set.

All of the 93 participants were low-income black mothers. Their average age was 25 years old. Twenty-three of the participants were under the age of twenty. Some were unemployed, while others had part-time or full-time jobs, mostly as domestic workers, farmworkers or factory workers. Their education ranged from Grade 7 to Grade 12. Participants had between one and four biological children, with the average number of children 1.73. The average birth weight of their babies was 2.985 kilograms.[18]

Ethical approval for the study was obtained from Stellenbosch University. Strict confidentiality was maintained. If necessary, women who were not in treatment were referred to a free treatment facility. Participants received a grocery store voucher of about R100 (slightly more than US$10) as compensation when they completed the last interview.

### The nurse study

Preliminary findings of the larger Maternal Mental Health Project study strongly indicated that poor women who were participants in this study often experienced the nurse-patient relationship in the maternity ward as highly compromised – an experience that certainly impacted on their health-seeking practices. Many women reported instances of abandonment, neglect or abuse at the hands of nurses. Given research on the impact of stress on nurses and the nurse-patient relationship, it seemed important from a mental health perspective to also focus on the emotional experiences of the maternity nurses themselves.[19] It was assumed that such a focus would provide information that could be utilised by mental health workers (psychologists and social workers) in their efforts to provide appropriate support for these health-care workers, which would ultimately also be beneficial for patients. The team consequently decided to also conduct a study focused on the experiences of the nurses of the maternity ward of the local state hospital.

All eight of the participants who participated in the nurse study self-identified as coloured and were middle class (in terms of socio-economic status). All were Afrikaans-speaking females. With regard to rank within the hospital, five of the participants were sisters, two were staff nurses and one was a nursing assistant. Sisters occupy the highest rank in the nursing hierarchy, followed by staff nurses and then nurses. The eight participants represented two-thirds of the maternity ward nursing staff at the time. One of the remaining four (a nurse) declined to take part (she did not want to give a reason for non-participation) and the remaining three members of staff (one sister, one nurse and one staff nurse) were unavailable during the two-week period of interviewing. After these two weeks, the researchers were clear that no new categories were emerging and that theoretical saturation seemed to have been achieved.[20]

The interviewers were both white, middle-class students, one male, aged 25 and one female, aged 21. The female interviewer interviewed six of the participants, four of them in individual interviews and two in a joint interview. The male student interviewed the remaining two participants.

Semi-structured interviews were used in this study. A basic interview schedule was agreed on beforehand. Open-ended questions were used. The goal was to allow the nursing staff as much freedom as possible to articulate their psychological experience of being a nurse. All interviews were conducted in the maternity ward of the hospital, during their working hours, since it was felt that this setting would be the most conducive towards allowing the participants to articulate their professional identities.

Ethical considerations were kept at the forefront throughout this study, which adhered to the requirements of the Subcommittee A of the Research Committee of Stellenbosch University. A long period of time was spent obtaining official permission from the hospital's management. Informed consent was obtained from all the nurses and participation was strictly voluntary. Pseudonyms were used for all the nurses and all references to real names during the interviews were omitted during transcription in order to ensure confidentiality.

## Mothering as a three-generational process

In rural and semi-rural South African communities, where affordable and accessible childcare is almost non-existent, low-income mothers often have no alternative but to rely on their own mothers for childcare.[21] In her qualitative investigation of childcare in one low-income South African community, Suzanne de Villiers explored the complexity of being a poor mother in South Africa. In her doctoral dissertation (I was her supervisor) she highlights how the existence of powerful gender and motherhood ideologies, ambivalent intergenerational psychodynamics and the harsh reality of mothering with very limited means impact in conscious and unconscious ways on how low-income mothers make decisions, how they cope and how they raise and relate to their children.[22]

Data from the study was generated by qualitative interviews conducted with the participants by De Villiers herself. The study consisted of eight participants, all of whom were mothers between the ages of 19 and 39. Participants were all women of colour from the local primary health-care clinic.

The interviews were semi-structured and comprised of a number of open-ended questions. The Women's Mental Health Research Project interview transcripts were used to construct an interview schedule, which facilitated two loosely structured in-depth interviews with each participant.

The research investigation abided by the ethical principles and guidelines specified by the University of Stellenbosch and the Psychology Board of the Health Professions Council of South Africa, in terms of informed consent (written in Afrikaans), privacy and confidentiality. In terms of privacy and confidentiality, participants were given the option of choosing a pseudonym or using their own name or preferred nickname. Additionally, participants were offered R50 (approximately US$5) as remuneration for their role in the study.

## Infant observation study

In this single case study, Jana Lazarus (then a doctoral student) considered the contribution that psychoanalytic infant observation might make to a needs assessment process within the community psychology paradigm.[23] I was also her research supervisor. At the time of her study, infant observation was predominantly used for training psychotherapists and other professionals in Western contexts. The goal of her research project was to conduct a 'classical' observation of a mother and child in a low-income South African community in the first year of the infant's life, in order to ask what kind of description it would yield. The question was whether such a description is useful for the needs assessment process and, ultimately, whether infant observation is a viable tool for psychologists working in low-income communities in South Africa.

In her dissertation Lazarus writes about a case study approach using infant observation techniques:

> A case study has been defined as a 'situation-analysis'.[24] The case study, Bromley noted, can take many forms. A case study is not of itself a research method, but rather a way of focusing upon a particular unit of analysis, which can be one or several cases.[25] The case study is characterised by an 'in-depth, intensive and sharply focused exploration' of a natural occurrence with defined boundaries.[26] A case study can focus on an individual, a social situation or process, or any major event that is interesting in its own right.[27] In other words, it is a good way to study a phenomenon in a particular context in some depth.[28] Its methodology is similar across disciplines: 'A particular set of events and relationships is identified. This "case" is then described, analysed, interpreted, and evaluated within a framework of ideas and procedures appropriate to cases of that sort.'[29] The case study method is 'the bedrock of scientific investigation'[30] and has been consistently used in the field of clinical intervention.[31] The choice of a case study method for the present study is based on its pervasive use in many areas, including psychoanalytic, community and anthropological practice.[32]

Infant observers enter the family home, where they can potentially see how group and social processes work. There is an accepted and well-valued tradition within community psychology of intervening with children through the adults that surround them.[33]

The participant in this study was Eve, a mother of two. She had her first child, Natasha, by a farmworker when she was staying at her mother's place of employment. At the time of the study, Eve had just married Piet, just before the birth of their child (Maria, the infant being observed). Piet was much older than Eve, possibly twice her age.

The data-collection methods and methods of analysis that informed the case study were diverse.[34] Several strategies and sources were used in collecting data to answer the research questions posed in this study: (1) observation, (2) interview and (3) data in the form of documents from other community sources, partly in response to the developments within it. Lazarus justified her choice of methodology as follows:

> It is proposed that the kind of psychodynamic practice involved in an infant observation can assist in gathering unspoken, unspeakable and unconscious information about the client group. It is felt, in the psychodynamic tradition, that multiple layers of meaning exist in any situation. For example, an expressed meaning may be contrary to a deeper, unconscious one. A simple act may need to be read for its true meaning. This may be particularly true in the complex setting of community work. A major contribution that infant observation can make, then, is a particular way of analysing situations, behaviours and events, aimed at extracting deeper meanings. There are bound to be many hidden meanings in interracial, cross-cultural contacts in low-income community settings following apartheid. Infant observation could extend its use to uncover the multiple layers of meaning in community work. This premise is also useful where power issues arise such as whose meaning predominates and which meanings may not be spoken. Psychoanalytic infant observation can help us to think more deeply about what the participants' experience was in a research project. What infant observation may offer is, as it were, 'new ways of seeing', on a number of levels.[35]

Lazarus engaged very seriously with the ethics of infant observation:

> While the ethics of not doing (of thinking) were raised at proposal level, I could not predict what a core issue this was to become.

The position of watching is always potentially an uncomfortable one to some degree, but possibly even more so in a severely deprived community. The participating mother approached me for money for the baby. Boundaries were challenged and were considered carefully in supervision. It was difficult not to respond with action, and to stay in a thinking space about what I was doing. Part of the rationale was that endless need could not be filled by charity, but that a rigorous study could result in interventions that address problems at their root in the longer-term. Buying a present to mark the baby's birthday at the end of the observation took on enormous significance and the question of what was appropriate arose. Infant observers traditionally do not give gifts of food to thank their subjects, but participants in WMHRP [Women's Mental Health Research Project] projects do receive supermarket vouchers in thanks. Even issues such as receiving scholarship money to conduct the research became an ethical issue. It was difficult to find a way to end the observation without feeling I was abandoning the family.[36]

### Women and depression study

In a follow-up study to the Maternal Mental Health Project, the women and depression study, we utilised a multiple case study design, drawing on interviews with 26 women.[37] Participants were recruited using convenience sampling. Nursing staff at the primary health clinic in the valley were requested to refer women who had been diagnosed with major depressive disorder as potential participants. Subsequent to the analyses of the early interviews, theoretical sampling was employed to further develop and saturate theoretical categories.[38] No women who had also been diagnosed with schizophrenia or schizoaffective disorder were included, but women with anxiety disorders and substance use disorders were not excluded.

Potential participants were told that the study was aimed at gaining an in-depth understanding of depression in low-income women. All participants were low-income, black mothers. Some were unemployed, while others had part-time or full-time jobs, mostly as domestic workers, farmworkers or factory workers. Their education ranged from Grade 7 to

Grade 12 and all of them identified themselves as Christians. Participants had between one and four biological children, ranging in age from 1 to 43.

Participants were interviewed by four graduate students, all of whom were registered mental health professionals, about their emotional distress. Semi-structured interviews were conducted in either Afrikaans or English. All interviews were video- or audio-recorded, transcribed and (if necessary) translated into English by the research team. The data was first analysed using an abbreviated version of social constructionist grounded theory, a data analytic strategy that facilitates the identification of both implicit and explicit categories.[39] Thereafter, underlying discourses were also analysed.[40]

Ethical approval for the study was obtained from Stellenbosch University and the South African Department of Health. Participation was voluntary. Strict confidentiality was maintained. If indicated, women who were not in treatment were referred to a free facility. Participants received R100 (slightly more than US$10) as compensation.

This study was subsequently extended to include women being seen in psychotherapy at Welgevallen clinic in Stellenbosch. Ethical clearance was once again obtained from the university and from the clinical manager.

Although we took all the steps required by formal ethical guidelines, these steps failed to address certain unpredictable and complex ethical dilemmas. For instance, we had difficulty with physical punishment of children, even though this is not against South African laws and in many South African communities is the norm. The South African Children's Act provides a vague definition of child abuse, stating that abuse entails 'any form of harm or ill-treatment deliberately inflicted on a child', including 'exposing or subjecting a child to behaviour that may harm the child psychologically or emotionally'.[41] In instances when physical punishment seemed to constitute abuse, we experienced tension between our duty towards research participants and the integrity of the research and the legal requirement to report abuse.

Our research participants, in general, were committed mothers and they described incidents of extreme violence as problematic and with much guilt and shame. Participants expressed the need and willingness to change their behaviours. The research team, after difficult reflections and deliberations, and in discussion with consultants, dealt with disclosures of extreme violence by discussing them with the participant after the interview and by arranging professional support for participants and children when indicated. With the permission of participants, counsellors were briefed about our concerns and asked to conduct follow-ups.

### Listening to the voices of women and girls

Another research study in which data was generated for this book was titled 'Listening to the voices of women and girls'. [42] This study was conducted as part of a community mental health intervention of graduate students in clinical psychology.

While a few interventions were conducted and generated data as part of this study, in this book I often refer to the group process from a feminist psychodynamic group therapy intervention, which was conducted with thirteen- to fourteen-year-old girls. This intervention was informed by various theoretical orientations:

- A local, personal growth and psycho-educational intervention, the Jamestown Girls' Programme;[43]
- The Respect4U project, which is a structured intervention used in life orientation classes for Grade 8 students in South Africa;[44]
- Yalom's principles of group psychotherapy;[45] and
- James Gilligan's accounts of work with young adolescent girls.[46]

In this psychotherapeutic group intervention, which was mainly aimed at providing a space for open-ended discussions, sessions focused on developmentally important topics, such as intimate relationships, menstruation, substance abuse, bullying, depression and gossiping. These topics were chosen on a yearly basis, depending on what the girls themselves identified as important issues. In this research we took 'advantage of one of the greatest resources at our disposal, clinical practice, which can and should serve as a natural laboratory for both generating and testing hypotheses'. [47]

The girls who participated in the psychotherapeutic group intervention were in Grade 8 in the local secondary school (thirteen or fourteen years old), classified as 'coloured' and generally from low-income backgrounds. As participants were selected on the basis of their willingness and availability to participate, convenience sampling was employed.[48] The girls were divided into two separate psychotherapy groups that consisted of approximately five members each.

The psychotherapeutic group sessions were led by Master's students in clinical psychology and community counselling and other psychology graduate students. Group sessions were conducted on a weekly basis after school hours. The sessions on the various topics simulated focus group discussions.[49] Journals of the group leaders were also consulted, as the immediate observations of the group discussions and group dynamics yielded important data. All group sessions were audiotaped.

Upon request of the school, these group therapy sessions subsequently also ended up including male learners. In later years the school also made it possible to run the groups during school hours, as part of their life orientation programme.

Women's groups were also conducted for a few years. These groups varied in terms of how successful they were.[50]

Ethical clearance for conducting this research was obtained from Stellenbosch University and the Department of Education. Informed consent was obtained from the learners who participated in the group and their parents.

# Notes

## Notes to Prologue

1. For a discussion of the 'power of girls' gossip', see Hamman and Kruger, 2017.

2. Literally translated, the name 'Dwarsrivier' means across or cross the river. However, the word '*dwars*' in Afrikaans also is used for people who are contrary, crabby, difficult or wrongheaded.

3. The term '*ordentlik*' is very important in this community and denotes a certain kind of moral superiority, linked to respectability, presentability, good manners, politeness and a certain kind of humility (Van der Westhuizen, 2018). For a general discussion of *ordentlik*, see Salo, 2009 and Ross, 2002, 2005, 2010, 2015. For discussions of the importance of *ordentlikheid* in the valley, see Pfigu, Gabriel and Van der Waal, 2014.

4. In a four-year period that we monitored birth records at the clinic, there were a total of 41 teenage mothers (mothers younger than twenty) giving birth out of a total of 276 births, meaning that 15 per cent of all births recorded were to teenage mothers.

5. It is widely assumed that the social and economic conditions of poverty can be linked to common mental disorders in low-, middle- and high-income countries, with numerous studies indicating complex associations between various poverty indicators and mental health (for reviews of the literature, see Hanandita and Tampubolon, 2014; Lund, 2014; Lund et al., 2010). For a discussion of different theories explaining the link between depression and poverty – namely, social causation and social drift, see Abrahams et al., 2018; Gibbs et al., 2018; Lund and Cois, 2018. Research has consistently shown that women's vulnerability to depression is heightened by poverty and economic hardship (Belle and Doucet, 2003; Burdette, Hill and Hale, 2011; Campbell et al., 2009; Coast et al., 2012; Connolly, 2000; Dukas and Kruger, 2016; Hwa-Froelich, Loveland Cook and Flick, 2008; Kiernan and Huerta, 2008; Manuel et al., 2012; Rodrigues et al., 2003; Silverstein et al., 2010; Simmons, Huddleston-Casas and Berry, 2007; Stewart et al., 2010). Literature also suggests that low-income coloured and African South African women are more likely than other groups to develop mental health problems such as depression (Pillay and Kriel, 2006; Stein et al., 2008).

6. Since 1998 this semi-rural area, with its seemingly disparate units, has been managed by the Stellenbosch Municipality as one region, the Dwarsrivier Valley. While this concept of a specific spatial identity was created in the post-1994 context for promotional and planning purposes, Van der Waal (2005) points out that the unifying name is important in that it does suggest that much is shared by the localities in the area: a uniquely bounded geographical character, an agricultural history of interdependence between landowners, factories and workers and the emergence of villages with strong local identities. '*Inkommers*' (new people coming in) are regarded with suspicion and often blamed for problems in the valley.

7. The Dwarsrivier Valley recently has also started publicising itself as a tourist destination. On the tourism website, it says: 'The Dwarsriver Valley serves as a triumphant example of the way forward. Here we can experience a unique balance between pure historical Cape Culture and modern-day lifestyles of wellness, gourmet foods and fine wines. The valley has what it takes to satisfy the humanitarian, the socialite, the nature lover, the historian, the adventurous spirit and certainly the connoisseur' (https://dwarsriviertourism.org.za/).

8. Most of the inhabitants of the towns of the valley are classified as 'coloured'. The Population Registration Act of 1950 required that each inhabitant of South Africa be classified as white, black, coloured or Indian. The Act defined the races as follows:

> A white person is one who in appearance is, or who is generally accepted as, a white person, but does not include a person who, although in appearance obviously a white person, is generally accepted as a Coloured person.
>
> A native is a person who is in fact or is generally accepted as a member of any aboriginal race or tribe of Africa.
>
> A Coloured person is a person who is not a white person nor a native (Posel, 2001: 56).

While the Population Registration Act was repealed by the South African Parliament on 17 June 1991, the racial categories defined in the Act remain ingrained in South Africa and still form the basis of some official policies and statistics aimed at redressing past economic imbalances (see, for instance, the Broad-Based Black Economic Empowerment Act, 53 of 2003 and the Employment Equity Act, 55 of 1998). In the words of Posel (2001: 68), 'Previously the locus of privilege, race has now become the site of redress.' However, Posel also highlights how ubiquitous race still is in post-apartheid South Africa:

> Constructs of race, which imagined its imprints in an elastic matrix of biological and social factors, were insinuated ubiquitously into the everyday lives of apartheid subjects, in ways that were enabled and reinforced by the materialities of apartheid's social geography and economic structure. Large chunks of this order remain in place, with the large majority of the black population still impoverished, economically

excluded and consigned to geographically separate and under-resourced residential areas. The majority of whites too are still confined within apartheid borders of thought and experience. To this extent bioculturalist conceptions of race may retain their purchase in ways that continue to reinforce apartheid modes of racial reasoning, in the lived experience of thoroughgoing difference and separateness (Posel, 2001: 69).

For a critical discussion of the notion of 'coloured', see the chapter on *Home*.

9. Despite the Basic Conditions of Employment Amendment Act of 2002 ostensibly aiming to improve the lives of farm labourers, their position remains precarious and seems to have worsened. Farm labourers and former farm labourers are particularly vulnerable to unemployment, poor housing, occupational health issues and a lack of access to essential services. According to a 2011 Human Rights Watch report, 'farm workers are among the most vulnerable people in South African society' (Randle, 2014: 50).

10. Cordes, Baldwin and Mthathi, 2011.

11. According to the *Webster Dictionary*, marginal can be defined as:
    1. Written or printed in the margin of a page or sheet
    2. Of, relating to, or situated at the margin or border
       (1) occupying the borderland of a relatively stable territorial or cultural area
       (2) characterized by the incorporation of habits and values from two divergent cultures and by incomplete assimilation in either
    3. Located at the fringe of consciousness
    4. Close to the lower limit of qualification, acceptability or function.

    The term 'marginal' seems important in this book; in fact, the first working title was 'Marginal Maternities'.

12. Randle, 2014; Robins, 2014.

13. Robins, 2014: 221.

14. Millen, Irwin and Kim, 2000.

15. Nobel-prize winner Joseph Stiglitz (2013) describes the unevenness of development in the United States as follows – this description is also applicable to the South African context:

    For years there was a deal between the top and the rest of our society that went something like this: we will provide you jobs and prosperity, and you will let us walk away with the bonuses. You all get a share, even if we get a bigger share. But now that tacit agreement between the rich and the rest, which was always fragile, has come apart. Those in the 1 percent are walking off with the riches, but in doing so they have provided nothing but anxiety and insecurity to the 99 percent. The majority of Americans have simply not been benefiting from the country's growth.

16. Nixon, 2011: 1.

17. See, for example, Kruger 2014a, 2014b. I discuss the problem of writing about this work a little later in this *Prologue*.

18. See *Appendix: Some Notes on Method and Ethics.*
19. While poor mothers in the developing world are commonly thought to be at risk for mental disorders, the mechanisms by which the cycle of poverty and mental health is maintained are complex and multidimensional (Hanandita and Tampubolon, 2014; Lund, 2014). Another critical research question concerns the factors that protect people living in circumstances of multiple deprivations from developing mental health problems. Lund therefore emphasises the importance of also doing qualitative studies on the link between poverty and emotional well-being, stating that such studies 'are essential to understand[ing]' (Lund, 2014: 135).
20. What is 'the poor'? The *Oxford Dictionary* highlights two kinds of associations: being poor is associated with not having means, but the word also elicits associations of something that is not so good or something that is unfortunate (deserving pity and sympathy). Similarly, in academic and policy debates about poverty and defining poverty, at least two aspects of poverty are usually highlighted: there is an objective lack of access to resources and there is a subjective experience of suffering and pain (Alcock, 1997; Belle, 1990; Belle et al., 2000; Du Toit, 2002; Lott and Bullock, 2001; Myers and Gill, 2004; Narayan, 2000; Schein, 1995). The term 'poverty' thus always includes an economic element and a moral or political element (Alcock, 1997). Within the technical discourses of economics these two sides of poverty are talked about in terms of the relationship between wealth and health: the assumption often being that income is the prime determinant of health (also mental health) (Deaton, 2004). This assumption of an income-to-health mechanism becomes the basis for the argument that economic growth or development will benefit population health or well-being (Deaton, 2004; Feachem, 2001). In such a discourse, the emotional suffering of the poor is assumed. It is also assumed that poverty will be addressed by development and globalisation. It is important here to understand that when I refer to 'the poor', I am not referring to an ontological category, but rather to a historical and political category. I am interested in historicising the production and reproduction of poverty in the valley. It may be that 'impoverished' is a more apt term than 'poor'.
21. Geertz, 1995: 3.
22. For a discussion of the importance of case studies in psychology, see *Appendix: Some Notes on Method and Ethics.*
23. Farmer, 2004: 305–25.
24. Farmer, 2005: 31.
25. Cited in Farmer, 2005: 43.
26. Farmer, 2005: 41.
27. Farmer, 2005: 30.
28. Farmer, 2005: 43.
29. As in the epigraph at the beginning of this book, Sen (2005: xi) writes in the foreword to Farmer's *Pathologies of Power*:

> It may be difficult for us to imagine how restricted a life so many of our fellow human beings lead, what little living they manage to do. There is,

of course, the wonder of birth (impossible to recollect), some mother's milk (sometimes not), the affection of relatives (often thoroughly disrupted), perhaps some schooling (mostly not), a bit of play (amid pestilence and panic), and then things end (without a rumble). The world goes on as if nothing much has happened.

The chapter headings in this book are inspired by the aspects of life identified in this extract. Nussbaum's catalogue of the ten central human capabilities are also relevant:

> For Nussbaum, being human means 'being able to move freely from place to place . . . Being able to use the senses; being able to imagine, to think, and to reason and to do these things in a "truly human" way, a way informed and cultivated by an adequate education . . . Being able to form a conception of the good and to engage in critical reflection about the planning of one's own life . . . Being able to live for and in relation to others, to recognize and show concern for other human beings, to engage in various forms of social interaction; being able to imagine the situation of another and to have compassion for that situation; having the capability for both justice and friendship . . . Having the social bases of self-respect and nonhumiliation; being able to be treated as a dignified being whose worth is equal to that of others . . . being able to participate effectively in political choices that govern one's life . . . being able to hold property . . . being able to work as a human being, exercising practical reason and entering into meaningful relationships of mutual recognition with other workers.' Anything less and the life under consideration is no longer a human life (Nussbaum, cited in Long, 2019: 17–18).

30. In reviewing the literature there are many studies concerned with the narratives of 'voices' of the poor. In fact, it is very difficult to systematically review this literature, because it is so vast and certainly not confined to one discipline. Most of the qualitative studies concerned with the emotional experience of poverty are in fact not psychological studies.

The vastness of this literature is quite daunting. For instance, in probably the biggest study of its kind conducted at the end of the 1990s, Narayan (2000) and a team of researchers reviewed 81 participatory poverty assessment (PPA) reports conducted under the auspices of the World Bank. These reports were based on discussions with 40 000 to 50 000 poor men and women from 50 different countries. The first sentence of the first book in the series, *Voices of the Poor*, proclaims, 'Poverty is pain' (Narayan, 2000: 3).

Looking at the qualitative literature on poverty, one can say that the voices of the poor have become audible in social scientific research and also, perhaps to a lesser extent, in psychological research. However, this literature seems to have its own problems.

It is remarkable that the studies reviewed seem to describe, rather than to analyse, the psychological experience of the poor; it was difficult to find studies that included in-depth analyses of the psychological experience of being poor. It seems that often, or more typically, the voices of the poor were presented as if they were transparently meaningful in themselves – taken at face value, without an awareness that the stories of the poor are socially constructed too – 'textual artefacts, themselves the products of conflicts, antagonisms and other encounters that are shaped by social power relations and concrete social interests' (Du Toit, 2006: 16). In participatory research studies concerned with poverty there seems to be very little reflexive awareness of the process of research itself and how this shapes the way qualitative data is produced, analysed and interpreted (Du Toit, 2006: 15).

The questions that should be asked about these large bodies of participatory research are: Under what conditions do the poor speak? What are they really able or permitted to speak about? What do they say and to whom? What gets reported about what they speak? Who will listen to what they say? What will be done with what is heard? Foucault helped us to understand that while what counts as true knowledge is ostensibly defined by the individual, what is permitted to count is defined by discourse. What is spoken, and who may speak, are issues of power – and it is this that should also be included in analysis (Parker, 1989).

If this does not happen, it means that even when, as has been the case more recently, spaces have been created for the 'voices of the poor', these voices are added to an analysis that is essentially unchanged (Du Toit, 2002). Du Toit asserts that, on the whole, qualitative data regarding the poor has been seen as having an essentially supplementary and illustrative role in accounts of poverty, still essentially shaped by the econometric imaginary. This assertion is supported by a fascinating volume reflecting on the opportunities and risks of doing participatory poverty research in which the contributors critically analyse their involvement in the World Bank's 'voices of the poor' project. Brock (2002: 2), the editor of that volume, cites the scathing words of Cornwall about participatory research:

> For some, the proliferation of the language of 'participation' and 'empowerment' within the mainstream is heralded as the realization of a long-awaited paradigm shift in development thinking. For others, however, there is less cause for celebration. Their concerns centre on the use of participation as a legitimating device that draws on the moral authority of claims to involve the poor to place the pursuit of other agendas beyond reproach. According to this perspective, much of what is hailed as 'participation' is a mere technical fix that leaves inequitable global and local relations of power, and with it the root causes of poverty, unchallenged.

It seems, then, that in qualitative research concerned with the well-being of the poor, much is being obscured – perhaps in the service of specific development and economic agendas.

While the importance of individual narratives is often highlighted in feminist scholarship, feminist scholars have also highlighted that narratives should not be regarded as transparent. They do not speak for themselves; they have to be attended to and analysed. It is in this process of making sense that the importance of theory becomes apparent. The researcher needs theory or to theorise in order to understand how the personal narrative is related to the material and ideological conditions within which it is constructed (Walby, 2001). Harding (2001: 517) emphasises the importance of using women's stories about their everyday lives as starting points, 'in order to identify sources of their oppression to be found in the conceptual practices of power that are embedded in institutional cultures and practices'. Storytelling may be crucial in the feminist demand for recognition of suffering, of strengths and of differences, but feminists need theory if stories are to become more than simply 'a gesture towards transformation and redistribution' (Felski, 2000: 228). Indeed, storytelling is not enough (Walby, 2001).

Flax also highlights the importance of studying and understanding the need for narrative. She sees narrative as a quest for closure and coherence: 'Feminist theories . . . should encourage us to tolerate and interpret ambivalence, ambiguity, and multiplicity as well as to expose our needs for imposing order and structure no matter how arbitrary and oppressive these needs may be' (Flax 1990: 56). See also Kruger, 2003a.

31. Nixon, 2011: 135.
32. Nixon, 2011: 3–4.
33. Butler, 2004.
34. Nixon, 2011: 8.
35. See also section on 'Writing' in chapter on *Distress*.
36. Frosh, 1999, 2006; Huffer, 2009.
37. Butler (2004: 170) refers to a 'Foucauldian perspective within psychoanalysis'. Frosh and Saville Young (2017) highlight 'the potential richness of results' when such an approach is used.
38. Frosh, Phoenix and Pattman, 2000: 227.
39. For other books concerned with motherhood that have similar approaches (in that they involve qualitative data, make use of a case study approach, use different kinds of data and different kinds of data analysis strategies and engage overtly in self-reflection), see Baraitser, 2009; De Marneffe, 2009; Hollway, 2015; Thomson et al., 2011.
40. Foucault (1988: 9) states: 'People will say, perhaps, that these games with oneself need only go on behind the scenes . . . But what, then, is philosophy today – philosophical activity, I mean – if not the critical labour of thought upon itself?'
41. The South African author Ivan Vladislavić (2006: 58), in a different context, also comments on the irony regarding what we write about in South Africa. He writes a paragraph called 'Excess (roll 3)':

the shoes, the socks, the button-down collars, the corduroy jackets. the tables, the chairs. the pavements, the grass on the verges, the flower beds, the impatiens, the Barberton daisies. the street names on the kerbstones, the white lines, the street lights, the bulbs in the sockets. the buckets, the spades. the cars, the caravans, the motorboats. the sheepskin seat covers, the halogen spotlights, the retractable aerials, the loudspeakers, the rubber mats. the driving, the parking, the driving back. the money in the parking meters. the walking in the parks, the drinking in the bars, the talking, the laughing, the eating in the restaurants, the glasses, the wine in the glasses, the knives, the forks, the plates, the food on the plates, the baby potatoes, the stuffed trout, the chocolate mousse, the brandy snifters. the reading, the writing. the paper, the pen, the ink in the pen. the books, the books, the books.

How to avoid myself and my privilege? A somewhat disdainful American reviewer comments on one of my papers:

> For this reviewer a much stronger sense emerged of the detail of the lifeworld of the author (choice of music, perfume etc) than of the patients. That would not be a problem if this work was framed as an auto-ethnography, but it is not. The author may find Pierre Bourdieu's argument about how the performance of taste classifies the classifier to be useful in contrasting this with the author's own declaration of her taste for Mahler, Isey Miayke etc.

I have no interested in writing an auto-ethnography.

I know, however, that there is no way in which I can objectively capture the lifeworlds of others. I can only describe encounters and what emerges in the encounters. In these descriptions I have to juxtapose my middle-class mentality (even if I try to be ironic about it) with the concerns and the preoccupations of the people that I work with in the valley. In writing about others, the act of reflexivity is deemed crucial. Myerhoff (1992: 309) says:

> Narcissus' tragedy then is that he is not narcissistic enough, or rather that he does not reflect long enough to effect a transformation. He is reflective, but he is not reflexive – that is, he is conscious of himself as an other, but he is not conscious of being self-conscious of himself as an other and hence not able to detach himself from, understand, survive, or even laugh at this initial experience of alienations.

Flax (1993: viii) quotes Foucault: 'There are times in life when the question of knowing if one can think differently than one thinks and perceive differently than one sees is absolutely necessary if one is to go on looking and reflecting at all.'

Merely holding up a single mirror is not adequate to achieve this attitude. The mirrors must be doubled, creating the endless regress of possibilities, opening out into infinity, dissolving the clear boundaries of a 'real world'.

If the reflexivity is a dialogue, an open conversation, it will not be paralysing, but empowering. If it means absolute transparency, such conversations can enrich, refine and even change positions.

42. Lady Anne Barnard was the wife of a British colonial officer at the Cape in the late 1700s. She was somewhat implicated in colonialism, but being a woman complicated her position by ensuring that she was 'on the fringe of colonial policymaking'. She also negotiated 'her position through the different roles that she [assumed], such as writer, artist, wife, adventurer and colonial agent [which allowed her to fluctuate] between the positions of centre and margin within colonial discourse' (Collins, 2007: 7).

43. Fairbridge, 1924: 39.

44. Pausanias, *Description of Greece (Greek travelogue, circa 2AD)*. https://en.wikipedia. org/wiki/Helicon_%28river%29.

45. Kolb, 1967: 50.

46. Krog, 1989: 79.

47. Coetzee, 1998.

48. Van Niekerk, cited in West, 2005.

49. Letter written in November 1797. https://digital.library.upenn.edu/women/ barnard/letters/letters.html.

50. Hoagland, 2010: 45.

51. Swartz, 2012: 197.

52. Swartz, 2012: 202.

53. Erasmus, 2001. In the words of another South African psychologist: 'My skin colour spoke before I could open my mouth . . . Throughout my life . . . I have had a feeling akin to what Bion terms "nameless dread"' (Esprey, 2013: 47). Each encounter inevitably becomes a microcosm of the larger socio-cultural context (Altman, 2004).

54. Trantraal, 2018: 112–13. The original Afrikaans text is as follows:

*VH1 Classics is oppie TV. Mrs Kamfer vacuum die voorhys waarie TV staan.*

*Mrs Kamfer stop die vacuum cleaner, en staan en lag skielik, 'n weggooi laggie. En dan sê sy half vi my en half vi haa self: ''n Wit man sal alles doen, behalwe ophou wit wies. Wat wiet 'n sak van sy tou af?'*

*Ek wiettie wat 'n sak van sy tou af wiettie, soe ek skryf it nee, soedat ek haa wee kan vra oppe anne tyd.*

*Mrs Kamfer, my vrou, Ronelda se ma, was 'n chronic white person roaster. Ronelda het vi my eenkee gesê haa ma wasse meid met guerilla tendencies.*

*Haa ma is nou ses jaa oorlede en ek het nooit gevra nie. Sy sê haa ma het altyd sukke gesegdes opgemaak, issie soot ding wat plaas mense doen.*

*Sy het oek gewonne wattit bedoel en haa ma gevra, en haa ma het vi haa explain wat sy mean mettie tou ennie sak. Wit mense exist in 'n sak, soes 'n shield soes 'n safe space, die res van ôs wattie wit issie, issie tou offie strap en ôs dra die sak whiteness rond en die sak dink hy is die belangrike een.*

55. The problems of whiteness and white writing specifically have been very prominent in the social sciences and humanities internationally, as well as in South Africa. I am not going to attempt to review this substantial literature or to engage with the issue theoretically. See Bhabha, 1988; Coetzee, 1998; Cuomo and Hall, 1999; Frankenberg, 1997; Hill, 1997; Nakayama and Martin, 1998; Van Robbroeck, 2006; West, 2009; Young, 2004.
56. Bhabha, 1998: 21.
57. *Merriam-Webster Dictionary.*
58. Byatt, 2001: 236–7.
59. Byatt, 2001: 101.
60. Byatt, 2001: 101.
61. Attwell (2015: 27) beautifully articulates the balance that great authors succeed in achieving when writing (in the third person):

    It is not a simple repudiation in the name of art; on the contrary, it involves an instantiation of self, followed by an erasure that leaves traces of the self behind . . . we continue to read biographically, not in order to limit the truth of the work to its biographical sources, but in order to understand how the self is written out, leaving its imprint as a shadowy presence.

62. In her book *White Women Writing White: Identity and Representation in (Post-) Apartheid Literatures of South Africa*, Mary West (2009: 25) distinguishes between confessional white writing and anti-confessional white writing. She says that in confessional and reconciliatory texts, women writers seem to consciously or unconsciously still write with 'the assumptions of white normativity' and rely on stereotypes in their depictions of black people. West (2009: 4) shows how white women writers are deeply concerned with race, but much of their work is also characterised by 'residual assumptions of entitlement'. She argues that guilt seems to get in the way of more progressive forms of representation and action and modes of action.

    A good example of the paralysis caused by guilt is Antjie Krog's (1996) writing about the personal toll of reporting on the Truth and Reconciliation Commission:

    I can talk about nothing else. But I don't talk about it at all . . . I wake up in unfamiliar beds with blood on my frayed lips . . . and the soundbites screaming in my ears . . . My hair is falling out. My teeth are falling out. I have rashes. After the amnesty deadline I enter my house like a stranger. And barren. I sit around for days. Staring. My youngest walks into a room and flinches: 'Sorry, I'm not used to your being home.'

    South African journalist Haji Mohamed Dawjee is scathing about tortured white writers: '*Al die wit trane en wit weerloosheid en broosheid . . . Ek verstaan dit tot 'n mate en miskien kan hulle nie daarvan wegkom nie, en maar ek voel: Bly nou net stil daaroor; ek is moeg daarvoor*' (All the white tears and the white vulnerability and brittleness . . . I understand it to some extent and maybe they can't get away from it, but I feel: Just keep quiet about it, I am tired of it) (La Vita and Dawjee, 2018). See also Dawjee, 2018.

63. Flax, 1993: 4.

64. Feminism has compelled me to do research and writing that are orientated towards social change. Research can be useful in direct and in indirect ways. It can be directly useful, in that knowledge that is useful can be generated; that is to say, the results can be useful. It can also be indirectly useful, in that the process of knowledge construction can be useful as well. If it is clear that research is conducted 'to be of use', it can also be stipulated what the standard is against which to measure research. In research where there is an emphasis on social change and usefulness, the idea that advocacy and scholarship are not compatible is of central importance. In such research, 'knowing will be judged by ethical as well as epistemological ideals. I evaluate ways of knowing and the knowledge they produce in the light of the good to which they lead and that they yield' (Ruddick, 1996: 267).

65. Steinberg (2015a: 326–7) writes about the value of his biography in the epilogue of *A Man of Good Hope*: 'I have spent a couple of years memorialising his life. But there is no intrinsic value in remembering . . . The book is for me and those who read it. It is of no value to him but for the money that will come his way.'

    Ruth Behar, an anthropologist, who in her ethnographic study of Esperanza, a Mexican woman, went to great trouble to foster a mutual relationship with her respondent and to make her, in a sense, a co-author. She worked hard at taking her own subjectivity and that of her respondent seriously. Behar wished for her 'wickedness' to be taken away by her research, but no one could respond in the way that she hoped. She expected her research to be liberating, but instead it was painful:

    > It pained me to discover that I had alienated my parents by writing about them in ways they found disturbing. Anguished about my 'wickedness' I returned to Mexico, hoping to be vindicated by giving the book I had written about her to my *comadre* Esperanza. But there was no redemption; my *comadre* told me she did not want to keep a text she would never be able to read. Writing hurts (Behar and Gordon 1995: 23).

    Similarly, Attwell (2015: 23), in his literary biography of J.M. Coetzee says in his preface that he 'was uncertain whether the book was a tribute or a betrayal, infinitely wishing that it were the former'.

66. Derrida, cited in Brault and Naas, 2003: 5.

67. Hornstein, 2005: 53.

68. Scheper-Hughes and Bourgois (2004: 318), in a critical reading of Farmer's work, say:

    > We need to specify empirically and to theorize more broadly the way everyday life is shaped by the historical processes and contemporary politics of global political economy as well as by local discourse and

culture. To be useful ethnography must be attuned to the local without predetermination. We have to be ready to see what we do not expect and what we do not want – irrespective of our political faiths and theoretical armature.

69. Farmer, 2004: 308.

70. 'The relations of anthropology and psychology are not easy to deal with. Psychologists began by taking their own culture for granted, as if it were uniform and universal, and then studying psychic behaviour within it' (Kroeber, cited in Farmer, 2004: 308).

71. Chodorow, 1999: 221.

72. I feel fragmented when I try to write, perhaps as a result of modern society (academic world, political world and professional world; academic disciplines; paradigms within one discipline, and so on) and the fact that I am almost forced to pluck out different aspects of myself in different contexts.

73. Geertz, 1973.

74. Foucault, 1980: 79.

75. Flax, 1993: 4.

76. Jackson, 2011: 190.

77. Woods (2017) writes about W.G. Sebald and says: 'Because we are not God, our narration of another's life is a pretence of knowledge – simultaneously an attempt to know and a confession of how little we know.'

78. Foucault, 1980: 79. See also Geertz, 1973.

79. Jackson, 2011: 191.

80. Sen and Hulme, 2006: 4.

81. Jackson, 2011: 191. Als (2017) writes as follows about 'Richard Avedon and James Baldwin's joint examination of American identity':

> What Avedon and Baldwin shared from the start, as creators, long before *Nothing Personal* was conceived, was an imagination that was not so much informed by reality as inseparable from it: they saw the exceptional in the real. Not the 'sublime' or transcendent, but the brutality, theatre, innocence, and confusion that made up their racist, sexist, sexy, and impossible city of love and lovelessness.

This seems to be the type of imagination that is necessary here.

82. Flax, 1993: xiii.

83. Flax (1993: 133) says:

> Postmodernism calls into question the belief (or hope) that there is some form of innocent knowledge possible . . . By innocent knowledge I mean the discovery of some sort of truth that can tell us how to act in the world in ways that benefit or are for the (at least ultimate) good of all. Those whose actions are grounded in or informed by such truth will also have their innocence guaranteed. They can do only good, not harm, to

others. They act as the servant of something higher and outside (or more than) themselves, their own desires, and the effects of their particular histories or social locations.

Rather, it is self-reflection on every level of research that is important. Self-reflection, or reflexivity, here means to be continuously reflective about process, methods, results, analysis, the impact of subjectivities and context. In other words, rather than saying that self-reflection is what may lead to paralysis, I am saying that it is too little self-reflection that leads to paralysis.

84. Myerhoff, 1992: 307.
85. Jackson, 2011: 195–6.
86. Hoagland, 2010: 71.

## Notes to Home

1. The original Afrikaans text is as follows: '*Ek het alle airs verloor; als. Ek het rêrig besef wie ek is, want dis die type of plek waar die internal word external. Alles wat op die bodem is, kom op en mense lewe tussen dit. Dis 'n baie weird plek. Dit maak jou alles gewoond.*'

2. Lazarus (2007: 9) describes infant observation as follows:

   Infant observation was introduced at the Tavistock Centre in London as part of the training course for child psychotherapists after the Second World War. It involves intently watching an infant (and her mother) in the home for an hour a week for the first one or two years of life. Notes about what transpired are written up afterwards.

   For a detailed discussion and critique of the practice of infant observation, see Lazarus, 2007: 65–127.

3. Calvino (1972: 4) describes Ersilia in his novel *Invisible Cities*:

   In Ersilia, to establish the relationships that sustain the city's life, the inhabitants stretch strings from the corners of the houses, white or black or gray or black-and-white according to whether they mark a relationship of blood, of trade, authority, agency. When the strings become so numerous that you can no longer pass among them, the inhabitants leave: the houses are dismantled; only the strings and their supports remain.

   From a mountainside, camping with their household goods, Ersilia's refugees look at the labyrinth of taut strings and poles that rise in the plain. That is the city of Ersilia still, and they are nothing.

   They rebuild Ersilia elsewhere. They weave a similar pattern of strings, which they would like to be more complex and at the same time more regular than the other. Then they abandon it and take themselves and their houses still farther away.

    Thus, when traveling in the territory of Ersilia, you come upon the ruins of abandoned cities, without the walls which do not last, without the bones of the dead which the wind rolls away: spiderwebs of intricate relationships seeking a form.

4. These are the lyrics that I wrote down in my notes. I have never been able to find a song with these lyrics. I must have made them up. The day before submitting this book to the publishers, I found a song that may have been the one. A song by Arlo Guthrie, 'Somebody Turned on the Light'. The line 'I just might be reborn' did not seem like a coincidence:

    I've been to wild Montana
    I went there in a storm
    My boots were Texas leather
    My Levis wet and torn

    I loved it in Montana
    Loved it in the storm
    I think I'm gonna cross that river
    I just might be reborn . . .

    If you never see the sun till '91
    Don't you ever give up the fight
    Sure be glad when you see the dawn
    Somebody, somebody turns on the light
    Somebody turns on the light.

5. Descriptions of the people and the place are loosely based on descriptions provided by Lazarus (2007: 172–88). Both Lazarus and I have changed details in the description to ensure the anonymity of the family.

6. '*Hebban olla vogala*', sometimes written '*hebban olla uogala*', are the first three words of an eleventh-century text fragment written in Old Dutch. The whole poem reads: '*Hebban olla uogala nestas hagunnan hinase hic enda thu uuat unbidan uue nu*', which translates roughly as: 'Have all birds begun nests, except me and you – what are we waiting for?' https://en.wikipedia.org/wiki/Hebban_olla_vogala. The fragment was discovered in 1932 on the flyleaf of a manuscript that was probably made in the abbey of Rochester in Kent and is kept in Oxford. An often-cited poem, it was long believed to be the only text remaining in Old Dutch.

7. In South Africa, 'Wendy houses are often a form of accommodation for low-income people. The structure is usually erected in someone's backyard. Although many people may view this as temporary accommodation, many families have lived in such structures for years. Among the more affluent population, Wendy houses are used as entertainment huts, children's playhouses, or for storage. Originally, a Wendy house or playhouse was a small house for children, large enough for one or more children to enter . . . Usually there is one room, a doorway with a window on

either side, and little or no furniture other than that which the children improvise. The original was built for Wendy Darling in J.M. Barrie's play, *Peter Pan, or The Boy Who Wouldn't Grow Up*.' https://wendy.co.za/.

'A prop house was created by Barrie for the first stage production of the play in 1904. It was constructed like a tent so that it could be erected quickly during a song which Wendy starts with:

I wish I had a darling house
The littlest ever seen
With funny little red walls
And roof of mossy green.'

See https://en.wikipedia.org/wiki/Wendy_house.

8. Beckett, 1958: 70.
9. The *Oxford Dictionary* defines 'demographics' as 'the study of statistics such as births, deaths, income, or the incidence of disease, which illustrate the changing structure of human populations'.
10. Flax (1993: 140) states in this regard: 'Knowledge constructors should seek instead to generate an infinite "dissemination" of meanings. They should abjure any attempt to construct a closed system in which the "other" or the "excess" are "pushed to the margins" and made to disappear in the interest of coherence and unity. Their task is to disrupt and subvert rather than (re-)construct totalities or grand theories.'
11. Szymborska, 1988: 205.
12. South African psychologist Wahbie Long, in a paper on shame, highlights Martha Nussbaum's emphasis on material space:

    . . . the freedom to move from one place to another, the reality of owning property. These are among the attributes that make us human. For the millions of disenfranchised South Africans, therefore, the question of landlessness is not only of practical importance: it is an existential question. To own land is to own oneself, to live with confidence in the world, to build communities of feeling, to pursue questions of meaning rather than survival, to have the sense that one is ontologically real. To deny a people their land, therefore, is to deny them their humanity (Long, 2019: 18).

13. Swartz, 2015: 184.
14. Kottler and Togashi, 2015: 170.
15. Winnicott, 1992; Motz, 2014. Motz explains:

    It is the sensitive interplay between mother (or other primary caregiver) and baby that enables the infant to develop a sense of itself; this includes the growing awareness of having an inner and outer being, a body with boundaries, and a mind with thoughts and feelings. In this way, a mind becomes 'housed' or contained (2014: 120).

16. Motz, 2014 cites Swinburne (2000: 224–5) on an inner sense of home of a 'home in the mind':

> It is the presence of a bounded internal space which is central to any individual's capacity to retain a sense of home within the mind . . . If we apply this theory to the idea of home, we see that the individual who is able to develop internal space with a containing object will then be able to function at the symbolic level. And will therefore be able to experience home in the non-psychotic sense – what we might call the home in the mind – the individual who fails to install a containing object and develop a sense of internal space will have no option but to project his feelings into containers which exist outside his own psyche.

17. Motz, 2001.
18. Du Plessis, 2016: 128.
19. Anker, 2018: 253.
20. Trantraal, in La Vita, 2014.
21. Lazarus, 2007: 191.
22. Bion' s notion of the maternal mind as container seems relevant here:

> Bion asserts that while projective identification is inevitable and an important way of communicating, the mother should, through her organizational capacities (maternal reverie) attempt to metabolize and reintegrate the child's (or group members') emotional states. In this process, unmetabolized affective experiences (beta elements) are transformed into thoughts that can be thought about (alpha elements). Such thought processes help the baby to cope with feelings and to deal with her frustration (Kruger, 2016: 51).

In psychoanalytic theory it is asserted that the central task of the mother is to take the infant's feelings and metabolise them for him or her, giving them back to the child in a more manageable way. In other words, the mother has the task of translating the child's (or, in the case of the analyst, the patient's) distress 'by giving names to its hardships and anxieties and thus calms and contains it' (Borgogno, Merciai and Talamo, 1998: 95). The maternal mind thus becomes a container for the projections of child. Normal development follows if the relationship between infant and mother permits the infant to project a feeling onto the mother and to reintroject it after it has been metabolised, detoxified and made tolerable to the infant psyche. The idea is that the child or the patient will eventually learn to carry out these transformations for themselves.

In contemporary psychoanalytic theory Winnicott's notion of holding and Bion's notion of containment are understood as the capacity to mentalise. In the words of Motz (2014: 120–1):

> In order to manage intense states of arousal and convert raw data in the basic building-blocks of thought, a child needs to have had the prior experience of another person doing this for them, reflecting back their mental states and also giving them words with which to define and communicate them. It is the mother's vital function of mirroring the

infants' feelings that allows babies to identify, experience and integrate powerful states of mind and bodily sensation and, ultimately, to develop a sense of themselves as the container within which they exist. The child then learns she has a mind housed within a body, with feelings and thoughts that can relate to other minds and other bodies.

There are many reasons why a mother may not be able to take on the emotional communication from the child. Hollway (2006: 51) writes about the different possible reasons:

> One is when the baby's carer is psychologically cut off from the baby's communications and so fails to respond with any vitality or recognition . . . for example, when mothers are depressed. Alternatively, a parent may be so distraught as a result of the baby's screaming that he or she abandons the attempt to help and even shakes or hurts the baby in anxiety and loss of control that has turned aggressive. In this case, the baby experiences its own negative feelings failing to be contained but rather re-projected; not only not detoxified but amplified.

If the mother is unable to name the infant's feelings and think about them, the infant is thought to be left with unthinkable or unbearable anxiety, a nameless dread (Bion, 1962a). This uncomfortable feeling of anticipating something with great apprehension or fear ('the world is a bad and unsafe place') can become too great and the infant will become psychotic or use other defences, such as acting out, to deal with the nameless or unknown dread.

But there is a third possibility:

> Less dramatically, reacting rather than reflecting, the carer may assume that she knows what is needed and impose this on the baby, irrespective of whether this turns out to be correct. If this happens too much, the absence of trustworthy recognition confuses the baby's grasp of reality, in which case, the baby's experience will be '. . . of being actively misunderstood . . . Such a baby will have more difficulty in getting to know and accept himself (Waddell 1998: 42)' (Hollway, 2006: 52; see also Bion, 1962a; Borgogno, Merciai and Talamo, 1998; Kruger, 2016).

23. Horizon, calm yourself, I have a house
    That liberates me; beneath its roof
    I am one who breathes freely (Geerds, 1992).
    See https://www.gedichten.nl/nedermap/gedichten/gedicht/219906.html.
24. Winnicott, 1960: 587.
25. Lazarus, 2007: 185.
26. Lazarus, 2007: 193.
27. Also see the chapter on *Love*.
28. In psychoanalytic terms I would argue that the exposure to scolding can have adverse psychological effects, even if it is common. Constantly being exposed to the unmetabolised feelings of others may create the nightmare world of Melanie

Klein's paranoid-schizoid infant. The perceptual apparatus becomes damaged as the infant feels itself surrounded by disintegrated hostile objects. The infant's links with reality are either broken or very painful and its capacity to link and to integrate is disrupted. Conversely, we need to think of the internal world of the scolding women who are apparently splitting and projecting all their bad feelings, typically onto those they care about most (see Hughes, 1989). See also chapter on *Love*.

29. In a paper on gossiping among high-school girls, Hamman and Kruger (2017: 1) conclude:

> This research highlights that gossip, as an instrument of effective and prominent social control in the hands of these early adolescent girls from a low-income South African community, can function as a form of democratic and empowering surveillance, can be a secret weapon of envious undermining, and also has the potential to be destructive. As such, gossip cannot be regarded as either simply negative or simply positive. It was also found that the power of gossip is limited. Therefore, while gossip can be seen as a potential instrument for the questioning, subversion and undermining of existing hierarchies, its potential power is also compromised by existing social rules; often unspoken ones.

30. The information exchange and surveillance operative in gossiping can be described as being myopticon, as opposed to Foucault's (1995) panopticon. Instead of the hierarchical and totalising gaze of panopticon, gossip renders everyone in the community 'visible', but in the form of non-hierarchical and partial myopic surveillance. The seemingly myopic qualities of gossip, as described by the girls, suggest a democratic form of surveillance in this community. The potential of democratic surveillance to be used as an informal control mechanism lies in the uncertainty of being observed and talked about – or not talked about (Turgo, 2013). The uncertain threat of gossip often represents strong expectations placed on individuals in terms of how to act and live within small communities (Haugen and Villa, 2006).

31. *7de Laan* is a South African Afrikaans soap opera, which also includes some English and Zulu dialogue and has English subtitles. It started in 2000 and is broadcast on SABC 2 from Monday to Friday in the early evenings. Ratings are generally around the 2 million mark, according to http://www.tvsa.co.za. The soap opera is set in and around a fictional street in the fictional suburb of Hillside, Johannesburg. The programme is very popular in the valley, with many research participants, when choosing pseudonyms, choosing the names of characters from the series. For academic articles on *7de Laan*, see, for instance, Van Coller and Van Jaarsveld, 2009; Marx, 2008; Milton, 2008.

32. Hamman and Kruger, 2017.

33. Fleming and Kruger, 2013.

34. Marais, 2006: 324.

35. For discussions of coloured identity, see, for instance, Adhikari, 2008; Erasmus, 2017; Noah, 2016; Trantraal, 2018.
36. Kruger and Lourens, 2016: 125.
37. Transcribed from a television appearance; the programme and date were unfortunately not noted.
38. Long (2019: 14) writes about the dilemma of the coloniser:

    As the Fanonian scholar Hussein Bulhan explains, colonizers are tragic figures. On the one hand, they need the colonized to remain in their place, to serve as the repository of their projections, a fate that no human being will tolerate indefinitely. On the other – since the colonial relationship is a recapitulation of the master-slave dialectic – the colonizer never feels recognized as human because the act of recognition is made by a slave and is therefore worthless. It is this hapless situation that constitutes what Kojève calls the *existential impasse* of the master – a situation that I believe may apply to many white South Africans today.

39. See Adhikari, 2004, 2006; Dawjee, 2018; Erasmus, 2001, 2017; Noah, 2016; Petrus and Isaacs-Martin, 2012; Trantraal, 2018; Vollenhoven, 2016; Wicomb, 1998.
40. Willemse, 2011: 25.
41. The quote is from Willemse (2011: 25); the quote within this quote is from F. Fanon, *The Wretched of the Earth* (New York: Grove/Atlantic, 2007).
42. G.J. Gerwel, *Literatuur en Apartheid* (Kasselsvlei: Kampen, 1983), cited in Willemse (2011: 25).
43. D.J. Macdonald, 'Die Familie-lewe van die kleuring: Met 'n noukeurige ondersoek na die Stellenboche kleurling familie' (Master's thesis, University of Stellenbosch, 1933), cited in Willemse (2011: 29).
44. La Vita and Dawjee, 2018.
45. South African writer Zoë Wicomb (1998: 92) writes extensively about apartheid's strategy of naming 'coloured' as a race and how this means that shame has become central in discussions of a coloured identity:

    Miscegenation, the origins of which lie within a discourse of 'race', concupiscence, and degeneracy, continues to be bound up with shame, a pervasive shame exploited by apartheid's strategy of the naming of a coloured race, and recurring in the current attempts by Coloureds to establish brownness as pure category, which is to say a denial of shame. We do not speak of miscegenation; it is after all the very nature of shame to stifle its own discourse.

46. Cited in Kruger, 2016: 63–4.
47. Motz, 2001: 94.
48. Heinz Kohut asserts that some of the most painful feelings people are exposed to are related to their sense of not being human (Kottler and Togashi, 2015).
49. Hoagland, 2015: 74.
50. Kafka, 1970:14.

## Notes to Birth

1. Sister Joubert's comparison of expelling faeces and a baby is interesting and one that we often came across in birth narratives. Freud asserts that the function of excretion has everything to do with being out of control or in control (see Kruger 2003b, 2005; Kruger and Van der Spuy 2007).

2. Despite a proliferation of psychological research on pregnancy, the psychological discourse on pregnancy has been described by feminist researchers as a discourse that omits subjectivity. There still is a relative paucity of literature on the meaning of pregnancy for the pregnant woman herself (Burmeister-Nel, 2005; Johnson, Burrows and Williamson, 2004; Schneider, 2002). Psychologists have traditionally regarded pregnancy, like puberty and menopause, as a period of adjustment and even emotional crisis involving profound psychological and physical changes (Bibring, 1959; Bibring et al., 1961; Brockington, 1996; Burmeister-Nel, 2005; Lederman, 1984; Raphael-Leff, 1991; Reading, 1983). Pregnancy has been described as a transitional phase (Lederman, 1996), a time of adjustment (Miller and Shah, 1999) and increased risk for psychological illness (Kumar and Robson, 1984). In an analysis of the pregnancy literature, Heidi Burmeister-Nel (2005) showed that quantitative studies on Western, middle-class, pregnant women reflected seven broad themes/issues pertaining to the experience of pregnancy. These include experiences of loss and change (Lederman, 1996; Leonhardt-Lupa, 1995; Trad, 1991); ambivalence or emotional disequilibrium (Brockington, 1996; Leifer, 1977; Leifer, 1980; Leonhardt-Lupa, 1995; Norbeck and Peterson Tilden, 1983; Parker, 1995; Stainton, 1994; Trad, 1991); anxiety and fear (Arizmendi and Affonso, 1987; Bardwick, 1971, cited in Trad, 1991; Brockington, 1996; Erickson, 1976; Mrdjenović, Anton and Topuzović, 1999; Raphael-Leff, 1991); psychological distress (Miller and Shah, 1999); preparation during pregnancy (Lederman, 1996; Raphael-Leff, 1991); adjustment and acceptance (Lederman, 1996) and prenatal attachment (Brockington, 1996). See also Macleod, 2010.

   The literature on pregnancy clearly suggests that there is the potential for stress in all areas: in the endocrinological changes; in the concrete lifestyle changes that a woman starts to prepare for; in the activation of unconscious psychological conflicts pertaining to factors involved in pregnancy and in the intra-psychic reorganisation of becoming a mother (Bibring, 1959; Burmeister-Nel, 2005). However, the significance attached to motherhood, and therefore pregnancy, cannot be seen as universal. Pregnancy seems to mean different things for different women (Cosslett, 1994; Raphael-Leff, 1991; Ruddick, 1994). Regarding poor women specifically, it is generally accepted that women from lower socio-economic groups experience a greater number of stressors and higher levels of psychological distress during pregnancy (Sénuin et al., 1995). The literature suggests that they are more likely to engage in adverse health-related behaviours (Adler et al., 1994), to live and work in riskier environments (Anderson and Armstead, 1995) and to have fewer social resources that buffer stress during pregnancy (Sénuin et al., 1995). However, research on pregnancy and low-income women has been particularly scarce and biased, focusing more on 'problematic' behaviour of poor women during pregnancy than on their subjective experience of pregnancy. Accounts of how low-income South African women experience pregnancy are few and far between (Burmeister-Nel, 2005). For more recent examples of discussions on pregnancy in South Africa, see Branson, Ardington and Leibbrandt, 2013; Evens et al., 2015; Tomlinson et al., 2013; Toska et al., 2015.

3. The average number of children for new mothers in the four years that we reviewed clinic records was 1.74.

4. See Kruger, Shefer and Oakes, 2015; Shefer et al., 2015.

5. Jackson, 2011: xi. Jackson cites several definitions of hope: Hannah Arendt says: 'Hope is synonymous with the appearance of the new which has the character of startling unexpectedness – something that is inherent in all beginnings and origins and occurs despite the overwhelming odds of statistical laws and their probability, which for all practical everyday purposes amounts to certainty.' Gabrial Marcel refers to hope as 'enthusiasm for living', while Pierre Bourdieu equates hope with 'the forthcoming' (in Jackson 2011: vii).

6. Jackson, 2011: xii.

7. Jackson, 2011: xii.

8. Kruger et al., 2014.

9. Macleod, 2001, 2002, 2011.

10. It is increasingly acknowledged that adolescent girls sometimes choose to fall pregnant and that their choice to be pregnant may be a 'rational' response to their life circumstances. See, for instance, Arai, 2003, 2009; Coleman and Cater, 2006; Duncan, Edwards and Alexander, 2010; Macleod and Tracey, 2010; Naong, 2011; Udjo, 2014. For a discussion of teenage fathers in South Africa, see Hendricks, Swartz and Bhana, 2010.

11. Raphael-Leff, 1982: 8, 1991, 1993.

12. See Bester and Kruger, 2018, for a more detailed discussion of this case.

13. In psychoanalytic terms, depression is considered defensive, characterised by unremitting sadness, lack of energy, anhedonia (inability to enjoy ordinary pleasures) and vegetative disturbances (problems with eating, sleeping and self-regulating). Whereas this roughly coincides with the DSM-5 symptoms of depression, the DSM-5 leaves out the subjective experience of the patient, whereas in psychoanalysis the internal experience is considered of utmost importance and has implications for treatment. Hence, two versions of depression are identified within psychoanalysis. The patients may have the same symptoms, but their internal experience is different. There is the anaclitic depressive defensive style, which is more shame-based, and there is the introjecting depressive defensive style, which is more informed by guilt.

Anaclitic depression is more narcissistic and is characterised by feelings of emptiness, loneliness, neediness, hunger and meaninglessness. Introjecting depression is more melancholic and the person suffering from this kind of depression feels bad about herself – evil, flawed, self-indulgent and guilty.

The anaclitic depressed person feels depleted, palpably sad about an unjust world in which they experience themselves as chronically inadequate and filled with longing, but destined to a life of disappointment. They are more likely to suffer shame (because no one wants them) than to feel guilt. They bemoan the fact that fate has treated them badly and thus feel victimised, powerless and passive. Their passivity manifests in a belief that help must come from the outside, that they can't save themselves.

The introjective depressed person tends to takes responsibility for her own sadness and feels that the source of unhappiness lies within herself. She feels that if she can become a better person and improve, life will be better. She feels bad about herself, but powerful in that badness. The bad in the world and in other people is introjected, thus the world can be kept good and other people are idealised. By turning against herself, she has a sense of power and her anxiety is less. She also denies or represses her own anger and hostility (Blatt and Zuroff, 1992; Blatt, Shafar and Zuroff, 2001; McWilliams, 2011).

From within a psychoanalytic perspective, Janine will be described as having a anaclitic depressive defensive style.

14. Like so many women, Janine is concerned that history will repeat itself and that her daughter will end up like her. 'She is behaving in much the same manner as I was, so I guess that is kind of bothering me at the moment,' she says. 'She's quiet, on her own, ja. She's a good child, she does not like pets or anything, so she's not really affectionate. But ja, she's a good child, growing up, starting to misbehave every now and then, but essentially a good child. Being kind of drawn back and not being able to talk, and to say if something's bothering her or, whatever. Ja, I don't want to feel like she's not able to speak to anybody, or to feel like no one loves her or anything.'

15. Russell, 1998; Wallin, 2007.

16. Bester and Kruger, 2018.

17. Kruger, Shefer and Oakes, 2015.

18. In the region there has been substantial anecdotal evidence of low-income women obscuring other important 'facts' regarding their personal functioning. Health-care workers working in low-income communities have often mentioned their patients' failures to disclose important health-related information (such as that they are HIV-positive, they are sexually active or that they are pregnant) as one of the major problems they have to deal with. See Kruger and Van der Spuy, 2007.

19. Brockington (1996: 438) notes that 'the fact the pregnancy can be concealed, even from the mother herself, is well-known'. He claims that while failure to recognise pregnancy is common in the early stages, especially in those women who are pregnant accidentally for the first time, this state of affairs could continue until the end of pregnancy for some women. A distinction can be made between women who simply do not notice the pregnancy and those who conceal it, and women

who, against all the evidence, remain obstinately unaware of it (Brockington 1996). Raphael-Leff (1991: 47) writes that while some women deal with the complex experience of pregnancy by becoming more introspective and listening to the unconscious, others 'hurriedly dismiss [it] from awareness'. She reports that in her clinical work with pregnant patients she saw altered states of consciousness, memory lapses, as well as sudden flashes of insight.

Despite the agreement of experts that it is quite common for women to keep their pregnancies from their awareness, there is no significant empirical literature to support this claim. George M. Gould and Walter L. Pyle (cited in Brockington, 1996) describe twelve cases reported in the literature in their miscellany *Anomalies and Curiosities of Medicine*. Jens Wessel, in an article in *Geburtsh u Frauenheilk* (cited in Brockington, 1996), describes four cases and claims that he saw one case in 366 births. Brezinka et al., 1994 collected 27 instances at Innsbruck between 1987 and 1990 – about 1:400 births. In seven cases, denial lasted for 21 to 26 weeks, and in nine cases it lasted 36 weeks; eleven continued their denial until the onset of contractions and the rupture of membranes.

20. Given the paucity of literature dealing specifically with obscured pregnancies, there have been few focused or thorough attempts to understand this phenomenon. According to Brockington (1996), there are a number of physical, psychosocial and psychological factors that could account for a failure to recognise pregnancy. Cessation of menses, the first sign of conception for most women, may occasionally be absent or less obvious in certain mothers – for example, those who are breastfeeding, those with a history of scanty or irregular menstruation, or those with amenorrhoea as a result of anorexia nervosa or menopause. Other physical symptoms of pregnancy – for example, nausea or cravings – may be absent or less marked. Weight gain can be minor and there may be little change in physical appearance. Social factors that might account for a failure to recognise pregnancy include isolation (in that there are no close friends or relatives to notice and comment on the change in appearance) and a moral climate antagonistic to extramarital sexual relations, with its fear of disclosure. The psychological mechanisms that enable pregnancy to remain unacknowledged include denial and dissociation. See also Mkhwanazi, 2010; Shefer, Bhana and Morrell, 2013.

21. The phrase 'kept at bay' is from Raphael-Leff (1991: 49). Feminist writers have argued that the maternal body may be seen as abject in a number of different ways. In the societal response to the maternal body there is a clear 'obsession with concealment, control, and cleanliness . . . to keep the event invisible and "sanitary"'. Or, in the words of Davis (1997: 5): 'The female body is always the other: mysterious, unruly, threatening to erupt and challenge the patriarchal order . . . the female body represented all that needed to be tamed and controlled.' Dimen (1992: 44) comments on the fact that reproductive matters – periods, pregnancies, unruly children, and so forth – are regarded by society as 'female matters'. They are

seen to be chaotic, crude, even ugly – especially unfitting in the organised world of
work. She states: 'In our culture, reproductive matters are to the politicoeconomic
domain what, in symbol, the vagina is to the neat penis – messy.'

22. Faced with the tremendous external and internal pressure that accompanies their
pregnancies, many women consciously and/or unconsciously choose to obscure (to
forget or deny or repress) the knowledge of their bodies. Julia Kristeva argues that
it is exactly through psychological mechanisms such as repression and dissociation
that individuals and society respond to the abject. This, she claims, is how identity
is fixed and the social order maintained. Kristeva's notions of the 'abject' and
'abjection' may be useful here. She describes the abject as 'that which is threatening,
fearful, incomprehensible, or vile' (cited in Rogers, 1997: 226). Abjection is
'a reaction to the recognition of the impossible but necessary transcendence of
the subject's corporeality, and the impure, defiling elements of its uncontrollable
materiality' (Gross, 1990: 87–8). Kristeva's notion of 'abjection' is useful, in that it
describes how the individual and society respond to the processes of the body and
the borders of the body. The process of abjection (expelling or repressing the abject)
is conceptualised as a prerequisite condition for the formation of the sexual and
psychological identity of the individual and of the construction of a social order.
The abject has to be rejected in order for the subject to achieve an identity and
for the social and political order to be maintained in society. 'It is thus not lack of
cleanliness or health that causes abjection but what disturbs identity, system, order.
What does not respect borders, positions, rules? The in-between, the ambiguous,
the composite' (Kristeva, 1982: 4).

23. It is in the experiences of some pregnant women that we can hear that the
postmodern mantra to celebrate the multiplicity of the self is as of yet an impossible
one. If the pregnant woman is the most concrete example of the split subject, it
seems clear that society is not yet able to tolerate the multiplicity: it demands of
certain women to obscure, to deny, to repress, to suppress, to dissociate, to keep
secrets. The argument is that some disempowered women do not acknowledge
their pregnant bodies or their identities as pregnant women because it is difficult
to deal with the fluidity or multiplicity that such recognition would entail. In the
words of Jane Flax (1990: 219–20):

> It is possible to construct views of self in which it does not experience
> difference as irreconcilable . . . To glimpse such a self is to confront a
> paradox: It cannot fully exist within contemporary culture. The forces
> of repression here are not only within the individual, metaphysics,
> metanarrative, or discursive formations, but in social relations as well.
> These social forces are too powerful, too fragmented, and too pervasive
> for any individual or individual analysis to comprehend or overcome.
> The existence of asymmetric gender relations and the asymmetries of
> race encourage and reinforce the splitting and disavowal of parts of the
> self.

24. I would suggest that a psychoanalytic understanding of identity, order and the abject might be useful in illuminating not only women's failure to disclose their pregnancies, but also their failure to report or seek help for bodies that are beaten and bodies that are ill (for example, with HIV or AIDS). In other words, if there is indeed a more pervasive tendency in low-income communities to not acknowledge feelings, thoughts, actions, decisions and conditions that can be construed as problematic (particularly those related to the body), this tendency may also not simply be related to a conscious decision to keep secrets, but may also have to do with what can be understood as an almost unconscious survival strategy of the disempowered. The tendency to not talk about or report or acknowledge problems has severe consequences for health decision-making, help-seeking behaviours and treatment adherence – for example, contraception, HIV and AIDS testing, coping with an HIV or AIDS diagnosis (breastfeeding when positive, having unprotected sex when positive), substance use during pregnancy, staying in violent relationships, not reporting child sexual abuse, getting help for depression, and so forth.

25. Jolly, 1998: 2.

26. Larger discourses (bodies of knowledges and accompanying material practices) have been constructed around moments in the reproductive cycle of women, and more specifically around the moment of birth. This means that all women's experiences of their bodies during pregnancy and birth are mediated by their interactions with institutions and discourses, even if in very different ways. These discourses then serve to produce and sustain the female reproductive body in particular ways, highlighting certain experiences by setting up particular understandings, subject positions, power relations and material practices. Simultaneously, however, some experiences or some women's experiences are marginalised and become silenced. See, for instance, Kruger, 2006a.

27. In contemporary psychological literature about childbirth there is much discussion about women's psychological experience of childbirth (see, for instance, Bryanton et al., 2008; Conroy and Cottrell, 2015; Dannenbring, Stevens and House, 1997; Dunn and O'Herlihy, 2005; Gizzo et al., 2014; Gungor and Beji, 2012; Hodnett, 2002; Langer et al., 1998; McKay and Barrows, 1992; Melender, 2002; Melender and Lauri, 1999; Pinto et al., 2016; Salmon, Miller and Drew, 1990; Simkin, 1991, 1992; Waldenstrom, 1999). Mostly these discussions focus on the issues of maternal satisfaction and childbirth pain, some studies treating them as variables that are closely associated with each other, other studies claiming that levels of pain experienced are not related to maternal satisfaction (Salmon, Miller and Drew, 1990). The notion that women should be 'satisfied' with childbirth is a relatively new idea and is related to a new interest in the psychology of women and an increased awareness of how maternal well-being is related to the well-being of an infant and child. The question then is what constitutes a 'satisfying' birth? Who decides? And is it possible that all women will define satisfaction in the same way?

What is striking about the quantitative and qualitative studies that have been conducted in this area is, firstly, that the list of variables is usually endless and, second, that there is hardly ever any conclusive finding that confirms the findings of previous studies. A meta-analysis of such studies suggests that the reason for a lack of conclusive results seems to be that while different researchers work with different models of what constitutes maternal satisfaction, different respondents or groups of respondents also have different ideas of what a 'satisfying' birth experience should look like. Empirical researchers typically do not reveal the models within which they operate and also do not interrogate the responses of respondents to determine the discourses within which they respond to standard questionnaires and open-ended questions.

In reviewing the literature (see, for instance, Bryanton et al., 2008; Chistiaens and Bracke, 2007; Hodnett, 2002; Hotelling, 2004; Kornelsen, 2005; Meyer, 2008), specific aspects of labour and childbirth, such as duration, the nature of interventions or type of delivery, appear to be unimportant. However, perceptions of support from partner and staff, perceptions of control and patterns of blaming, together with factors such as trait anxiety and past mental health problems do appear to act as predictors.

This notion of maternal satisfaction, and how it is tied to the expectations that women have of childbirth, highlights the fact that childbirth is a physical and social event and, like most aspects of the social and physical world, deeply embedded in discourse. In other words, while women's experiences of childbirth are shaped by their expectations, their expectations, in turn, are informed by dominant discourses of childbirth. Large discourses have been constructed around the moment of birth – as is true for all important moments in the reproductive cycle of women. These discourses then serve to produce and sustain the female reproductive body in particular ways (highlighting certain experiences by setting up particular understandings, subject positions, power relations and material practices). Simultaneously, however, some experiences or some women's experiences are marginalised and become silenced.

In reviewing these studies, it seems clear that there always seems to be some unspoken ideal of childbirth against which individual women's experiences are measured. Even in the qualitative studies researchers fail to reveal their own assumptions of what birth should be like and the reader is left to read between the lines that the researchers expected birth to be satisfying, fulfilling, an accomplishment, and so on. It is not surprising then that a critical reading of recent studies suggests that there is one variable that is always operative in women's experience of childbirth – the extent to which it matches their expectations. Remarkable also is that most studies that focus on women's satisfaction during childbirth focus on women opting for natural childbirth: the question of satisfaction is not so pertinent in births where there is maximum medical intervention.

Given this substantial literature, it is striking that in the birth narratives we have encountered in the valley, women's endurance is more of an issue than maternal satisfaction.

For more literature on maternal satisfaction, see Edwards, 2018; Erenoglu and Baser, 2019; Tasseau, Walter-Nicolet and Autret, 2018.

In so-called birth plans women are encouraged to write down (in detail) their expectations and preferences for the management of labour. This is often regarded as a routine part of the antenatal care process in the developed world (see, for instance, Blomquist et al., 2011; Carty and Tier, 1989; Cook and Loomis, 2012).

Much has been written about how a birth plan is the way in which the discourse on natural birth becomes embedded in the lived experience of labouring women (Frost et al., 2006). Frost et al. specifically researched the tension between natural labour discourse and actual labour experiences in a group of British women. They found that women resolve this tension in three ways: acceptance, challenge or reinforcement. The first response was acceptance, to simply be grateful for the safe delivery of the baby. Others responded to the discrepancy by challenging the natural birth discourse. The authors were surprised to find that a substantial number of respondents actually ended up reinforcing the discourse, notwithstanding the huge discrepancies between the discourse and their own experiences.

The whole problem with the notion of choice in relation to childbirth is that it deflects attention from the social relationships within which the supposed choice is made, which are irrevocably unequal (for example, the obstetrician or the obstetric nurse, with more knowledge, is more powerful).

28. See also Kruger and Schoombee (2010).

29. Kalmanofsky (2008: 66) asserts that the image of the labouring woman is depicted in the Old Testament as an image that expresses horror and elicits horror. The labouring woman, she states, expresses physical and emotional vulnerability, trembling both from pain and panic. She experiences fear, confusion and futility. This is contrary to how contemporary Western women conceive of childbirth: 'For us, living in an age of prenatal care and epidurals, it is easy to associate childbirth with strength and to focus on the immense power of women who birth babies'. The book of Jeremiah (6:22–4) has this to say:

Thus said the Lord:
'See, a people comes from the northland,
A great nation is roused
From the remotest parts of earth.
They grasp the bow and javelin;
They are cruel, they show no mercy;
The sound of them is like the roaring sea.
They ride upon horses,
Accoutered like a man for battle,
Against you, O Fair Zion!

We have heard the report of them,
Our hands fail;
Pain seizes us,
Agony like a woman in childbirth.'

30. The Afrikaans translation is even more frightening. The word 'pain' is not used, the word *'smart'* is – literally, in English, 'misery': *'Aan die vrou het hy gese: Ek sal grootliks vermeerder jou moeite en jou swangerskap; met smart sal jy kinders baar; en na jou man sal jou begeerte wees, en hy sal oor jou heers.'* In misery you will bear children.

31. The English word 'horror' comes from the Latin *horrere*, meaning 'to bristle' and the old French *horror*, meaning 'to bristle' or 'to shudder'. So there is both a physical and emotional dimension to horror. Kalmanofsky (2008) cites Noël Carroll's *The Philosophy of Horror, or Paradoxes of the Heart* for a list of the most common physical sensations associated with horror: muscular contractions, tension, cringing, shrinking, shuddering, recoiling, tingling, frozenness, momentary arrests, chilling, paralysis, trembling, nausea, a reflex of apprehension or physical heightened alertness, involuntary screaming. The *Oxford Dictionary* online defines horror as 'a painful emotion compounded of loathing and fear; a shuddering with terror and repugnance; strong aversion mingled with dread; the feeling excited by something shocking or frightful. Also in weaker sense, intense dislike or repugnance.'

32. Kalmanofsky, 2008.

33. The idea of regaining control over one's body became popular among educated, middle-class women and ultimately became a major tenet of feminism (Wertz and Wertz, 1977. In its most extreme form, this discourse of natural childbirth upholds the idea of ecstatic, drug-free, painless, natural birth and is dependent on ideas of primitive, essential motherhood.

  In *The Woman in the Body: A Cultural Analysis of Reproduction*, Emily Martin (1987) juxtaposes this way of thinking about childbirth with the medical discourse on childbirth. She criticises the fact that the medical model is based on an analogy between the production of goods and the production of babies. She says that there is a 'compelling need for new key metaphors, core symbols of birth that capture what we do not want to lose about birth' (Martin, 1987: 157). She discusses the notion of 'purebirth', as developed by Lois J. Estner and Nancy Wainer Cohen: 'Birth that is completely free of medical intervention. It is self-determined, self-assured, and self-sufficient, without necessarily being solitary . . . purebirth has no stages. Rather, it is a continuation of creative energy that began with conception and will grow through years of nurturing.'

  According to this childbirth discourse, women have to learn how to give birth, just as they had to learn how to read. Birth is a 'performance' for which one 'rehearsed' or a 'competition that you are going to win'. Early French reports presented the method as a series of challenges to be met with courage and skill. The method shifted emphasis from the doctor to the woman, who was to control her own labour. Childbirth 'is not something that you simply let happen to you . . . it is something that you do'. Above all, the woman does not need to be passive; autonomy is the key to this method. The woman regains control of birth; the doctor is simply there to assist. The woman is the star and will deliver the baby (Wertz and Wertz, 1977: 193–4). See also Kruger, 2006a.

34. See chapter on *Love* for more discussion of the connection between cruelty and care.

35. In an early analysis of the medical discourse used in obstetrics and gynaecology textbooks, Treichler (1990: 122) points out how the focus in such texts was on the foetus and physician, with the woman often erased altogether:

> [Normal] labour is the physiologic process by which the uterus expels, or attempts to expel, its contents . . . through the cervical opening and vagina to the outside world. Normal labour is characterised by periodic, involuntary uterine contractions which produce gradual cervical effacement and delatation, as well as descent of the fetal presenting part.

She discusses how, in medical dictionaries, birth was typically defined as 'an accomplishment of the fetus (and/or physician) rather than of the mother' (135) – for example, in phrases such as 'the emergence of a new individual from the body of its parent', 'the act or process of being born' and 'the offspring's emergence from the womb of the mother'.

36. The average birth weight of babies in the four years that we surveyed clinic records was 2.975 kilograms. According to Wikipedia, 'the average weight of babies of European heritage is 3.5 kilograms, though the range of normal is between 2.5 kilograms and 4.5 kilograms'. See https://en.wikipedia.org/wiki/Birth_weight.

37. Discussing different ways of giving birth, most women said that if they had a choice, they would have a vaginal birth without painkillers. The notion seems to be that this is the best way to give birth. A caesarean was regarded as more painful. It is not clear that the women of the valley, giving birth in local public hospital, ever could choose how they wanted to give birth.

38. In the psychological literature on childbirth and pain, it is typically asserted that physical factors, psychosocial factors and environmental factors all have an impact on the experience of pain. Physical factors include: age (older women have less pain), menstrual difficulties, ratio of weight to height, onset of labour, mode of delivery, frequency of contractions, gestational age at delivery, induced labour, assisted delivery and fetal weight. The psychosocial factors that have been discerned in the literature are fear, anxiety, expectations about experience, perceived personal control, sense of self-efficacy, confidence in coping skills, lower socio-economic status, childbirth preparation training, previous experience of pain, strategies to cope with pain, communication during birth and cultural differences. Environmental factors that are thought to have an impact on how pain is experienced in childbirth include caregivers, philosophy and practice policies of care facility, quality of care, degree of strangeness, noise, lighting and temperature and restrictiveness of

environment. See, for instance, Callister et al., 2003; Cook and Loomis, 2012; Hall et al., 2018; Käll, 2013; Kruger, 2007; Leifer, 1980; Melender and Lauri, 1999; Scott-Palmer and Skevington, 1981; Van der Gucht and Lewis, 2015.

39. Despite the consensus that the pain was beyond words and descriptions, there were attempts to describe it. There were attempts to describe the exact location of the pain and its significance: 'It was pains that I had on my bladder that moved around. The cross of my back. With my two girlchild's birth it was not the same. Everything came from the back. The son's pain was on my bladder' and 'My stomach started aching lightly.'

    The duration of the pain was also emphasised: 'Then I rest first and when I got up I thought the pain will go away, but it was still there. But after that the pain took me again and it took me until 11 o'clock.' Another woman said: 'And the pain started from there and it never paused. It was a constant pain. I gave birth at 11 o'clock. But it was all the time yes, and it was very bad.' And this from another woman: 'The pains were very sore so I walked up and down. Then I started bleeding and then I had pains the whole day, the whole day I had pains. I ate nothing and only that evening, the Thursday evening, ten past eleven, I finished.'

40. The pain is described as burning: 'It was just the pains that were so sore, just the pains. But when I felt burning, they said that I should start pushing because the head came through already and I must now start pushing.' Another woman said: 'Then I had to go and take a bath and so, and then you now feel the burning pain afterwards.' One woman described the severity of the pain by saying: 'For me it felt as if the veins in my head are going to explode.' A few women described the pain as so severe that they thought they were seeing red: 'And if you start seeing red, as they say . . .'. It was also experienced as hot and cold flushes: 'It was pain, then it was there, then it was gone. Then I was too hot, then I was cold.'

41. See chapter on *Home*.

42. For many middle-class women, birth is seen as a site of control (Kruger, 2005, 2006a).

43. This mantra is also prominent in the discussion of the pain of intimate relationships (see the chapter on *Love*).

44. This breakdown of narrative in the face of vulnerability, especially embodied vulnerability, should not be surprising. Elaine Scarry (1985), in her book *The Body in Pain: The Making and Unmaking of the World*, talks about pain as the shattering of language. She describes how physical pain does not only resist language, but actively destroys it, bringing about an immediate reversion to a state anterior to language, to the sounds and cries a human makes before language is learned. Other observers have remarked on how the physical condition of maternity (the body) challenges all our cultural scripts – including the dominant scripts of childbirth. In some of the articulations of childbirth, the actual form of the talk may suggest something about the experience of the body – it is fragmented, disorganised, chaotic (Adams, 1994).

Odent (1984: 12), who is heralded as a champion of natural childbirth in Europe and the United States, describes what happens to women during childbirth as a return to an animal-like, childlike state (this made him very unpopular with some of the feminist proponents of natural childbirth):

> Women seemed to forget themselves and what was going on around them during the course of an unmedicated labour . . . they get a faraway look in their eyes, forget social conventions, lose self-consciousness and self-control. Many let out a characteristic cry at the moment of delivery . . . I have found it very difficult to describe this shift to a deeper level of consciousness during labor. I had thought of calling it 'regression'.

In a study investigating women's responses to viewing videotapes of their second stage of labour, McKay and Barrows (1992) found that many women did not recall details. The language women used to describe what they were seeing when they watched themselves again suggests something about the impossibility of being articulate about the experience of birth. They used words such as 'weird' (the most common adjective), 'embarrassing', 'gross', 'yucky', 'comical', 'exciting', 'surreal', 'interesting', 'neat', 'unreal', 'wild', 'intense', 'amazing', 'vivid', 'strange', 'pride-evoking', 'dramatic' and 'fun'. The 'weirdness' of the videotape viewing seemed related to their feeling 'this is me, this isn't me', which was a common theme when women discussed what it was like to relive their labour.

In the writings of Kristeva, there are numerous references to the 'primal regression' of giving birth. The mother who comes to us in Kristeva's discussion of pregnancy is not a writing or speaking one: 'She is the model of a split and divided identity, a catastrophe that threatens the illusory coherence of the paternal order' (Walker, 1998: 157). During birth, Kristeva says, there is a clear descent into the semiotic, a regression during which the woman loses access to the symbolic. When she uses the term 'symbolic' (a term roughly coinciding with Lacan's mirror stage), she uses it to refer to the modality of truth and meaning, implicated in the acquisition of language (Grosz, 1990). It is identified with consciousness, the transcendental ego – the paternal order. The semiotic is the pre-Oedipal, pre-linguistic modality. It is the domain of rhythm, intonation and gesture. It 'precedes evidence, verisimilitude, spatiality, and temporality' (Kristeva, *Powers of Horror*, cited in Adams, 1994: 21). Kristeva suggests that the pregnant and birthing woman enjoys a privileged relation to the maternal body. As a result, she renews connection to the repressed, pre-conscious, pre-symbolic aspect of existence. Instead of being a unified ego, the subject of the paternal symbolic order, the pregnant subject straddles the sphere of language and instinct.

What is essentially feminine, in Kristeva's view, is the inarticulate cry (Adams, 1994). 'In "woman" I see something that cannot be represented, something that is not said, something above nomenclatures and ideologies' (Kristeva, *Powers of Horror*, cited in Rowley and Grosz 1990: 194). Although Kristeva associates the semiotic with the feminine, with the moment of birth being in some sense the moment of the feminine, she also regards the feminine as something not specific to women, but a psychic position. Both the semiotic and the symbolic constitute the subject – whether a masculine or feminine subject. The symbolic is established through the repression of the semiotic, but the semiotic emerges continually in the symbolic, challenging it, undermining it, and keeping it open (Rowley and Grosz, 1990: 194). The semiotic (or the feminine position) of any person is therefore seen as heightening creativity, an approach to the mystical, a fuller knowledge of the self and the realisation of the absurdity of 'communital meaning' (Adams, 1994: 32). Or, in the words of Kristeva herself: 'It is the place where the speaking subject is both generated and negated, the place where his unity succumbs before the process of charges and stases that produce him' (Kristeva, *Powers of Horror*, cited in Adams, 1994: 21).

It is perhaps Mary Douglas (1966: 95), in her classical text *Purity and Danger: An Analysis of Concepts of Pollution and Taboo*, who most succinctly articulates the creative potential of the inarticulateness of disorder:

> Granted that disorder spoils pattern; it also provides the materials of pattern . . . disorder by implication is unlimited, no pattern has been realised in it, but its potential for patterning is indefinite. This is why, though we seek to create order, we do not simply condemn disorder.
>
> We recognise that it is destructive to existing patterns; also that it has potentiality. It symbolises both danger and power. In these beliefs there is a double play on inarticulateness. First there is a venture into the disordered regions of the mind. Second there is the venture beyond the confines of society. The man [or woman] who comes back from these inaccessible regions brings with him [or her] a power not available to those who have stayed in the control of themselves and society.

Kristeva asserts that for most women childbirth represents a 'descent into the semiotic' (where there is no access to the symbolic or the paternal order) (Adams, 1994: 15) or, in Douglas's (1966: 95) words, the 'inarticulateness of disorder'. It is suggested here that some birth stories are formulated within certain medical and feminist discourses where control and maternal fulfilment are prioritised. In such birth stories (examples are cited above), there are coherent ways of describing and categorising that help women to make sense of the experience of childbirth (Lupton, 1994). One can detect certain patterns of words, figures of speech, concepts, values and symbols in talk about birth.

This kind of discourse can be contrasted with dominant discourses, within which such moments of vulnerability are framed by so much certainty that the meaning of the moment is determined and prescribed, sometimes even before it has happened. Instead of highlighting the moment of vulnerability, it is obscured. Kristeva (1980: x) stresses the importance of holding the tension between two types of discourses, one in which the symbolic is prioritised and another where there is more emphasis on the semiotic:

> The daily attention given to the discourse of the other confirms, if need be, that the speaking being maintains himself or herself as such to the extent that he/she allows for the presence of two brinks . . . if the overly constraining and reductive meaning of a language made up of universals causes us to suffer, the call of the unnameable, on the contrary, issuing from those borders where signification vanishes, hurls us into the void of our universe, saturated with interpretation, faith, or truth.
>
> In other words, there is a problem with the fact that large discourses distance people from their own pain and suffering, reducing it to the universal. There is, however, also a problem with staying too close to the unnameable pain and suffering – to not be able to create meaning at all. Kristeva's emphasis on the moment of vulnerability as a moment of tremendous potential suggests that it is important to pay attention to such moments. This does not necessarily mean that there should not be narratives or closure of meaning. It simply means that it is problematic if the closure is premature, predetermined or permanent. See chapter on *Distress* on the importance of both mindfulness and mentalisation (Wallin, 2007).

45. Hyde et al., 2006; Kabakian-Khasholian et al., 2000; Weaver, 2000.

46. Adams (1994) uses Foucault's notion of an 'anatomo-chronological schema of behaviour' in the military (a schema in which each step is broken down into a series of precise and minute components) to illuminate the medicalisation of birth. In hospitals this means in practice that nurses have a body of knowledge that informs certain practices and disciplines through which they 'govern'. In this process the female body becomes a 'docile' body – a body that, through the organisation and regulation of time and space, is externally regulated, subjected and transformed (Foucault, 1989). See also Adams, 1994; Cosslett, 1994; Davis-Floyd, 1994; El-Nemer, Downe and Small, 2006; Kruger and Schoombee, 2010; Marshall and Woollett, 2000; Treichler, 1990; Wall, 2001.

47. Foucault (1989: xvi) refers to the patient's bed as a 'field of scientific investigation'. In this South African state hospital, the patient is systematically and literally kept out of the hospital bed and thus out of the medical gaze until she is fully dilated and the baby's head has started to emerge. The patient only qualifies for surveillance and intervention when certain 'signs' appear, when true labour has started and the appeal for help is deemed to be 'legitimate'. Through the clinical gaze, the body becomes an 'object of inquiry' and the individual becomes a 'case' (Henderson, 1994). Conversely, in the absence of the gaze, the body is not an object of inquiry and the individual is not yet a case.

48. Other researchers writing about childbirth in developing countries also comment about the prevalence of nurses being absent (El-Nemer, Downe and Small, 2006) or negligent (D'Oliveira, Grilo Diniz and Blima Schraiber, 2002) in maternity wards, stating that this is often the most distressing part of women's experiences of childbirth. See also Chadwick, 2017; Hastings-Tolsma, Nolte and Temane, 2018; Sen, Reddy and Iyer, 2018.

49. The data here seem to suggest that being admitted to this state-funded hospital does not automatically make a patient the subject of surveillance (the 'medical gaze'). Writing about the ideal of the panoptical gaze in South African state hospitals, Gibson (2004: 2014) describes instances of patients who were 'forgotten' or 'lost' while in foyers, in waiting bays and between wards. This kind of neglect seems to remain part of the experience of women in South African maternity wards. For instance, in an article published in November 2018 a story is related of a woman who was physically abused by nurses while in labour and subsequently left alone to give birth (Mahopo, 2018).

50. One way for the women to deal with childbirth was to simply start moving. This impulse to move was very much accommodated by the nurses' instructions for women to walk up and down the hospital corridors when they were experiencing contractions. Most birth stories include accounts of pacing up and down in the hospital corridors ('*die gange geloop*'): one woman recalled: 'No, I was lying in the bed and then I decided, yes, no, the pain is too terrible, I am going to get up.' Another said: 'You have to walk the corridors the whole time. You can't just lie down.' One woman said: 'Your hours you have to sit through and curl here from the pain and run there from the pain.'

51. D'Oliveira, Grilo Diniz and Blima Schraiber (2002) state that many studies in developing countries suggest that neglect is used as a systematic punishment and deterrent for non-compliance within the obstetric system. Although the gaze of the nursing staff is very much what women want once they are in hospital, it seems also clear that the attention of the nurses is not simply experienced as being positive. Being visible and being under surveillance does not necessarily mean being visible as a person (Foucault, 1989). Crowe (2000) uses Foucauldian theory to show how nurses employ disciplinary procedures to demonstrate their alignment with more dominant discursive constructions of nursing work, ensuring bodies that are docile, obedient and useful. The other instruments of control that nurses used during this stage of labour were verbal and physical abuse.

52. The Afrikaans word *gelos* (translated as 'left') literally means 'let go of' or 'dropped'.

53. The reality may be that shortage of staff makes it impossible for nurses to always be present – even during the later stages of labour. In such circumstances, it seems likely that nurses have to make conscious decisions as to who will receive care (Terreblanche, 2007). This may mean that certain kinds of patients ('difficult', 'disobedient' and 'undeserving' patients) will systematically not be attended to (Schoombee, Van der Merwe and Kruger, 2005).

54. D'Oliveira, Grilo Diniz and Blima Schraiber, 2002.

55. Other researchers have also reported the same procedures for women in other developing countries (D'Oliveira, Grilo Diniz and Blima Schraiber, 2002; El-Nemer, Downe and Small, 2006; Frenkel, 2002) or low-income women. Adams (1994) describes some health-care providers as unkind, rude, brusque, unsympathetic and uncaring – attitudes that are typically expressed in shouting or scolding.

56. See Kruger, 2006a.

57. These stories were collected at a time when reports of problems in maternity wards in state hospitals in South Africa were rife (Strydom, 2007; Terreblanche, 2007). The narratives seems to suggest that despite the fact that the South African government claimed in an advertisement in a popular Sunday newspaper that it 'made extra efforts to ensure that health services respond to the needs of women including making reproductive health services available and accessible to all women', maternal health services in this country are still severely compromised. See also Chadwick, Cooper and Harries, 2014; Jewkes, Abrahams and Mvo, 1998; Kruger and Schoombee, 2010. For a discussion on obstetric violence, which includes physical, emotional and verbal violence as well as non-dignified care, unnecessary medical technologies and structural violence, see Chadwick, 2017.

58. I try to understand the underlying mechanism of how such problematic interactions became an integral part of medical care in this particular maternity ward and can therefore be described as having been ritualised, sanctioned, normalised and ultimately institutionalised (Jewkes, Abrahams and Mvo, 1998). Listening to how patients and nurses talk about their experiences in a maternity ward in a state hospital, we hear how women themselves (nurses and patients) maintain and support discourses within which women are objectified and abused, and contest and undermine them. It is also important to understand how hospital hierarchies impact on nursing staff, who are usually looked down upon (Schoombee, Van der Merwe and Kruger, 2005). I am arguing therefore that nurses and patients, who seem powerless in the midst of social constraints, actually also have agency – even if it is limited (Ceci, 2004). While both nurses and patients normalise some of the harsher aspects of the interaction, it is clear from the interactions that there are instances in which they question it, resist it, subvert it and ultimately do tell the stories (Jewkes, Abrahams and Mvo, 1998; Kabakian-Khasholian et al., 2000). Foucault's (1977) notion of the agency of the seemingly powerless in the midst of social constraints seems relevant here when it becomes clear that even docile and passive subjects are not solely constructed by disciplinary techniques external to themselves, but exercise power by listening to their conscience and undertaking an intimate exchange with the power that is exercised.

59. The abuse of women by health-care workers has been documented in research conducted by universities, non-governmental organisations and government agencies (see, for example, Davis-Floyd, 2000; D'Oliveira, Grilo Diniz and Blima Schraiber, 2002; Kabakian-Khasholian et al., 2000; Koblinsky et al., 2006). Researchers and activists have claimed that the 'important' and 'disturbing' problem of disrespectful, exploitative and inhumane maternity care is particularly pertinent in developing countries (Davis-Floyd, 2000; D'Oliveira, Grilo Diniz and Blima Schraiber, 2002; Koblinsky et al., 2006). Compromised maternity care in South Africa has been a topic in the popular press for decades (see, for example, Jewkes, Abrahams and Mvo, 1998; Marks, 1994; Strydom, 2007; Terreblanche, 2007)

and remains a major issue of concern. Research in South Africa has highlighted the turbulent nature of nurse-patient relationships, specifically within the field of obstetrics (Chadwick, 2017; Chadwick, Cooper and Harries, 2014; Fonn et al., 1998; Jewkes, Abrahams and Mvo, 1998, 2001; Kruger and Schoombee, 2010; Myburgh, 2006; Penn-Kekana and Blaauw, 2002; Schoombee, Van der Merwe and Kruger, 2005). In their seminal article Jewkes, Abrahams and Mvo (1998: 1781) argue that contrary to the 'discourse of caring' that is thought to be dominant in the nursing profession, patient treatment in South Africa seems to be more strongly characterised by the 'humiliation of patients and physical abuse'. See also Frenkel, 2002; Walker and Gilson, 2004.

60. Truyts, 2016: 9–11.
61. Truyts, 2016: 10.
62. See, for instance, Dunne, Fraser and Gardner, 2014; Howell-White, 1997; Lane and Garrod, 2016; Nolte, 1998; Wilson and Sirois, 2010; Wolman et al., 1993.
63. Winnicott, 1992.
64. Winnicott (1992) would call this the 'maternal preoccupation'.
65. See Kruger, 2003b.

## Notes to Love

1. Kunitz, 2000: 183.
2. Tolstoy, 1877: 13.
3. Sweet, 2012: 16. On the front cover of Sweet's book there is quote from the renowned neurologist Oliver Sacks: 'Required reading for anyone interested in the "business" of healthcare – and especially those interested in the humanity of healthcare.'
4. Capogrosso et al. 2013.
5. As a psychodynamic therapist I pay attention not only to what is explicitly said, but also the implicit and the non-verbal. What happens in the therapeutic relationship (transference and countertransference) is crucial in directing us to what is salient in the patient's experience (Wallin, 2007). See also the section 'The Relationship: The Intersubjective Space' in the chapter *Distress*.
6. In a paper since submitted for publication Kruger and Marquard (2018) summarise the literature as follows:

> Intimate partner violence is one of the most common forms of violence experienced by South African women (Kaminer et al., 2008; Vetten, 2014). Studies have consistently found that more than half of female homicide deaths are caused by intimate male partners (a phenomenon known as 'intimate femicide'), making it the leading cause of female homicides in South Africa (Abrahams et al., 2013; Abrahams et al., 2012; World Health Organisation, 2012). One study suggests that a woman dies every six hours at the hands of an intimate partner

(Abrahams et al. 2012). While homicide rates have reportedly declined recently, intimate femicide appears disproportionately resistant to change and rape homicides have increased (Vetten, 2014). It has been said that violence against women and girls (including domestic violence, rape, sexual assault, child sexual attack, witchcraft harassment murders, sexual harassment and intimate femicide) creates 'a deeply insecure environment for South African girls and women' (Mkhize et al., 2010: 4).

Intimate partner violence exposes women to severe physical and psychological harm, as has been widely documented both globally (Black, 2011; Boonzaier, 2008; Crofford, 2007; Dekel and Andipatin, 2016; Johnson and Ferraro, 2000; Towns and Adams, 2009; Abrahams et al., 2012) and in the South African context (Gass et al., 2011; Peltzer et al., 2013; Marais, 2009; Jack, 2014). The impact of intimate partner violence has resulted in women suffering from long-term psychological reactions (for example, post-traumatic stress disorder [PTSD] and depression) in addition to the physical injuries sustained from the abuse (Marais, 2009; Mechanic, Weaver and Resick, 2008; Scheffer Lindgren and Renck, 2008; Dekel and Andipatin, 2016). Despite the destructive impact of intimate partner violence on women, research in South Africa and elsewhere suggests that women often stay in abusive relationships (Bell and Naugle, 2008; Marais, 2009; Hayes and Jeffries, 2013; Sideris, 2013; Jack, 2014; Hayes, 2015). It is estimated that a woman leaves her abusive partner between five to seven times before she leaves for the final time, or is killed (Handsel, 2007). Even when they do seek help, more than 50 per cent of women return to their partners after interventions (Seeley and Plunkett, 2002; Stark and Flitcraft, 1995; Strube and Barbour, 1983). Often, upon the return of the women to their partners, they face even more severe abuse (Jack, 2014). Mathews et al. (2004) report that the most volatile period for a woman in a violent relationship is just prior to her leaving. Furthermore, McCue (2008) has found that women who have separated from their violent partners are fourteen times more likely to report incidences of abuse by a spouse or ex-spouse.

Several international (Heim et al., 2018; Kiss et al., 2012; Peterman, Bleck and Palermo, 2015; Rose, 2015; Vyas, Mbwambo and Heise, 2015) and South African (Boonzaier, 2003; Dekel and Andipatin, 2016; Jack, 2014; Mathews et al., 2004; Marais, 2009) empirical studies have examined the structural and cultural factors influencing women's decisions to stay in violent relationships. The reasons for this decision seem to include socio-cultural norms of submission to men's authority; economic security and dependence; perceived risk to children; fear of reprisal by society; fear of further abuse; and the normalisation of abuse by the society (Dekel and Andipatin, 2016; Jack, 2014; Marais, 2009; Tshifhumulo and Mudhovozi, 2013).

For a discussion of intimate partner violence and rural, low-income mothers, see Burnett et al., 2016.

7. Boonzaier, 2003; McWilliams, 2011; Young and Gerson, 1991.
8. Motz, 2014: 38.
9. Motz, 2014.
10. Motz, 2001: 18.
11. McWilliams, 2011.
12. Gilligan (2003:1168) defines 'guilt' as follows:

> Guilt can be thought of as a defence against active aggressive wishes
> . . . When people who have developed a capacity for guilt feelings find
> themselves hating another person and experiencing wishes and impulses
> to injure them, those feelings and wishes stimulate feelings of guilt. The
> guilt feelings inhibit them from expressing or acting out those wishes,
> and motivate them to introject the anger instead, directing it against
> themselves, as a result of which they experience a need for punishment,
> which may manifest itself in masochistic or even suicidal behavior. The
> fear that underlies guilt feelings is the fear that one will kill a person
> whom one not only hates but also loves (the capacity to love others
> being a precondition for the capacity to feel guilty). Related to this is
> the fear that one will be punished by one's own conscience, or superego,
> because of having had such a guilty wish.

13. Successive waves of feminism have engaged with women's 'choosing' to stay in abusive relationships. This phenomenon, called 'adaptive preferences' or 'deformed desires', has been described as women's unconscious responses to oppression – a 'troubling, dangerous, seemingly intractable, phenomenon' (Walsh, 2015: 834). Prominent feminist philosophers such as Catherine MacKinnon and Martha Nussbaum have insisted that feminism needs a paradigm that both recognises the power of such choices and explains how oppression permeates the behaviour and consciousness of women, thus implicating the victims of patriarchy in their own oppression (Walsh, 2015). Nussbaum specifically highlights the fact that in considering why women stay in abusive relationships, attention should be paid to the reality of asymmetrical power relationships, relationships of mutual dependence and socially constructed preferences (Nussbaum, 2005). More recently, feminist scholars (Sperry, 2013; Van Schalkwyk, Boonzaier and Gobodo-Madikizela, 2014) have emphasised the importance for feminism to be 'sensitive to empirical investigation into the actual choice-making of oppressed persons in their sociotemporal context' (Sperry, 2013). If this is not acknowledged, there is the risk of 'recapitulating women's oppression by unfairly regarding such women as dupes of patriarchy' . . . To the extent that there is a choice to stay in abusive relationships, the preference is always socially constructed, as dominant discourses determine not only what a good woman is,

but also that a woman is determined by relationship (Nussbaum, 2005). When thinking about women who stay, individual women and their 'choices' should not be pathologised. Rather, it is the discourses that should be critiqued and subverted. In the words of Spivak (1998: 342–3): 'But the real force of the struggle comes from the actual players contemplating the possibility that to organize against homeworking [or trafficking/rape/domestic violence?] is not to stop being a good woman, a responsible woman, a real woman [therefore with husband and home], that there are more ways than one of being a good woman.'

14. Poststructuralist feminists working in the field of intimate partner violence have emphasised how women in abusive relationships fluctuate between positions of power and powerlessness in relation to their abusers (Enander, 2010, 2011; Hydén, 1999; Van Schalkwyk, Boonzaier and Gobodo-Madikizela, 2014).

15. Motz (2014: 38) explains:

> The awareness that there are fears and terrors that can drive people to control others so wholly, is another factor that can stop women from leaving violent men . . . Like good therapists, they understand that underneath the aggression there is so often fear, isolation and emptiness, and that violence is the way in which such people communicate this need without losing face. There can be the feeling that to transcend one's own pain and humiliation, to forgive and understand the violent partner, is the best way to act. When this self-sacrificing attitude is socially sanctioned and the partner also offers affection, attention and even care, at some times, it can be hard, if not impossible, for a battered partner to find a different voice, and to allow their own sense of outrage to surface.

16. Gilligan (2003: 1172) argues that one only has the capacity to feel guilty (a more advanced feeling than the feeling of shame) if one is aware of one's own strengths and skills. He says:

> It is only those who continue to see themselves as weak and incompetent who do not develop the capacity for guilt feelings. These are not just words or theories, nor do the examples given apply only to children. I was amazed to discover how many violent criminals still wet the bed, for example, over which their feelings of shame are almost unlimited.

There are many synonyms for being shamed: 'being slighted; insulted; disrespected; dishonoured; disgraced; disdained; demeaned; slandered; treated with contempt; ridiculed; teased; taunted; mocked; rejected; defeated; subjected to indignity or ignominy; feelings of inferiority, inadequacy, incompetence; feelings of being weak, ugly, ignorant, or poor, of being a failure; "losing face" and being treated as if you were insignificant, unimportant or worthless, or any of the numerous other forms of what psychoanalysts call "narcissistic injuries"' (Gilligan, 2003: 1155).

17. Gilligan, 2003.

18. The word 'mortification', which means 'overwhelming humiliation', comes from Latin roots that mean 'to make dead' (*mortis*, dead, and *facere*, to make).

19. Long (2019: 1) states:

   > But in the intervening centuries, that belief has evolved into something
   > we can all appreciate today: the idea that *all* human beings deserve to be
   > treated with dignity. In his new book on identity, Francis Fukuyama goes
   > as far as positing the universal existence of something the ancient Greeks
   > called *thymos* – 'the part of the soul that craves recognition of dignity'.
   > Human beings, that is, seek recognition from their peers, and when they
   > do not receive it, one of two things happens. If they feel undervalued,
   > they become resentful, and if they reckon within themselves a failure to
   > meet the standards of others, they feel ashamed. Human beings are not
   > satisfied with only food and shelter: they also want *respect*.

20. Gilligan, 2003: 1153.

21. Gilligan, 2003: 1167–8.

22. Gilligan, 2003: 1168–9.

23. N. Fraser and A. Honneth, *Redistribution or Recognition? A Political-Philosophical
    Exchange* (London: Verso, 2003), cited in Long, 2019: 17.

24. In the words of Gilligan (2003: 1157):

   > Recognition, *re-cognidon*, is both etymologically and psychologically
   > related to *re-spect*; the former derives from Latin words meaning
   > to 'know again', to 're-know', so to speak, and the latter from words
   > meaning to 'see again', to 'take a second look'. Both words imply that
   > the person is important enough to be worthy of a second look, and well
   > known enough, renowned enough, to be worthy of being re-known, ac-
   > knowledged, re-cognized.

   In another context Long (2019: 2–3) writes:

   > Human beings are first and foremost social beings, and when social
   > formations compromise the dignity of marginalized groups, the
   > consequences can be devastating, involving either self-hating shame or
   > envious resentment. For Hegel, therefore, the history of our species is
   > a history of the struggle for recognition. Human beings only become
   > conscious of themselves when recognized by others, and the failure
   > to attain this recognition must eventuate in conflict. History begins,
   > therefore, with warriors who risk their lives in order to compel their
   > adversaries to recognize them. If they succeed, they become masters
   > who are recognized without having to reciprocate, but if they fail, they
   > become slaves who must recognize their vanquishers without themselves
   > being recognized. Inside this matrix of unreciprocated recognition,
   > Hegel's famous *master-slave dialectic* takes shape, the master affirmed in
   > his dignity and the slave deprived of his humanity.

25. When love is considered, recognition and respect are central. Kohut's (2009)
    concept of mirroring is relevant here. In Nicole Krauss's novel *The History of Love*

the main character, an elderly man, poignantly talks about the very human need for recognition:

> I try to make a point of being seen. Sometimes when I'm out, I'll buy a juice even though I'm not thirsty. If the store is crowded I'll even go so far as dropping my change all over the floor, the nickels and dimes skidding in every direction . . . All I want is not to die on a day when I went unseen (Krauss, 2005: 3).

26. Farmer, 2005: 41.
27. Gilligan, 2003: 1164.
28. See, for instance, Moffett, 2006.
29. Anderson, 1999: 75.
30. Anderson, 1999: 75.
31. Gilligan, 2003: 1161; Anderson, 1999: 119.
32. See chapter on *Home*.
33. Winnicott, 1984: 125.
34. Anker, 2014: 277; English translation is from Anker, 2018: 274.
35. Smith, 2003: 138.
36. Euripides, 2002: 31.
37. In the early days of feminism Adrienne Rich (1986), a feminist poet, wrote about the invisible violence of the institution of motherhood. The anthropologist Sarah Blaffer Hrdy, in her book *Mother Instinct: A History of Mothers, Infants, and Natural Selection*, a meticulous historical, biological and psychological investigation of the idealisation of motherhood and the myth of mother instinct, writes:

    > From the 1980s onward, however, there was increasing awareness that infant abuse, neglect, abandonment and infanticide were far more widespread than even those of us who studied such phenomena had realized. I already knew that abandonment – both in humans and other animals – stretched far back in evolutionary time. I just had not realized the magnitude of what was going on (Hrdy, 1999: 25).

    She cites George Eliot: 'Mother Nature – who by the bye is an old lady with some bad habits.'

    One day, in the year 2000, Pumla Lolwana walked into a train on the Cape Flats with one child in her arms, two holding on to her hands. Athol Fugard wrote a play about this incident called *The Train Driver* and says: 'I think all of my writing life led up to the writing of "The Train Driver" because it deals with my own inherited blindness and guilt and all of what being a white South African in South Africa during those apartheid years means' (in Johnson, 2010).

38. Langenhoven, n.d. The lullaby in Afrikaans is as follows:

    *Siembamba, mamma se kindjie,*
    *siembamba mamma se kindjie,*
    *draai sy nek om, gooi hom in die sloot,*
    *trap op sy kop dan is hy dood.*

*Siembamba, ek is 'n baba,*
*Siembamba, ek is 'n baba*
*– pas my veilig op in die nood,*
*sus my liefies op die skoot.*

*Siembamba, ek is 'n seuntjie,*
*Siembamba, ek is 'n seuntjie*
*maar jy sal sien ek is net nou groot;*
*slaan maar orige kêrels dood.*

*Siembamba, ek is 'n jonkman,*
*Siembamba, ek is 'n jonkman*
*–tel my nou maar af van die skoot;*
*ek slaan self die kêrels dood.*

*Siembamba, ek is getroud nou,*
*Siembamba, ek is getroud nou*
*– maar sy dink ek is nog op die skoot,*
*wil nie glo nie ek is groot.*

*Siembamba, almal babas.*
*Siembamba, almal babas*
*– al die mans is danig groot –*
*almal babas tot hul dood.*

39. The original Afrikaans in the poem 'Lae Lewens' reads:
    *sy was my ma*
    *en sy het my geleer*
    *hoe om nie lief te wees*
    *vir myself nie* (Kamfer, 2016: 20).

40. From the Afrikaans poem 'antie Gerty, suster Kamfer, antie Trui':
    *die vrou wat haar siek*
    *leave gehou het*
    *vir wanneer iemand*
    *anders in die huis siek raak* (Kamfer, 2016: 74).

41. Currier, 2004. I am more than ever aware of the complexity of violence and the shameful secrets of violence we all carry within ourselves and our societies and how we desperately defend against this darkness by dichotomous thinking, simplification, vilification, idealisation and fierce denial. As a feminist, it was very tempting not to write about violent women – for political reasons, but also deeply personal ones.

42. Naylor, 2001.

43. Delize seems to suffer from introjective depression.

44. Kruger and Lourens, 2013. Typical symptoms of depression include depressed mood, low energy, low appetite, low libido, inability to concentrate, hopelessness, listlessness, sleep disturbance (American Psychiatric Association, 2013). See also chapter on *Distress*.

45. We write about this extensively in academic articles (Kruger and Lourens, 2013, 2016; Kruger et al., 2014) Other researchers and clinicians also acknowledge a relationship between anger and depression (Newman et al., 2006), but anger is not recognised as a symptom of adult depression in most formal diagnostic systems. Epidemiological studies investigating a link between anger and depression have found gender to be a key variable (Hill and Needham, 2013). It is more acceptable for a woman to be depressed than to be angry (Currier, 2004; Jack, 1999; Motz, 2001). Newman et al. (2006: 161) hypothesise: 'The seeming compatibility of depressive symptoms and the corresponding incompatibility of anger symptoms with the feminine gender role may greatly increase the likelihood that psychological distress in women is manifested in depression rather than anger, regardless of underlying aetiology.' The biomedical framing of a diagnosis of depression and the subsequent obscuring of anger can serve an important (if problematic) protective role in women's constructions of self (Lafrance and McKenzie-Mohr, 2013).

    The only diagnosis in the *Diagnostic and Statistical Manual of Mental Disorders* that includes anger as a symptom is intermittent explosive disorder, a diagnosis that cannot be made before the age of six or after the age of eighteen. This diagnosis includes the following criteria:
    - Severe recurrent temper outbursts manifesting verbally or behaviourally that are grossly out of proportion in intensity or duration to the situation or provocation;
    - temper outbursts inconsistent with developmental level;
    - occur on average two or three times a week;
    - mood between temper outbursts is persistent irritability or anger most days;
    - symptoms have been present for twelve months, never three months without symptoms;
    - symptoms present at least two of three settings (home, school, peers) (American Psychiatric Association, 2013).

46. Jack, 1991; Newman et al., 2006.

47. Jack (1991: 169) claims that the division between an outward self that is conforming and an angry and resentful inner self is 'the core dynamic of female depression'. Depressed women are likely to internalise anger and articulate it as self-blame and self-doubt. Other feminist psychologists assert that both suppressed anger (anger-in) and anger expressed in verbal and physical aggression (anger-out) are implicated in women's depression (Sperberg and Stabb, 1998). Blum (2007: 54) asserts that 'although overcontrol of anger, with repression of it and/or guilty self-reproach for it, is a problem, loss of control is an opposite risk . . . Occasionally loss of control threatens to follow from overcontrol, as internal pressure builds up.'

Anger also seems to play an important part in maternal depression. For instance, depressed mothers often experience recurring obsessional thoughts of harming an infant, even though they are horrified by those thoughts and keep them secret (Barr and Beck, 2008; Murray and Finn, 2012).

48. S. Freud, 'Femininity', in *Standard Edition*, 22, 112–185 (London: Hogarth Press 1964), cited in Raphael-Leff, 2010: 2.

49. Raphael-Leff, 2010: 3.

50. Dawes et al. (2005) found that 57 per cent of adults with children in a national sample reported that they had smacked their children in the past year. Of the parents, 60 per cent said that they had used a belt or another object to beat a child in the past year (33 per cent of the total sample). Women smacked children more frequently than men (70 per cent, as compared to 30 per cent). These findings suggest that females are more likely to use physical violence against children than males – perhaps not surprisingly, given that women typically spend much more time with children than men do. Although men are generally more violent than women, women tend to aim their violence at their own bodies and those of their children (Motz, 2001). Working in low-income communities, we have frequently heard accounts of women who lash out at their children in states of agitation and rage. Anecdotal reports of mothers who kill their children are not infrequent (Kruger, 2012). Recent statistics suggest that at least 40 per cent of adolescents have experienced violence (Richter et al., 2018).

51. Kruger and Lourens, 2016. See also chapter on *Hunger*.

52. Low mutuality is associated with more anger suppression and/or less control over expression of anger. As Swartz (2013) states, although the relational difficulties of volatile, angry and demanding women are often attributed to internal instability, women are often reacting to a disturbed and disturbing intersubjective field, which is situated in a specific context. See also the chapter on *Death*.

53. English translation provided by Antjie Krog, email to the author. The original Afrikaans poem reads:

> *en ek word mal*
>> *die kinders rand my aan met hulle luidrugtigheid*
>>> *selfsugtigheid*
>>> *astrandheid*
>>> *vernielsugtigheid*
>> *hulle vrese komplekse onsekerhede dreigemente node*
>> *kap my 'beeld as moeder' steaksag op die plankvloer* (Krog, 1981: 39).

54. English translation provided by Antjie Krog, email to the author. The original Afrikaans poem reads:

> *ek ruik na kots en kak en sweet*
>
> . . .
>
>> *ek is dikbek soos 'n meelsak*
>> *afgechip soos 'n melkbeker*

*my hande ouer en droër as gisteroggend se toast*
*deel slae uit halfhartig teen die kabaal* (Krog, 1981: 39).

55. See section 'The anger of melancholia' in the chapter on *Death*.

56. English translation provided by Antjie Krog, email to the author. The original Afrikaans poem reads:

*gaan sit dan hierdie sondagmôre op die treetjie*
*neither nugter nor verleë*
*en wonder*
*hoe en waarmee oorleef mens dit* (Krog, 1981: 39)?

57. Psychoanalyst Hans Loewald (1980: 393) claims: 'Without the guilty deed of parricide there is no autonomous self.' He explains that development is an ambiguous process for both children and parents. While children strive to kill their parents by 'usurping their power, their competence, their responsibility for us . . . In short, we destroy them in regard to some of their qualities hitherto most vital to us' (Loewald, 1980: 390), they feel guilty about the destruction. 'Parents resist as well as promote such destruction, no less ambivalently than children carry it out.' The only successful way in which a child can go through this inevitable process is if he/she acknowledges the guilt, bears its burden and therefore masters it. 'What will be left if things go well, is tenderness, mutual trust, and respect, the signs of equality.'

58. Stiver, 1991.

59. Stiver, 1991: 110.

60. Duras, 1985: 55.

61. Rich, 1986: 165.

62. Chodorow, 1995.

63. J. Kristeva, 'I Who Want Not to be', in *About Chinese Women*, edited by T. Moi, 138–59 (New York: Wiley-Blackwell, 1986), cited in Adams, 1994: 48.

## Notes to Labour

1. https://www.bergzichttraining.com/.

2. Foucault, 1977.

3. Kristeva, 1982.

4. Lorenz and Watkins, 2001.

5. Connolly, 2000; Lorenz and Watkins, 2001; Nichols, 1993.

6. Foucault (1980) would claim that in their larger manifestations these techniques of exclusion or mechanisms of power become economically advantageous and politically useful. Sen and Hulme (2006) cite Kristeva's work to understand social exclusion and social violence. They state that given the growing multiplicity, contingency and apparent fungibility of the identities available to individuals in the contemporary world, there is a growing sense of social uncertainty about people, situations, events, norms and even memories.

7. Williams, 1988: 11.
8. Lorde, 1984: 120.
9. See Kruger, 2005.
10. Crossley, 2007.
11. Foucault, 1980: 98.
12. Goudini is a holiday destination in Rawsonville in the Western Cape.
13. Jansen, 2015: 464.
14. Lenta, 1989: 241–2.
15. Cock, 2011: 132–3.
16. As domestic workers, women work on a full-time or part-time basis and may be employed by a single household or by multiple employers. Some domestic workers live in the household of the employer (live-in worker), but mostly the women in the valley live in their own houses (live-out). Their work includes tasks such as cleaning the house, cooking, washing and ironing clothes, taking care of children, or elderly or sick members of a family, gardening, guarding the house, driving for the family, and even taking care of household pets. Domestic workers comprise a significant part of the global workforce in informal employment and are thought to be among the most vulnerable groups of workers.
17. Maboyana and Sekaja, 2015: 114.
18. Joubert, as cited in Graham, 2014: 180–1.
19. Jansen, 2015.
20. See, for instance, Archer (2011); Cock (2011); Gama and Willemse (2015); Jansen (2015); Maboyana and Sekaja (2015); Phillips (2011); Shefer (2012).
21. Ally, 2011: 1.
22. Ally, 2011: 3.
23. Jansen, 2015.
24. Shefer, 2012.
25. Nuttall, 2009: 1.
26. McWilliams (2011: 132) defines 'splitting' as a a defence mechanism 'in which a person segregates experiences into all-good and all-bad categories, with no room for ambiguity and ambivalence'.
27. McWilliams (2011: 144) defines projection as follows:
    Projection is the process whereby what is inside is misunderstood as coming from outside. In its benign and mature forms, it is the basis for empathy. Since no one is ever able to get inside the mind of another person, we must use our capacity to project our own experience in order to understand someone else's subjective world. Intuition, leaps of nonverbal synchronicity, and peak experiences of mystical union with another person or group involve a projection of the self into the other, with powerful emotional rewards to both parties. People in love are well known for reading one another's minds in ways that they themselves cannot account for logically.

In its malignant forms, projection breeds dangerous misunderstanding and untold interpersonal damage.

28. Shefer, 2012: 314.
29. Shefer, 2012.
30. Koos Kombuis, 'Kytie', from the album *Elke Boemelaar se Droom*, 1994. The original Afrikaans lyrics are as follows:

    *Ek onthou haar nog soos gister*

    *Vandat ek so klein was, was sy daar gewees*

    *Met haar oë soos kafferbier laat sy jou dink die Mona Lisa was dalk bruin gewees*

    *Kytie Adams was die vrou geinstalleer in ons kombuis*

    *Sy kon dishes doen en klere was, die kinders oppas en vir ons maniere wys, maniere wys*

    *Kytie, Kytie, Kytie, jy't nie verniet vir 20 jaar by ons gebly*

    *Kytie, Kytie, Kytie, jy was nie net 'n meid nie, maar 'n ma vir my* (as cited in Jansen, 2015:18).

31. The original Afrikaans poem is as follows:

    *my auntie Katie was sestien toe sy in service begin*

    *werk het sy net tot standert 5 skoolgegaan*

    *my ouma auntie Katie se ma was ook 'n huishulp*

    *my auntie Katie was 'n baie glamorous vrou haar*

    *hare het altyd blonde streaks in gehad sy het net*

    *goue jewellery gedra en het nêrens sonder haar musky*

    *perfume en rouge lipstiffie gegaan nie*

    *behalwe*

    *werk toe 'n mens moet altyd jou werk met pride doen*

    *het my ouma haar gesê maar sy kon nie het sy geantwoord*

    *sy wou lyk soos*

    *sy voel het sy gesê soos die meid* (Kamfer, 2011: 38).

32. Jansen, 2015.
33. D. Cornell, 'The Ethical Affirmation of Human Rights: Gayatri Spivak's Intervention', in *Reflections on the History of an Idea: Can the Subaltern Speak?*, edited by R. Morris (New York: Colombia University Press, 2010), as cited in Krog, 2014: 60).
34. The original Afrikaans reads:

    *Die vrou langsaan bêre haar polony slices in ons fridge dis okay is dit jou dogter wat nou afgeklim het? ja, sy gaan die kind se grant haal 'n ander vrou sien gisteroggend die hond eet iets in haar jaart toe sien sy dis 'n fetus die hond was besig met die arms die oë het nog so geroer maar daar was niks meer geluid nie* (Krog, 2014: 65).

35. Long, 2017: 71.

36. Roodt, 2012.
37. Light, 2007: 4.
38. See the chapter on *Love*.
39. Dookoom, 'Larney Jou Poes', from the album *A Gangster Called Big Times*, 2014. The original Afrikaans lyrics are as follows:

   > *Ek is keelvol*
   > *Want voel ek is te keelvol, te veelvol*
   > *My siel en my liggaam, ek voel gebreklik*
   > *Ek sê net voetsek, ek brand jou*
   > *plaas af*
   > *Nou kan jy soos ek werk.*

   A literal translation of '*keelvol*' in lines 1 and 2 is 'throat-full', 'had it up to here (throat)', which gives a sense of choking.
40. De Villiers, 2011.
41. Long (2019: 15–16) says:

   > Kojève explains how the master realizes that he is on the 'wrong track [yet he] has no desire to "overcome" . . . himself as master . . . he cannot be transformed, educated . . . Mastery is the supreme given value for him, beyond which he cannot go.' Without the prospect of redemption, the master can only continue as before. Kojève again: 'The Master . . . does not work, [he] produces nothing stable outside of himself. He merely destroys the products of the Slave's work [by consuming them]. Thus his enjoyment and his satisfaction remain purely subjective: they are of interest only to him and therefore can be recognized only by him; they have no "truth", no objective reality revealed to all. Accordingly, this "consumption", this idle enjoyment of the Master's, which results from the "immediate" satisfaction of desire, can at the most procure some pleasure for man; it can never give him complete and definitive satisfaction.'

## Notes to Hunger

1. The original Afrikaans reads:

   > *As jy swaa grootwôd, slaap jy baie soedat daa minner ure innie dag moet wies. My uncle kan heeldag slaap. Toe my ma hom eendag vra hoekom hy soe slaap, antwoord hy: 'Ek is vrek honge, as ek slaap droem ek van hoe lekke ek iet dan kom maak jy my wakke. Ek was noggie ees klaa geëet'ie . . .' Honge ly kannie digter in jou ytbring én'it kan jou mal maak.*

2. Truyts, 2016: 40–3.
3. When research is conducted about food, it is clear that at least three issues relating to food and gender are prominent. First, the responsibility of feeding (food provision and preparation) is still relegated to women. Second, men and women eat

differently and are entitled to different kinds and amounts of food. Third, women, particularly in Western societies, engage in dieting and disordered eating behaviour (Caplan, 1997; Matthee, 2001).

4.  In the global mental health literature, the term 'food insecurity' is used to refer to hunger, food insecurity being defined as 'the state of being without reliable access to a sufficient quantity of affordable, nutritious food', with a substantial literature confirming that food insecurity is one of the factors operative in the association between poverty and mental health, especially in developing countries (Cole and Tembo, 2011; Maes et al., 2010). Several studies specifically link food insecurity with maternal depression (Dewing et al., 2013; Grisaru et al., 2011; Maes et al., 2010; Siefert et al., 2007).

5.  Scheper-Hughes, 1992: 130.

6.  Scheper-Hughes, 1992: 128; see also Keys, Henschel and Brožek, 1950.

7.  Scheper-Hughes, 1992: 138.

8.  Orr, 2013: 702.

9.  In the *Oxford Dictionary*, the word 'hungry implies both distress (caused by lack of food) and desire (a desire to eat). The word 'hunger' refers to a person's uncomfortable or painful experience of not having something or an adequate amount of food to eat (see also McIntyre et al., 2002; Quandt et al., 2006).

10. Devereux and Roelen, 2016: 1.

11. Matthew 6:9–13, New International Version.

12. Truyts, 2016: 119.

13. Truyts, 2016: 117–18.

14. Truyts, 2016: 119.

15. Truyts, 2016: 136.

16. Devereux and Roelen, 2016: 1.

17. Devereux and Roelen, 2016: 1.

18. Burman, 2011, 67, 68.

19. Dermott, 2012; Gillies, 2007; Jensen, 2010; Nouvet, 2014.

20. 'In this neo-liberal [Western] discourse women are expected to have what some have termed "relational autonomy", an autonomy that is already woven into relationships and forms of social belonging and points to the importance of being able to deal with everyday emergencies and sustaining the social world: "Relational autonomy can thus also be conceived as an art of living through the precarious present, as that which makes possible a continued shared existence in delicate times" (Millar, 2014: 48). The lack of relational autonomy and the distress that inevitably accompanies it has been described by Peacock, Bissell and Owen (2014: 174) as a discourse of "no legitimate dependency", in which everything is "deemed to be the responsibility of the individual, who alone should be able to manage whatever was happening to them, and where turning to others, or even acknowledging the need for help, was seen as weak and unacceptable". In their study of "lone mothers" and dignity, Wright et al. (2014: 232) found that one of the main themes emerging in

relation to the impact of poverty on dignity was women's impeded role as caregivers and how the women struggled to meet their own and their children's material needs – specifically the lack of access to adequate food for their children. They also emphasised the prominence that women gave to their role as caregivers and the negative impact on dignity when they are unable to fulfil such roles. There is a clear need to acknowledge and deal with the stigma of dependency and to acknowledge that poor people are and will be dependent on others: "The question ought not to be whether they are dependent, but rather on whom and under what conditions."' (Kruger and Lourens, 2016: 136–7).

21. With regard to the wide range of emotions elicited by hunger (and specifically by hungry children), our findings were similar to those of Nouvet (2014: 93), who found that the impoverished residents of Barrio los Heroes in Brazil were 'often visibly and sensibly agitated – angry, anxious, sad, pain-ridden, desperate, depressed – as they negotiate the hardships of their lives'. Similarly, Wright et al. (2014) describe the expressed despair of South African 'lone mothers' who struggled to meet the material needs of their children and themselves. Pike and Patil (2006: 317) also identified hunger as a major concern for women in northern Tanzania, who were very likely 'to cite fears of hunger owing to the pivotal role they play in provisioning of food in the household'.

22. Youngleson, 2007; De Villiers, 2011.

23. Raphael-Leff, 2010.

24. See chapter on *Distress*.

25. Similar feelings of guilt and shame are described in the literature. See, for instance, Wright et al. (2014), who describe how participants in their study articulated how poverty caused damage to self-esteem and led to shame.

26. 'The "good mothering" discourse of developmental psychology impacts profoundly on how governments, psychologists and mothers themselves evaluate mothering practices. This "good mothering" discourse legitimises a kind of surveillance that involves both the monitoring of how mothers care for their foetuses, infants and children and how fulfilled and happy they are while being involved with this care work. They are thus continuously faced with "the very real threat of being situated as a bad mother, arguably one of the most vilified identities possible" (Lafrance and McKenzie-Mohr, 2013: 129). If they have failed as mothers, they have also, in their own eyes and in the eyes of others, failed as women and citizens' (Kruger and Lourens, 2016: 138).

27. The association of anxiety and hunger, not surprisingly, is also consistent with the international literature on food insecurity and mental health. See, for instance, Hadley and Patil, 2006; Whitaker, Phillips and Orzol, 2006; Ivers and Cullen, 2011; McLaughlin et al., 2012.

28. Wright et al. (2014) similarly describe how impoverished women in their study stated that they feel like rejecting their children and how their participants described fantasies of infanticide.

29. Refer to chapters on *Labour* and *Love*.

30. Scheper-Hughes, 1992: 141.
31. Lubbe, 2014: 71.
32. Lubbe, 2014: 74.
33. The feelings of despondency and defeat are similar to those described by Wright et al. (2014) and Nouvet (2014), who also refer to the disengagement and paralysis of their participants.
34. Standing, 2011: 20.
35. Nouvet, 2014: 89.
36. See section on 'Discourses' in chapter on *Distress*.
37. Reid and Tom, 2006.
38. Orr, 2013: 706.
39. Pike and Patil, 2006: 317.
40. Devereux and Roelen, 2016.
41. In a chapter titled 'Smoke and Mirrors' in his book *Life within Limits: Well-Being in a World of Want*, Jackson (2011: 59) writes about being reprimanded for thinking about hunger as a metaphor. He concedes and writes about the hungry time or rainy season, but then ends the chapter looking at the metaphor of hunger – significant even in a 'world of want'.
42. According to Lyman (1989: 3), in psychology a lot of attention has been paid to eating disorders, but 'of all the activities in which we normally engage in on a daily basis, eating and the psychological effects of food has been almost totally ignored by psychologists'. This may have to do with the mind-body split and psychology traditionally being more concerned with matters of the mind, but it also may be that food and eating are associated with the feminine: 'Philosophy is masculine and disembodied; food and eating are feminine and always embodied.' See also Lupton (1996: 3); Matthee (2001).
43. Freud, 1989: 123.
44. Klein, 2011: 245.
45. Power and control, ambivalence and contradiction are always already inscribed in women's everyday relationships with food. In the words of Charles and Kerr (1986: 571), 'women's problematic relationship with food is not something peculiar to those who suffer from one or other of the eating disorders ... the characteristics of these disorders are a product of women's structural position in society and are common to almost all women'.
46. Seuss, 1990: 2.
47. https://allpoetry.com/Love-After-Love.https://allpoetry.com/Love-After-Love.
48. Klein, 1975.
49. Jackson, 2011: 60.
50. See chapter on *Labour*.
51. See chapter on *Distress*.
52. See chapter on *Distress*.
53. American Psychiatric Association, 2013.

## Notes to Distress

1. American Psychiatric Association, 2013.
2. Taylor, 2011.
3. DSM-5 criteria of major depressive disorder. See American Psychiatric Association (2013).
4. See *Prologue* and *Epilogue* (Wendy); chapter on *Home* (Eve); chapter on *Birth* (Karesha); chapter on *Love* (Delize); chapter on *Labour* (Wilmien) and chapter on *Death* (Lettie).
5. 'If we are to talk sensibly about depression, one must explicitly acknowledge that the term itself captures a very heterogeneous group of experiences . . . A major challenge to acknowledge this fundamental diversity of the experiences of depression is the current approach to the classification of the condition, which is, inadvertently, contributing to the large "treatment gaps" and the clash of ideas' (Patel, 2017: 2).
6. My pseudonym, of course, refers to Freud's Wolf Man, arguably his most famous case. Freud (1989: 403) describes the Wolf Man as follows:

   > The patient with whom I am here concerned remained for a long time unassailably entrenched behind an attitude of obliging apathy. He listened, understood, and remained unapproachable. His unimpeachable intelligence was, as it were, cut off from the instinctual forces which governed his behaviour in the few relations of life that remained to him.

7. Standard descriptive diagnostic systems such as the DSM-5 (or the ICD-10) are informed by the biomedical model. Psychoanalyst Glen Gabbard (2014: 6–7) says that practioners of this approach

   > categorize patients according to common behavioural and phenomenological features. They develop symptom checklists that allow them to classify patients according to similar clusters of symptoms. The patient's subjective experience is peripheral to the essence of psychiatric diagnosis and treatment, which must be based on observable behaviour . . . the descriptive psychiatrist is primarily interested in how a patient is similar to rather than different from other patients with congruent features.

   The psychologist working within this biomedical model will typically attempt to objectively measure the number and severity of signs and symptoms at the beginning of psychotherapy, make a diagnosis and use a prescribed treatment for that diagnosis, with 'the imperative to rely to a much greater extent on empirically supported treatments for specific disorders at the level of clinical practice' (Kagee, 2006b: 234) and, after a predetermined time period, again try to objectively measure how symptoms have improved. Treatments that lead to the improvement of symptoms as objectively measured in clinical trials are deemed to be based on objective evidence and therefore empirically supported. This focus on the biomedical model has been ostensibly informed by 'a need to ensure that the interventions rendered by clinicians have the highest chances of therapeutic success' (Kagee, 2006b: 244).

This need has been specifically emphasised in the context of developing countries such as South Africa, where it is argued that given the scarce financial resources for many users of mental health services, a low ratio of mental health professionals to the population, cultural barriers that inhibit the use of psychological services and the increasing costs of clinical training, developing countries 'can ill afford to continue to entertain the use of costly and time-consuming interventions of which the effectiveness is unknown'. With the emphasis on evidence-based therapies, data obtained from studies involving experimental designs, such as randomised controlled trials, quasi-experimental designs and time series designs, are considered to be most valid in supporting claims about therapeutic effectiveness. See Kagee (2006a, 2006b); Kagee and Breet (2015).

8. Clinicians, specifically in South Africa, have been severely criticised for their resistance to so-called evidence-based therapies, therapies that can be manualised and outsourced to non-psychologists (Kagee, 2006a, 2006b).

9. It has been suggested that the movement to establish evidence-based practice, or empirically supported therapies, as the 'gold-standard' status of practice for the medical sciences, as well as the psychological sciences, is faltering because not enough effort has gone into understanding why clinicians often do not adhere to this idealised model of using the best evidence (Gabbay and Le May, 2011; see also Patel, 2017).

10. Gabbay and Le May (2011) coined the term 'practice-based evidence' to refer to this kind of knowledge. See also Patel (2017).

11. Several psychological traditions present alternative approaches to psychiatric classification and diagnosis. These approaches have in common that humans are viewed as active agents and meaning makers, with personal meaning arising in the context of social worlds. These approaches include cognitive approaches, radical behaviourism, the interpretive or hermeneutic approach, constructivist approaches, social constructionism, critical realism, process philosophy, systemic approaches, spiritual perspectives, liberation and social justice approaches, feminist perspectives, indigenous psychology, narrative approaches, cross-cultural approaches and psychoanalytic approaches (Johnstone and Boyle, 2018).

In 2018 the Division of Clinical Psychology of the British Psychological Society, critical of the biomedical model and its philosophical assumptions ('deeply embedded in fundamental Western philosophical assumptions'), published an extensive document titled *The Power Threat Meaning Framework*, an attempt to develop an alternative to psychiatric diagnosis and classification. These problematic assumptions, they say, include, but are not limited to

the separation of mind from body, thought from feeling, the individual from the social group, and human beings from the natural world; the privileging of 'rationality' over emotion; and a belief in objectivity or the possibility of partialling out values, ethics and power from theory and practice in human systems (Johnstone and Boyle, 2018: 5).

Furthermore, 'these worldviews can broadly be described as positivism, which tends to promote a view of human beings as objects acted on by causal forces rather than agents who have reasons for their actions' (Johnstone and Boyle, 2018: 5). The document calls for approaches to psychological distress 'which allow us to see humans as active, purposeful agents, creating meaning and making choices in their lives, while at the same time subject to very real enabling and limiting factors, bodily, material, social and ideological' (Johnstone and Boyle, 2018: 6). The implications of such an approach are to acknowledge that 'patterns underpinning individual and group experiences of distress will be inseparable from their material, environmental, socio-economic and cultural contexts, and that alternatives to diagnosis need to recognize the centrality of meaning, narrative, agency and subjective experience'.

Clinicians' resistance to a rigorous and systematic adherence to a biomedical model is also based on substantial political and ideological concerns. Other examples of critiques include Bass, Bolton and Murray (2007); Fernando (2012); Myers and Gill (2004); Orr (2013); Patel (2014b, 2017) and Summerfield (2008). Feminist scholars, in particular, have been critical of the biomedical model. See, for example, Chesler (1972); Lafrance and McKenzie-Mohr (2013); Stoppard (2010); Ussher (2010).

There has been questioning of this kind of thinking not only in critical psychology, but also in the global mental health literature and the literature concerned with evidence-based treatment.

In the evidence-based treatment literature the move away from discrete diagnostic entities, as conceptualised in psychiatric diagnostic systems, can be seen, for instance, in the United States of America's National Institute of Mental Health's project, called Research Domain Criteria (RDoC). The RDoC arose from the increasing recognition of psychiatric researchers' failure to move beyond the level of subjective complaints, their failure to describe patterns that are more valid than committee-generated clusters of behavioural 'symptoms' (Insel, 2013; Insel et al., 2010; Johnstone and Boyle, 2018).

The aim of the RDoC project is to produce a diagnostic system based on underlying neurobiological and biobehavioural mechanisms of 'mental disorders' that will eventually lead to definitive treatments. In what has been termed the 'transdiagnostic conceptualization of psychopathology', there is an emphasis on identifying the core biological and psychological processes that are at the basis of clinical dysfunction, thus a new focus on aetiologies, paths and critical characteristics and how they merge and emerge (Kazdin, 2016).

Kazdin (2016) identifies several factors underlying the impetus for a transdiagnostic conceptualisation of psychopathology: There are high rates of comorbidity so that individuals (children or adults) who meet criteria for one disorder are likely to meet criteria for at least one other disorder as well; underlying processes that maintain 'different disorders' often are quite similar; several disorders share common biological underpinnings, as reflected in brain structures, neurotransmitters and genes; broad characteristics such as a general psychopathology factor (a 'p factor'), neuroticism, perfectionism and tolerance of uncertainty have been proposed as underlying factors mediating characteristics of many different disorders; a number of treatments are effective across a range of disorders, suggesting some common mechanisms or core processes in how changes occur; and when treatment focuses on a narrow and well-defined clinical problem such as depression, changes often occur across a broad range of symptoms whether or not they were targeted. See also Cuthbert and Insel (2013); Kirmayer and Crafa (2014).

The Division of Clinical Psychology of the British Psychological Society critiques the RDoC project for a number of reasons. These include its assumption that diagnosable mental disorders

> exist independent of species, time and place; its overestimation of the conceptual and methodological power of the 'tools of neuroscience' and of the data these have so far produced; its extremely limited conception and relative neglect of social context in favour of genetic and biological factors; its misunderstanding of the reciprocal and dependent relationship between brain functioning and the social world and, finally, the loss of distinctly human aspects of functioning such as language, metaphor, narrative and subjective experience (Johnstone and Boyle, 2018: 35).

Vikram Patel (2017: 2) suggests an alternative approach that takes both the dimensional approach of the RDoC project and the categorical approach of the biomedical model into account:

> Thinking dimensionally helps one understand problems, whereas acting categorically helps one solve them. Both matter to people who are experiencing depressive symptoms. One potential way forwards to find a balance between the two poles is by modifying the binary model into an ordinal one . . . from wellness through distress and disorder of increasing severity or chronicity.

12. For instance, Patel (2014b: 19), psychiatrist and global mental health expert, asserts that the biomedical model is particularly problematic when applied in the developing world. He refers to what he calls a credibility gap, a yawning gap, between 'mental health specialist communities and the rest of the world'. This gap, he says, 'is one of the major reasons for the treatment gap everywhere' (Patel, 2014b: 17). According to Patel, mental health experts (with their nosology and their treatments) seem to have lost touch with the lived emotional suffering of real people in the world, especially people in the developing world. Patel problematises what he calls 'the deliberate tilt in the balance between the personal narrative and the biomedical concept, toward the latter', arguing that 'adopting an increasingly arcane jargon of diagnostic categories to communicate with each other . . . we have lost the ability to communicate with virtually everyone else in our communities'.

His point is not that diagnostic categories are useless or that the neurobiology of emotions is not important, but he suggests that the use of such labels and their associated biomedical explanations may be unnecessary or even counterproductive. He talks about the fact that 'certain mental illness categories, such as depression, in particular, do not travel well across cultures. The critique is that the use of such labels represents a medicalisation of a social condition where the solutions lie not within a medical approach, but more likely within the social or political sphere (Patel, 2014a: 44). Patel advocates for

> the replacement of rigid diagnostic systems . . . much more suited to psychiatry and the specialized mental healthcare systems you might encounter in developed countries, with broader, more public health-oriented and contextually appropriate labels and diagnostic systems that communicate better to local policymakers, primary care workers and most importantly, to local communities (Patel 2014a: 44).

Patel's (2014b: 17) argument that 'diagnostic categories [can] reflect a medicalization of normative phenomena' that may impose 'artificial dichotomies imposed on naturally occurring dimensions of psychological responses to common human life experiences' is not a new one. Very important, however, is that he highlights the danger of adopting this approach in the developing world, where emotional suffering is perhaps even more 'inextricably linked to powerful social and cultural determinants and with a person's own identity of oneself'. He states:

> A key lesson from programs seeking to enhance access to care and the acceptability of psychological treatment for depression in the global context is that most innovators avoid psychiatric labels in favour of contextually informed metaphors and explanations. Idioms . . . are less stigmatizing and widely understood, and they seamlessly capture the continuum of distress and disorder. Such approaches, which are aligned with the idioms of distress, can lead to a dramatic increase in demand for care, an essential prerequisite to ensuring that people move from more severe stages to milder ones and ultimately towards wellbeing (Patel, 2017: 6).

This concern is even more relevant when it comes to women in the developing world. While the movement for global mental health has identified women as a group of focus, critics have pointed out that the biomedical model adopted by this movement has served to silence women's voices in various ways (Burgess, 2016: 79).

First, if psychiatric diagnosis is used as the lens when women are asked about their distress, certain aspects of women's lives are left out and not considered worthy of treatment. This is particularly true if structured diagnostic interviews or questionnaires are used, but it is also true if qualitative data is approached with a diagnostic lens (Kruger et al., 2014; Stoppard, 2000).

Second, the medicalisation of women's distress situates the problem in the individual, rather than in social processes and thus reduces the complexity of stark social realities to biomedical conditions (Burgess and Campbell, 2014; Kruger et al., 2014; Stoppard, 2000).

Third, in such approaches to distress, women who are already disempowered become the objects of treatment, rather than autonomous subjects. In the words of Burgess (2016: 92): 'Furthermore, women have very limited spaces to contribute to the shape of services, or engage in action on the issues they identify as problematic in their lives, as treatment approaches are narrowly defined prior to their exposure, often linked to interventions designed in high-income country settings.'

13. Of course, this is not to imply that the biomedical model is not useful for communication between health professionals, patients and their families. The biomedical model is also useful in allowing for third-party reimbursements, labelling in legal proceedings and, in some cases, treatment planning.

14. Freud, 1989: 732.

15. McWilliams, 2011.

16. Gabbard (2014: 70) highlights several differences between psychodynamic assessment and psychiatric or medical assessment. In medical interviewing, physicians pursue a direct course from the chief complaint to its aetiology and pathogenesis, while psychologists 'who attempt to steer a linear course in the clinical interview will encounter potholes and detours at every turn'. This, Gabbard asserts, has to do with the fact that people often don't know what is really bothering them; they may feel ambivalent about what bothers them or even embarrassed or ashamed.

The interrelationship between diagnosis and treatment is different in psychodynamic assessment. In medical interviewing, diagnosis precedes treatment. In psychodynamic interviewing, the distinction is thought to be artificial. The initial interview and the way it is conducted may of itself be therapeutic. Gabbard (2014: 3) cites Karl Menninger as saying, 'The patient comes to be treated and everything that is done for him, so far as he is concerned, is treatment, whatever the doctor may call it. In a sense, therefore, treatment always precedes diagnosis.'

While a patient, to a large extent, is a passive participant in the medical assessment process, the psychodynamic approach 'involves actively engaging the patient as a collaborator in an exploratory process' (Gabbard, 2014: 71). Gabbard (2014: 77) states:

> If a patient begins an interview with anxiety, the psychiatrist does not try to eliminate it to facilitate the interview. On the contrary, the psychiatrist might attempt to engage the patient in a collaborative search for the origins of the anxiety with such questions as: 'What concerns about this interview might cause you to be anxious right now?' 'Does this situation remind you of any similar anxiety-provoking situations in the past?' or 'Have you heard anything about me or about psychiatrists in general that might contribute to your anxiety?'

The psychodynamic assessment process does not stop with the collection of signs and symptoms. The intrapsychic life of the patient is a crucial part of the data pool. For the therapist to get to know the patient as a person, the establishment of the therapeutic relationship is as important as getting to know the signs and symptoms.

In psychodynamic assessment, there is an emphasis on the clinician's feelings. For the therapist, her feelings about the patient constitute crucial information, as they tell the clinician what reactions the patient elicits in others. Countertransference is therefore of central importance.

17. McWilliams, 1999. Depending on their theoretical paradigm, clinicians have different questions that they want to answer when assessing a patient to determine how they will treat them. While psychological signs and symptoms are the main focus in psychiatric diagnosis, practising clinicians often have more complex assessment strategies. The assessment strategy outlined here is informed by psychodynamic theory, loosely based on McWilliams's (1999) approach. She proposes the following assessment areas: assessing what cannot be changed; assessing developmental issues; assessing defences; assessing affects; assessing identifications; assessing relational patterns; assessing self-esteem; and assessing pathogenic beliefs.

18. Ivey, 2006: 325.

19. Gabbard, 2014: 7.

20. Orange, 2005: xii. The British Psychological Society strongly recommends that the question at the heart of medicalisation ('What is wrong with you?') should be replaced with five others: 'What has happened to you?' 'How did it affect you?' 'What kind of threats does this pose?' 'What sense did you make of it?' and 'What did you have to do to survive?' (Johnstone and Boyle, 2018: 27).

21. Gabbard, 2014.

22. Bantjes and Swartz, 2017: 516–17.

23. These include intersubjective psychoanalysts (for example, Orange, Atwood and Stolorow, 1997), relational psychoanalysts (for example, Greenberg and Mitchell, 1983), self-psychologists (for example, Kohut, 1971) and feminist therapists (for example, Benjamin, 1988).

24. McWilliams, 1999: 103.

25. McWilliams, 1999: 103.

26. Much has been written about the exercise of mindfulness. Mindfulness refers to the concentrating of attention deliberately and non-judgementally on the breadth of experience in the present moment. It also facilitates disembedding and disidentification from problematic mental states (Wallin, 2007).

27. Wallin, 2007. Mentalisation refers to the capacity to think about one's own feelings and the feelings of others. The more one is able to think about feelings, the more agency and self-control one is thought to have.

28. Wallin, 2007.

29. Psychoanalytic theorists such as Bion (1967) and Ogden (2004) assert that countertransference does not only represent the activation of the therapist's

own unconscious archaic object relations, but is also a result of the projective identifications of the patient. Countertransference is thus thought of as an empathic regression on the part of the therapist, potentially facilitating emotional contact with the patient by enabling the therapist to understand much about the patient's unconscious fantasies and anxieties (Ogden, 2004).

For Bion (1967), 'normal projective identification' is not only the single most important medium of communication in infancy, it is also the most significant form of interaction between patients and therapists. Building on Klein's notion that projective identification impacts on the way the patient sees the analyst, Bion asserts that the patient's actions induce the analyst to feel what the patient unconsciously wants her to feel. Betty Joseph, extending Bion's understanding of projective identification, shows how the patient constantly but unconsciously 'nudges the therapist to act out in accordance with the patient's internal situation' (Spillius, 1992: 73).

30. Ogden (1994: 3) calls this mutuality and recognition the 'analytic third'.
31. Esprey, 2013: 45.
32. Dimen, 2011: 45.
33. Constructions of femininity dictate that 'good' women are calm, in control and self-sacrificing in relationships and that they engage in self-silencing feelings or behaviours in order to conform to these ideals (Jack, 1999; Newman et al., 2006).
34. McWilliams (1999) identifies typical unconscious phenomena: a sense of weakness (risk of psychic decompensation, fragmentation, annihilation), vanity (vulnerability to shame, aspirations to perfection, fantasies of omnipotence, specialness, and entitlement), conflict (tensions between wishes and prohibitions, ambivalence, pursuit of mutually exclusive aims), moral deficit (self-deception, temptation to be self-righteous, blindness to reality and consequences of actions), lust, greed, competition and aggression. See also Kruger (2006b).
35. Bion, 1962b: 183; Winnicott, 1992: 57.
36. Freud (with Marx and Nietzsche) has been called one of the masters of suspicion. They directed our critical attention to the seemingly transparent nature of consciousness, common sense, ordinary language and everyday structures. Freud's psychoanalytic theory pushes us in the direction of the gaps, urging us to focus on what has been left out, seducing me into what D.H. Lawrence called 'the cavern of dreams'. Psychodynamic therapists are suspicious of everything that is certain, proven and even empirically verified. We are interested in the holes, the openings, the breaks, the breaches, the cracks, the spaces, the pauses, the silences, the interruptions and the lulls. Consciousness (identity, a sense of coherence, mental well-being) is always unstable, always at risk of sabotage from the unacceptable feelings of loss and desire, which we have to repress in the unconscious to conform to culture (Greenberg and Mitchell, 1983: 21; see also Kruger, 2006b).
37. Important here is the difference between an anaclitic depressive defensive style (more shame-based) and introjecting depressive defensive style (more guilt-based) (Blatt,

Shafar and Zuroff, 2001; Blatt and Zuroff, 1992; McWilliams, 2011). Anaclytic depression is more narcissistic and is characterised by feelings of emptiness, loneliness, neediness, hunger and meaninglessness. Introjecting depression is more melancholic and the person suffering from this kind of depression feels bad about herself and evil, flawed, self-indulgent and guilty.

38. In this case the therapist is experiencing a lot first-hand, as the interview is conducted in Dora's house. Mostly we have to rely on the patient's descriptions of her external world. The point is not to get a photographic or objective glimpse of the patient's external world, it is to get a sense of how this world is internalised.

39. La Vita, 2014.

40. Bronfenbrenner's (1979) bio-ecological frameworks also emphasise interrelatedness of the individual and her environment. In his bi-directional model he identifies four systems: the micro-system, meso-system (family, school, peers), exo-system (neighbours, local politics and mass media) and macro-system (attitudes and cultural ideology). He argues that all these systems impact on how individuals understand themselves and their behaviour.

41. The British Psychological Society lists some of the most important contextual factors that play a role in the development and maintenance of psychological, emotional and behavioural problems: social class and poverty; income inequalities; unemployment; childhood neglect and sexual, physical and emotional abuse; sexual and domestic violence; belonging to subordinate social groups; war and other life-threatening events; bullying, harassment and discrimination and significant losses, such as the loss of a parent in childhood (Johnstone and Boyle, 2018: 92).

42. In the biomedical model, also sometimes referred to as the biopsychosocial model, there is also an acknowledgement that contextual issues are implicated in psychopathology. The difference here is that we are not focusing on how these factors impact on an individual. We are interested in how the outside world is internalised and becomes part of the psyche of the individual. The psychologist thus cannot pass on social and political problems to social workers and politicians, but has to work with the mental representations of these worlds in the patients and communities she works with.

43. https://www.poetryfoundation.org/poems/48419/this-be-the-verse.

44. In the biomedical model the interest is mostly in current symptoms and signs, a cross-sectional view of the patient. To the extent that there is an interest in history, it is mostly focused on the course of the illness, the history of the symptoms and signs. While in most psychiatric textbooks assessment includes taking a full developmental and familial history, it is asserted by some that 'the practice of conducting psychohistories also falls into the category of non-falsifiable activities, since a psychohistory, by definition, is *post hoc* activity that has no predictive component. Psychological analyses of this nature therefore can never be shown to be incorrect' (Kagee, 2006b: 236).

45. McWilliams, 1999.

46. See chapter on *Love*.
47. Lorde, 1973: 235.
48. Dawn Garisch (2012) titled her one of her books *Eloquent Body*.
49. Donna Wilshire describes a distinction in the Western positivist world between what she calls 'male knowledge' and 'female knowledge'. Male knowledge is 'true or higher knowledge', associated with words such as mind (ideas), head, spirit, reason (rationality), order, control, objectivity, public, detached, linear, permanent, changeless and immortal. Female knowledge, which is construed in binary opposition to this male knowledge, is lower knowledge and is associated with words like body, womb, nature, emotion, feelings, chaos, subjectivity, the private sphere and process. She focuses on how information that women obtain from their bodies (through the heat of the body, the blood of the body) should not be marginalised:

    > Women's blood is not a peripheral issue in devising a feminist epistemology . . . Respecting the 'private' and 'down inside' as places where knowledge is, respecting the minding body, respecting the way a woman 'is in the world', respecting being female as a method and technique for gathering and defining what can be or ought to be known, and respecting being female and the female body as a way of knowing . . . all these respects are essential ways in which humans know; they should be accounted for in an epistemology (Wilshire, 1989: 108).

50. Much has been written about somatisation, especially in non-Western cultures. Somatisation is defined as the 'cultural patterning of psychological disorders into a language of distress of mainly physical symptoms and signs' (Helman, 2001: 182) or the 'presentation of personal and interpersonal distress in an idiom of physical complaints together with a coping pattern of medical help-seeking' (Kleinman, 1986: 51). It is argued that in certain cultures this is the preferred 'idiom of distress' or 'language of distress', but as clinicians we see this in all contexts (Kadish, 2012).

51. Discourse refers to structures of knowledge that are embedded in particular historical and social relations of power (Squire, 1998). 'Identities are actively negotiated and transformed in discourse', meaning that language is the area where 'strategic construction and reconstruction of self occurs' (Marshall and Wetherall, 1989: 125).

    The individual is thus both a product of discourse and constitutive of it. Dominant discourses set an acceptable range of actions that are governed by the discourse. Self-surveillance and self-policing are central to this disciplinary process, in which individuals 'incorporate the "gaze" of external social structures, including dominant cultural ideas and practices, which embody certain prescriptions for thinking and living' (O'Grady, 2005: 18). The British Psychological Society (Johnstone and Boyle, 2018: 95) says about the contribution of Foucault:

    > His interest was in power as exercised rather than possessed, as relational rather than top-down, as pervading every social interaction and reaching 'into the depth of society – to the bodies, wills, thoughts, conduct and everyday life' of all of us (O'Grady, 2005: 18).

He saw language and the production of knowledge as inseparable from systems of power and, above all, saw these systems as creative and productive rather than repressive, in their ability to create norms, standards, identities and desires. This obviously overlaps with the notion of ideological power . . . both are crucial in shaping the meaning of events and experiences. The threats here are subtler – invalidation through imposition of others' meaning; shame and humiliation; loss of valued identities or imposition of devalued identities.

We therefore need to understand how individual subjectivities have been constructed by prevailing discourses and cultural practices. Discourse determines what can intelligibly be thought and said about the world.

All of this means that we have to pay attention to the underlying discourses that inform the emotions that our patients experience. In trying to understand the distress of our patients, we need to understand the dominant discourses that they compare themselves with and the shame caused by the failure to live up to the ideals.

52. I. Parker, 1997; Youngleson, 2007.

53. See also chapters on *Love* and *Birth*.

54. Although neo-liberalism involves a set of economic policies, like all economic systems it also makes strong assumptions about human behaviour, in that it requires people to behave in certain ways and believe certain things about themselves in order to function within the system. The interdependence between the political economy of neo-liberalism and psychology and psychiatry involves several processes. The first is placing a high value on hypothesised intrapsychic attributes (rather than social institutions or structures) said to be necessary and even sufficient for success, such as aspiration, motivation, internal locus of control, self-esteem, character and resilience (Johnstone and Boyle, 2018: 45). The second is encouraging people to find meaning in life through consumption and measuring their personal success by their income and material possessions. Last is hiding the damaging effects of economic systems by individualising and pathologising them in individuals. Neo-liberal policies have been associated not only with materialist attitudes, but also with greatly increased inequality, fragmentation of communities and damage to the environment (Chomsky and McChesney, 2011; Klein, 2007; Sayer, 2016). Inequality is associated with increased levels of emotional and behavioural problems at all levels of society, even the most privileged (Johnstone and Boyle, 2018: 46). Psychiatry has a long tradition of writers who have linked the medicalisation and individualisation of distress and 'deviance' to social control and social injustice (Cooper, 1971; Foucault, 1961; Ingleby, 1981; Laing, 1967; Rose, 1985; Scheff, 1966; Szasz, 1974).

55. Jo, 2013: 518–19.

56. Gilbert, 1998: 22.

57. Chase and Walker, 2013: 740.
58. Orange, 2009.
59. Orange, Atwood and Stolorow, 1997.
60. McWilliams, 2011.
61. Taylor, 2011.
62. McWilliams, 1999: 158.
63. 'This position is enabled by enduring and often limited views of women's agency and the agency of mentally distressed individuals. Within wider development discourse, women's agency has been problematically viewed as valid only in instances where it is in line with a neo-liberal logic: discrete, visible acts that reject social norms viewed as problematic by global, high-income partners' (Burgess, 2016: 92; see also Madhok, 2013; Mannell, 2014). Burgess continues:

    > Alternatively, further arguments seek to highlight the agency visible in the absence of action, or 'small wins', as they may be more accurate indications of how women are able to act within the realities of their social environments. When applied to the sphere of global mental health, neoliberal logic frames women as empowered agents when they engage in the project of improving their mental health through engagement and adherence to the services provided. This idea is supported by the emphasis on secondary prevention that promotes increased knowledge and training for local women about mental health issues within the Western framework of mental distress.

    Within the patient-practitioner dialogue, women's accounts are over-ridden by the expertise of the practitioner, who seeks to provide help within their own framework of understanding of the problem (Burgess, 2016).
64. Gabbard, 2014: 75; see also Langellier, 1989.
65. This conception of language is based on very specific epistemological assumptions in which knowledge is not equated to truth. In such a postmodern epistemology, the focus is language – in other words, the signifying activities of a collection of subjects. Ferdinand de Saussure's classic distinction in *Course in Linguistics* between the signifier (utterable words), the signified (lexically definable meaning) and the referents (the objects themselves) states: 'Without language, i.e. apart from its expression in spoken or written words, thought is only a shapeless and indistinct mass, a vague uncharted nebula' (Saussure, cited in Hudson, 1986: 4).
66. Bakhtin, 1981: 293.
67. Postmodern notions of subjectivity resist the idea of a unified subject, contesting the notion of one telling. The task of the therapist is not to explain the story or to find another master story, the task is to listen for what is left out, for unusual verbalisations and affect in order to find out what is obscured in the narrative:

    > The very breakdown of narrative order, the temporary chaos which is provoked, may, in itself, be vital to a creative process, a reorganization of experience into   far more complex and flexible patterns . . . I am

claiming that the real task in therapy is not so much making sense of the data as it is, but resisting the temptation to make sense of the data (Levenson, 1988: 193).

This take on narrative corresponds with how Freud approached narratives:

Freud . . . construed the patient's life not as a coherent narrative of unearthed historical facts, but as a subversive, overdetermined, and endlessly unfolding story – a narrative saturated with secrets, ambiguities, and multiple meanings. Viewing coherent narratives as the work of the censoring era, as a defence, Freud searched for the points of discontinuity where the narrative 'stumbles' or fails (Loewenstein, 1991: 24).

68. In psychoanalytic terms, another way of putting it is that we use language defensively, to defend ourselves against ourselves and our reality. The individual deals with her own 'polyvalence, multiplicity, fluidity, indeterminacy, open-endedness, fragmentation' by escaping into a coherent and sensible narrative (Hirsch, 1989: 39).

According to Mischler (1984), narrative can either be understood through a broad or pragmatic view or in terms of a narrow view. According to the broad view, narrative is understood as the way in which people transform knowing into telling. In the narrower view of narrative, it is regarded as one particular strategy or mode of telling. See also Kruger (2003b, 2005).

69. Hirsch, 1989: 9.

70. Schafer, 1992.

71. According to Foucault (2002: 88):

One no longer attempts to uncover the great enigmatic statements that lie hidden beneath its signs, one asks how it functions; what representation it designates, what elements it cuts out and removes, how it analyses and composes, what play of substitution enables it to accomplish its role of representation. Commentary has yielded to criticism.

72. Orange, 2011: 197.

73. Scarry, 1985.

74. See chapter on *Birth*.

75. The unspeakable is different from the unspoken. In psychoanalytic language it refers to the unconscious or the unthought known (Bollas, 1987).

76. Orange, 2011: 201.

77. See chapter on *Death*.

78. Frosh, 1989: 135.

79. See Hartley and Kruger, 2017.

80. Baldwin, cited in Als, 2017. In *Nothing Personal*, Baldwin also quotes the lyrics to an old Bessie Smith tune: 'It's a long road . . . I picked up my bag, baby, and tried again . . . / You can't trust nobody, you might as well be alone / Found my long-lost friend, and I might as well have stayed home!'

81. White, 2000.
82. Beutler, cited in Tong, 2010.
83. Freud, 1912.
84. Freud, 1912.
85. This includes classical Freudian theory, ego psychology, object relations theory, self-psychology, relational psychoanalysis and inter-subjective psychoanalysis.
86. Mitchell and Black, 1995: 206.
87. Mitchell and Black, 1995: 252.
88. Ogden, 1999: 197.
89. Ogden, 1997: 594.
90. Ogden, 1997: 567.
91. Ogden, 1997: 568.
92. Ogden, 2005: 6; see also Tronick, 2003. Co-creative processes produce unique forms of being together, not only in the mother-infant relationship, but in all relationships.
93. McWilliams, 1999: 2.
94. Orange, 2011.
95. Orange, 2006: 7.
96. Interestingly enough, in the global mental health field, with its emphasis on diagnosis and manualised treatments, it is also acknowledged by practitioners that certain common factors in psychotherapy are vital for successful treatment, regardless of the specific technique. Common factors refer to those practices assumed to be universal for delivery of any effective psychotherapy (Barth et al., 2012). Therefore, if one is starting with non-specialists, they need to be competent in these common factors first before teaching them the required treatment-specific skills. Competency in common factors contributes to phenomena such as the 'primary care paradox', the observation that some conditions can be well treated by generalists despite delivery of manualised care that is of lesser technical proficiency (Stange and Ferrer, 2009). Unfortunately, common factors have received limited attention in low- to middle-income countries (Jordans et al., 2013; Kabura, Fleming and Tobin, 2005) despite their importance for care delivered by non-specialists.

    Common factors have been categorised differently by scholars (Frank and Frank, 1993; Lambert and Bergin, 1994; Rosenzweig, 1936; Wampold, 2011), but the main domains relate to therapist qualities and therapeutic alliance, mobilisation of client and extra-contextual factors, promoting hope and expectancy of change, collaborative goal setting, ritualised procedures to work towards that goal, eliciting feedback, explanation for treatment grounded in a patient's belief system, and a healing setting.

    Kohrt et al. (2015) identify the following common factors that counsellors should be assessed for: non-verbal communication and active listening; eye contact; facial expression; body language and gestures; verbal communication skills; open-ended questions; summarising and clarifying statements; rapport building and appropriate self-disclosure; exploration, interpretation and normalisation of feelings; demonstration of empathy, warmth and genuineness; assessment of functioning and impact on life; exploration of patient's and social support networks explanation for problem; incorporation of coping mechanisms and prior solutions; assessment of patient's recent life events and acknowledgement of impact on psychosocial well-being; assessment of other mental health problems, alcohol/drug use and physical health problems; appropriate involvement of family members and other caregivers; collaborative goal setting and addressing patient's expectations; promotion of realistic hope for change; psychoeducation incorporating local (ethnopsychological) concepts and themes; use of problem-solving steps (problem formulation, prioritisation, solution generation and action planning); elicitation of feedback when providing advice, suggestions and recommendations; explanation and promotion of confidentiality; assessment of harm to self, harm to other, harm from others and developing a collaborative response plan.

97. Roth, 2000: 93–111.
98. See Hartley and Kruger, 2017. This take on psychotherapy corresponds with Bacal's (2017: 11) notion of 'specificity theory', which regards the effectiveness of psychodynamic therapy as 'fundamentally determined by therapeutic possibility that becomes available to a particular dyad in the moment and over time'. Bacal (2017: 13) continues:

> The *sine qua non* of psychoanalytic psychotherapy is not empathy culminated by verbal interpretation as the response . . . but the entire process that includes understanding the complex mental/emotional states of another, and discerning responses that may be therapeutic for the patient, and possible for that analyst, in the uniqueness of the unfolding process.

Generally, in contemporary psychoanalytic thinking, the uniqueness and the complexity of each individual patient is thought to imply that we need to be open to different psychoanalytic perspectives in order to best serve those we treat (Ivey, 2006; Kruger et al., 2014; McWilliams, 1999, 2011; Swartz, 1999; Teicholz, 2006; Wallin, 2007). It is also argued treatment is shaped not only by the dynamics of the patient, but also by what the therapist brings to the interaction. In other words, the analytic third (Benjamin, 2004; Ogden, 1994) or the intersubjective space (Orange, Atwood and Stolorow, 1997) will also determine what theory or theories will be useful for a particular therapist working with a particular patient. While it is acknowledged that mixing concepts from different psychodynamic schools without knowledge of the different nuances and assumptions of each theory and its unique language can be problematic and confusing conceptually, recognising complementarity of the theories means that therapists are able to select from a broader range of approaches for different patients and also to move between theories as our understanding of the patient and his/her needs shift (McWilliams, 2011).

99. However, if the projection is not accepted by the mother or therapist and the sense impressions are not digested by being named or thought about, they are not transformed and remain as beta-elements. The infant has to reintroject not a fear or anxiety made tolerable, but undigested elements that may potentially overwhelm her. This uncomfortable feeling of anticipating something with great apprehension or fear (the world is a bad and unsafe place) can become too great and the individual will either become psychotic or use other defences, such as acting out, to deal with the nameless or unknown dread. Similarly, in therapy, patients who do not feel contained will deal with the nameless dread by defending against it.

On a societal level, one can understand that in such unequal relationships where one party is expected to make themselves very vulnerable, both the carer and the one taken care of may end up with unmetabolised distress, which may be experienced as a kind of dread that is not named and not understood. This nameless dread, if not received and metabolised, will heighten the possibility of the other being experienced as persecutory, enhance the chances of a fight/flight response and thus destroy the potential for a caring relationship (Kruger, 2016).

100. Flyvbjerg, 2006.

101. In the words of Freud (1989: 375–6):

It is not difficult for the skilled analyst to read the patient's secret wishes plainly between the lines of his complaints and the story of his illness, but what a measure of self-complacency and thoughtlessness must be possessed by anyone who can, on the shortest acquaintance, inform a stranger who is entirely ignorant of all the tenets of analysis that he is attached to his mother by incestuous ties, that he harbours wishes for the death of his wife whom he appears to love . . . and so on . . . the truer the guess the more violent will be the resistance . . . Even in the later stages of the analysis one must be careful not to give a patient the solution of a symptom or the translation of a wish until he is already so close to it that he has only one short step to make in order to get hold of the explanation for himself.

102. I would argue that one way of excluding the painful experience of poverty is not to engage, not to apply our powerful theoretical tools to the raw data of qualitative investigations – to leave such data as if it spoke for itself: the 'voices of the poor' (Narayan, 2000), transparent, opaque, obvious, self-evident and innocent (Brock, 2002; Du Toit, 2002, 2004, 2005; Narayan and Petesch, 2002). One can perhaps say that what is common in quantitative and qualitative psychological research and psychological practice, is a reluctance – some would say a refusal – to engage psychologically with the complex subjectivity of the poor person herself. In an early commentary, Swartz (1991) comments on the fact that psychologists are racist and classist because when they deal with white, middle-class people they explore object relations, but if they deal with poor, black people they focus on

context. As my colleague Ronald Davis, clinical psychologist for the Department of Health, remarked: 'Where is the psychology in mental health?'

103. Wallin, 2007: 175. Wallin refers to the conflicting impulses in therapists and patients, which mean that while at times a new and needed relationship is activated, sometimes a relationship is repeated This activation of the repeated relationship often happens in implicit ways, through unconscious processes such as projective identification (Spillius and O'Shaughnessy, 2013).

Bion (1967) asserts that while projective identification is inevitable and an important way of communicating, the mother (or the therapist) should, through her organisational capacities (maternal reverie) attempt to metabolise and reintegrate the child's emotional states. In this process, unmetabolised affective experiences (beta elements) are transformed into thoughts that can be thought about (alpha elements). Such thought processes help the baby to cope with feelings and to deal with her frustration. In other words, the mother (or therapist) has the task of translating the child (or the patient's) distress by giving names 'to its hardships and anxieties and thus calms and contains it' (Biran, 2003: 491). The maternal mind (or therapist) thus becomes a container for the projections of child (or patient). Normal development follows if the relationship between infant and mother permits the infant to project a feeling into the mother and to reintroject it after it has been metabolised, detoxified and made tolerable to the infant psyche. The idea is that the child or the patient will eventually learn to carry out these transformations for themselves (Borgogno, Merciai and Talamo, 1998: 95).

104. Kruger and Lourens, 2016.

105. The original Afrikaans text is as follows:

> As daa niks daa geskrywe innie margins staanie issit ma net oo dai stories nooit geskryf wod ie, of truthfully geskryf wod ie . . . Daa is niks meer unimportant as die liewens van arm mense nie. As arm mense doodgan, los hulle niks agte nie, niks trace dat hulle exist et nie. Vi my is my writing history as told by the losers.

106. Farmer, 2005: 50.

107. Kohut, 1984: 200. Kohut says that 'an individual wants to be surrounded by humans whom she experiences as essentially human rather than as not-human or as things. If she is unable to experience them as human, she cannot experience herself as human' (in Kottler and Togashi, 2015: 18). Self-psychology asserts that 'a twinship self-object experience serves the function of humanization, that is, the developmental process of coming to feel human' (Kottler and Togashi 2015: 19). Writing about Kohut's notion of the importance of becoming human or experiencing ourselves as human, Bacal (2017: 14) writes about his own therapy with Kohut, saying that what is needed in therapy is 'acceptance and optimism, delivered with warmth and kindness'.

108. Certainly, this suggests that manualised care is highly unlikely to be effective, specifically in low-income contexts or 'low-resource settings' where the origins of pain are arguably more complex than in other settings.

109. Most clinicians will agree that symptom relief can be a goal of psychotherapy, but is often not the primary goal or the only goal. For instance, McWilliams (2011) identifies the following important outcomes of psychotherapy: symptom relief, insight, agency, identity, recognition and handling of feelings, ego strength and self-cohesion, capacity to love and work, mature dependency and pleasure and serenity. Psychodynamic therapist Samuel Roth (2000) does not even include symptom relief on his list of desirable treatment outcomes. He prioritises emotional stability, integrity, honesty, discretion, self-knowledge, insight, openness to others, ability to engage in human relationships, empathy and tolerance of feedback and criticism as desirable treatment outcomes.
110. See chapter on *Hunger*.
111. Kohut, 1984: 200.

## Notes to Death

1. Szymborska, 1988: 95.
2. Szymborska, 1988: 95.
3. In my experience of utter helplessness and shame, I probably felt something that she felt (concordant countertransference), as well as something felt by all those who interact with her (complementary countertransference) (Wallin, 2007: 271).
4. Steinberg, 2015a: 326.
5. The original Afrikaans text is as follows:

   *Ek wiet vanne familie waa die hele familie behalwe die een suste in een jaa dood gegan 'et, ek wiet van klomp broes wie 'n jaa offe paa maande ytmekaa doodgeskiet was. Die mense wat agtebly move an, accept 'it as 'n normal part vanne painful life, sonne om te acknowledge meeste vannie tyd dat 'it 'n painful existence is. Is soes fantasy en reality wat seamlessly begin melt met tyd* (La Vita 2014).

6. As discussed in some detail in the chapter on *Hunger*, in general, social and political inequalities are often implicated in women's distress, but 'these are often eclipsed from view when suffering and challenge are understood as psychiatric illness' (Lafrance and McKenzie-Mohr, 2013). The persistent finding that poverty is one of the most consistent predictors of depression in women (Belle and Doucet, 2003; Dermott, 2012) seems more complex in my work. Women do not seem to be distressed about being poor per se, they seem particularly distressed and angry at not being able to provide for their children. It is clear that the emotional experience of motherhood is profoundly impacted upon by the social reality of poverty (Collins, 1994a, 1994b; Gillies, 2007; Kruger et al., 2014). Implicit in the women's stories is the ideal of the all-providing, ever-giving, self-sacrificing mother (Bassin, Honey and Kaplan, 1994), an ideal that the women cannot live up to, given the context within which they are mothering. This ideal is also prominent in notions of best-practice parenting, prominent in developmental psychology, where the care

of children is often viewed as a 'classless activity' (Gillies, 2007: 7), which fails to recognise that there is a profound interaction between parenting and poverty (Dermott, 2012).

7. Raphael-Leff, 2010.
8. Blum, 2007.
9. Weissmann, Paykel and Klerman, 1972:106.
10. Motz, 2001.
11. Gillies, 2007; Stoppard, 2010.
12. Gillies, 2007.
13. Like the working-class mothers in Gillies's study (2007: 84), the low-income mothers in the valley do not buy into middle-class, Westernised notions of sensitive mothering and democratic parenting. Their focus is more on 'remaining in control and steering . . . children towards a respectable future'. They seek to control their children through surveillance and discipline, perhaps understanding that, for a working-class child, the values of trust, obligation and mutual responsibility are more crucial than a child's agency and uniqueness (Gillies, 2007). As Beverley Skeggs states: 'The ontological security of the working classes is more likely to lie in fitting in rather than standing out' (B. Skeggs, *Formations of Class & Gender: Becoming Respectable* (London: Sage, 1997), as cited in Gilles, 2007: 77.
14. Dermott, 2012; Jensen, 2010.
15. I have argued elsewhere that a diagnosis of depression does seem to obscure the more complex nuances of women's psychological distress. More specifically, it serves to obscure women's anger, which seems to be a very important aspect of women's psychological distress. In contexts such as the valley, this anger may manifest in violent behaviour specifically aimed at children. Not only does the diagnosis of depression serve to medicalise the distress of women, but it may serve to obscure their anger as well. See also Ussher, 2010.
16. Jack, 1991; Sperberg and Stabb, 1998; Swartz, 2013.
17. Sperberg and Stabb, 1998; Swartz, 2013.
18. Swartz, 2013: 46.
19. J. Bernard, *The Future of Motherhood* (New York: Dial Press, 1974), as cited in Bassin, Honey and Kaplan, 1994: 3. It is very important to stress that for most mothers anger is mostly not an ego-syntonic emotion.
20. The literature also strongly suggests that mothers who were neglected and abused themselves are likely to re-enact destructive patterns with their own children. This intergenerational transmission of neglect and abuse was apparent in my fieldwork, with many participants relating how they, in turn, were neglected and physically abused by their mothers. See Jack (1999); Motz (2001).
21. Motz (2001) contends that it often is a lack of separateness that puts the mother in an untenable state and can lead to her punishing her child. She says: 'Abusive mothers characteristically experience serious difficulties in separation and individuation, both in terms of their own relationships with their mothers and with their [children]' (Motz 2001: 78). Mills (1996) argues that in women who have

had rejecting or abusive mothers themselves, the wish for a child may reflect a wish to please internal objects – to have another opportunity to please the internalised critical mother. When the child then turns out not to be like the ideal child they longed for, they are deeply disappointed and angry, an anger that may manifest in violent behaviour. The mothers thus seem to relate their anger to seeing unwanted aspects of themselves in their children (Benedek, 1970; R. Parker, 1997). The angry reaction can be interpreted as being aimed, not so much at their children, but at the children as extensions of themselves. See also the chapter on *Love* and the chapter on *Distress*.

22. According to Motz, it is both 'the irrevocable link between the mother and her child, and the failure of psychic differentiation between them' and 'the identification of the mother with the terrifying parent that she has become' that are at the root of maternal violence (Motz, 2001: 91).

23. R. Parker, 1997: 32.

24. Ussher, 2010. I have written extensively about the anger of women who have been diagnosed with depression (see, for example, Kruger and Lourens, 2016; Kruger et al., 2014). In an unpublished preliminary overview of the literature Trish Blake wrote the following:

    Increased levels of depression have been associated with:

    - increased levels of anger and anger expression (Baeg, Wang, Chee, Kim, & Kim, 2011; Balsamo, 2010; Fava et al., 1993; Hur & Kim, 2009; Koh, Kim, & Park, 2002; Perlis et al., 2004; Shay & Knutson, 2008; Simon & Lively, 2010; M.K. Taylor, Larson, & Norman, 2013; Whiteside & Abramowitz, 2004);
    - hostility (Benazzi & Akiskal, 2005; Perlis et al., 2004);
    - aggressive and violent behaviour (Dutton & Karakanta, 2013; Moscovitch, McCabe, Antony, Rocca, & Swinson, 2008; Posternak & Zimmerman, 2002; Swanson, Holzer, Ganju, & Jano, 1990);
    - aggression toward partners (Feldbau-Kohn, Heyman, & O'Leary, 1998; Maiuro, Cahn, Vitaliano, Wagner, & Zegree, 1988; Marshall, Sippel, & Belleau, 2011);
    - and aggression toward children (Berger, 2005; Hien, Cohen, Caldeira, Flom, & Wasserman, 2010; Mammen, Kolko; & Pilkonis, 2002; Shay & Knutson, 2008).

    In a prospective, naturalistic investigation of patients with depression (N = 536), studied systematically at intake and during up to 31 years of follow-up, Judd, Schettler, Coryell, Akiskal, and Fiedorowicz (2013) found that irritability and anger were present in 54.5% of the sample. Depression with anger was associated with significantly increased depressive severity, longer duration of the index depressive episode, poorer impulse control, a more chronic and severe long-term course of illness, higher rates of lifetime comorbid substance abuse and anxiety disorder, more antisocial personality disorders, greater psychosocial impairment before intake and during follow-up, and a reduced life satisfaction. These results were not explained by manic spectrum symptoms or other comorbidity. Other studies have found depression with anger to be associated with an increased number of suicide attempts and suicidal ideation (Verhoeven, Booij, Van der Wee, Penninx, & Van der Does, 2011), and increased anxiety symptoms (Fava & Rosenbaum, 1998; Verhoeven et al., 2011).

Both suppressed anger (Kopper & Epperson, 1996; Rude, Chrisman, Burton Denmark, & Maestas, 2012) and expressed anger (Deffenbacher, Oetting, Lynch, & Morris, 1996; Koh et al., 2002; Terasaki, Gelaye, Berhane, & Williams, 2009) have been associated with increased levels of depression (Bridewell & Chang, 1997; Busch, 2009; Luutonen, 2007). With regard to gender, a significant association between anger and depression has been found among both men and women (Hien et al., 2010; Newman, Fuqua, Gray, & Simpson, 2006; Shay & Knutson, 2008; Simon & Lively, 2010).

Although researchers acknowledge a strong link between anger and depression for both men and women (Newman et al., 2006; Painuly et al., 2005) and anger is generally regarded as a factor in the onset and maintenance of depression (Judd et al., 2013), the nature of the link between anger and depression remains far from understood. A 2005 review of the literature on the relationship of depression and anger, also anger attacks, concludes: 'the occurrence of anger, irritability and hostility in depression have been known for many years, but the prevalence, significance for treatment and prognosis and the mechanisms involved remain poorly understood' (Painuly et al., 2005, p. 215).

This may, in part, be due to the fact that, while the DSM 5 includes anger in the diagnostic criteria of certain disorders . . . and acknowledges that individuals diagnosed with a Major Depressive Episode may 'report or exhibit increased irritability (e.g., persistent anger, a tendency to respond to events with angry outbursts or blaming others)' (American Psychiatric Association, 2013, p. 163), the diagnostic criteria for depressive disorders such as MDD and PDD do not include anger. This is also true for the International Classification of Diseases 10th Revision's (World Health Organisation, 1992) diagnostic criteria for a depressive episode. In general, it can be said that while the connection between depression and anger has received enduring attention from psychoanalytic theorists (Busch, 2009), and anger is considered to be a significant public health concern (Frumkin, 2002), the link between depression and anger has received little attention in formal psychiatric diagnostic systems (Anand & Malhi, 2009; Stein, 2013); systems which have widespread influence on all aspects of mental health, including research focus and development (Nemeroff et al., 2013).

25. Lafrance and McKenzie-Mohr, 2013: 136.
26. Jack, 1999:183.
27. Lafrance and McKenzie-Mohr, 2013.
28. Gillies, 2007: 8.
29. Blum, 2007: 54.
30. Trad, 1990.

## Notes to Epilogue

1. Wallin 2007.
2. See more about shame in chapter on *Love*. The inevitable shame of the patient is discussed later in this chapter under the subheading 'The boy with the shining shoes'.
3. Morrison, 2008.
4. Orange (2008) points out that although relational psychoanalysis has sought to minimise the shaming aspects of the therapeutic situation, there is no avoiding them completely.
5. Jacobs, 1996.
6. Javier and Herron, 2002: 157.
7. Again, Bion's 'nameless dread' (1962b: 183).
8. It is no coincidence that each chapter of this book starts with an arrival and a reaching out and ends with an almost violent or brutal departure.
9. Within all psychoanalytic traditions the fact that the therapist's countertransference is often characterised by ambivalence is emphasised. Freud describes the therapeutic relationship as one of love and hate, gratification and frustration, while Klein sees the therapist as both good and bad object (Mitchell and Black, 1995). Winnicott (1949: 69) refers to 'hate in the countertransference'. Kohut uses the term 'transmuting internalizations' to refer to the limits and imperfections of the therapist, 'who cannot (and indeed should not) always be perfectly attuned to the patient's needs . . . So the analyst like the adequate parent, fails the patient slowly and incrementally', so that the patient can develop 'a more realistic, but still vital and robust, sense of self and other' (Mitchell and Black, 1995: 162–3). Intersubjective therapists use the notions of rupture and repair to highlight the fact that psychotherapy typically assumes the form of a series of connections and disconnections. For instance, Wallin (2007) discusses in detail the importance of sequences of rupture and repair in the therapeutic relationship. He says that if the therapist is able to repair a rupture, it 'strengthens the patient's confidence that the relationship can be relied on to contain difficult feelings and help resolve them' (Wallin, 2007: 197). He adds: 'Successive episodes of repair tend, in addition, to disconfirm the patient's pre-existing transference expectations . . . that no one will ever take responsibility for problems they caused and that he alone would be held liable' (Wallin, 2007: 197–8).
10. Hollway, 2015: 191.

11. Seu, 2006: 288. Psychologists have written (but not enough) about the psychological experience of poverty and how the shame associated with it can be incorporated into identity. Historically speaking, Trevor's position as a coloured South African may also be associated with shame. See Altman (2004); Brown (2005); Charos (2009); Kruger (2012); Lazarus (2007); and the chapter on *Home*.

12. Gilligan, 2003: 1154.

13. Kohut (2009: 116) claims that every child needs a parent that admires and respects him and confirms his self-worth (mirroring transference). He also says that every child needs a parent or caretaker to idealise and admire (idealising transference). Should the child miss out on these experiences, she does not learn to love others and does not learn to love herself. Kohut says: 'The deepest level to which psychoanalysis can penetrate when it traces destructiveness [is to] the presence of a serious narcissistic injury, an injury that threatened the cohesion of the self.'

14. See the chapter on *Love*. Gilligan's (2003) notion of shame as a defence against both an unbearable longing and a ghastly fear seems relevant here.

15. The patient himself is also probably ashamed on many levels. The therapeutic situation is potentially more shaming for the patient than it is for the therapist. The patient usually needs the psychotherapist more than the psychotherapist needs the patient. A therapist is approached usually because a patient needs help or support or other inputs.

16. Tomkins, 1963: 192.

17. The white therapist is saddled with different levels of shame: shame of being afraid of her patient, shame of being a psychotherapist in this context, shame of feeling unable to help, shame of being a white, middle-class South African. South African author J.M. Coetzee (2007: 39) writes on 'national shame' in his book *Diary of a Bad Year* and cites Demosthenes: 'Whereas the slave fears only pain, what the free man fears most is shame . . . The generation of white South Africans to which I belong, and the next generation, and perhaps the generation after that too, will go bowed under the shame of the crimes that were committed in their name.' On a personal level, this particular therapist's shame may be exacerbated by the fact that she comes from a family well known for their efforts in the struggle against apartheid and for their commitment to not simply being bystanders. Her shame might also feel very old: in supervision she could talk about how ashamed she used to be as a child for resenting her parents' political work and specifically the impoverished foster children they took in on a regular basis. She is, like therapists everywhere, 'always unwittingly enacting scenarios with [her] patients that stem from [her] own unconscious needs, working models, defences and so on' (Wallin, 2007: 273). See also Kruger (2012).

18. In becoming part of the patient 's world through enactment, the therapist is able to experience and know the patient in an emotionally direct way that is unmediated by language. This gives the therapist access to the unverbalised and unverbalisable realms of the patient's experience.

19. Orange, 2005: xiv.
20. Morrison, 1994: 19.
21. Altman, 2004.
22. Charos, 2009.
23. In reviewing the literature, the mutual abandonment of patient and therapist seems not to be uncommon, both in individual therapy and in group therapy. There are many accounts in the South African literature of patients abandoning therapy unexpectedly and prematurely and of therapists leaving their patients, either emotionally or quite literally (Kadish, 2016; Kruger, 2012, 2016).
24. Gilligan discusses four different preconditions for shame to produce violence:

    First, either the individual has not yet developed the capacity for the emotion that inhibits violence toward others – namely, guilt and remorse – or the situational circumstances present at the time diminished or neutralised whatever guilt feelings the person would otherwise have felt. Second, the degree of shame and humiliation the person is experiencing is so intense that it is overwhelming, to the point that it threatens the cohesion and viability of the self (that is, it threatens to bring about the death of the self). Third, the individual perceives herself as not having sufficient non-violent means by which to save or restore her self-esteem. Most of us, when shamed or insulted, either by others or by some mistake we have made that we ourselves feel was foolish, have sufficient other sources of self-esteem, some degree of knowledge or skills or achievements, some standing in the community or esteem in the eyes of our friends, family, or colleagues, or just material status symbols that ourselves and our self-esteem are not wiped out even by a severe humiliation. But the violent criminals with whom I worked for the most part lacked all of these barriers against violence: most were uneducated or even illiterate, unskilled or unemployed, poor or even homeless, or members of ethnic or demographic groups that are subjected to systematic shaming by the rest of society; in short, they were almost all of the lowest social and economic status. I am not saying that one has to be poor or discriminated against to become violent and certainly being wealthy or belonging to the upper middle class does not prevent one from becoming violent, but statistics on the epidemiology of violence make clear the connection between poverty and marginalisation and violence. A fourth precondition that enormously increases the chance that shame will lead to violence exists when the individual has been socialised into the male gender role that, in our patriarchal culture, means he has been taught that there are many circumstances and situations in which one has to be violent in order to maintain one's masculinity or sense of masculine sexual identity and adequacy, and in which a non-violent man would be seen as impotent and emasculated, a coward,

wimp, eunuch, boy, homosexual, or woman, a man who has 'no balls'.
For men in a patriarchy, there are many situations in which violence is
honoured and non-violence is shamed (Gilligan, 2003: 1165–6).

25. Steinberg, 2005.
26. Wallin, 2007: 279.
27. See *Prologue*.
28. In thinking about why I agreed to drive Wendy to her dance and thus break the
frame of psychotherapy, I first told myself that there was no option to say no. I also
told myself that therapy was over – Wendy had terminated psychotherapy. I was
not breaking the frame.

On further reflection it is clear that I was enacting something. For me, and
perhaps for her, my driving her to the dance can be seen as a metaphor for me
facilitating her connection with her confidence and her ambition – in the Kohutian
sense of the words. In writing about enactment with a patient, Wallin (2007: 288)
says, 'In my response to her as a lovable and beautiful being, she had glimpsed a
new image of herself and a new sense of possibility.'

However, Wallin (2007) also reminds us that enactments happen at the
'intersection' of the unconscious needs and vulnerabilities of both the patient and
the therapist. I now also think that on an unconscious level Wendy must also have
responded to my sense of shame about my work in the valley: she must have known
in some way that I also needed acknowledgement and affirmation (a need that I
also feel ashamed about) – I needed to be rescued from my shame. By making me
the fairy godmother driving the princess to the ball, Wendy not only confirmed
that we did manage to co-create a new relational experience, she also succeeded in
consoling me: for a few moments I was really useful to her and not ashamed.

I have tried to argue that shame is an almost inevitable part of the
psychotherapeutic encounter. Therapist and patient are ashamed not only of what
they dread, but also of what they hope for. Shame is also inevitable in the new
South Africa, specifically in encounters between black and white, between rich and
poor.

When shame is present, it lingers over every encounter, often obscuring other
important aspects of the encounter. Shame is typically not spoken, but acted out.
It shuts people up and it shuts people out. Because of its very nature, shame is
very difficult to articulate, difficult to make explicit – even and especially in the
process of psychotherapy. Shame that is obscure and hidden – disavowed – leads
to substitute affect such as rage or depression. Shame may lead to anticipatory
rejection, abandonment, ostracism, relegation to inferior status. Tomkins (1963)
points out how shame may quickly turn to contempt or disgust if the subject
feels that identification with the other is unattainable. If love and recognition
seem impossible, the other may be rejected with extreme violence (Charos, 2009).
Furthermore, people may attempt to affirm their affective self-containment by
violently projecting the undesirable feeling of shame onto others.

In psychotherapy it is necessary not only to attempt to be emphatically immersed in the world of the patient, but also to be open to the unplanned and the unexpected as enacted by both parties (Teicholz, 2006). When shame is recognised and the reasons for the shame remembered and made explicit, there is potential for connection. The misattunement created by the fog of shame can become attunement exactly because the shame is recognised. Therefore, if we pay exquisite attention to the shame that is implicit (Beebe and Lachmann, 2002; Beebe et al., 2005; Bollas, 1987; Fonagy, 1999; Fosshage, 2005; Lyons-Ruth, 1998; Nahum, 2002), the shame that is evoked, enacted and embodied in and by us and our patients, it does not have to lead to rage and rejection (Wallin, 2007). It does not have to be paralysing or lead to silence, as Samantha Vice (2010) proclaimed in a controversial and widely cited paper (see also Barnard, 2012). Making the implicit explicit can be a key part of the recognition processes that heighten the probability that 'moving along' in psychotherapy will also be 'moving forward' (Wallin, 2007: 261).

Furthermore, if we were to acknowledge shame in the everyday, without stigmatising the feeling itself, we might be able to counteract many of the prejudices that inform discourses of 'othering', both within and outside the therapeutic encounter. Thinking about shame as truly human and as indicating our interest in communing with one another, can transform shame into a powerful and positive motivator of human interaction and engagement (Charos, 2009). 'Paradoxically,' Swartz (2012: 207) states, 'it is the resonance of shame that crafts the way forward . . . a shared experience of shame provides the vehicle for a slow movement.' This sharing of shame involves an acknowledgement that shameful feelings are still with South Africans after apartheid and that they might never go away.

Shame does not have to shut us up or shut us out. If shame is recognised, either explicitly or implicitly, 'moments of meeting' (Wallin, 2007: 125) become possible. Intersubjective psychoanalysis has helped us to understand that these 'now moments' do not come from the psychotherapist alone, but 'through a reconfiguration of what is brought to the encounter by each party, resulting in a third realm of meaning and experience, the realm of the intersubjective' (Teicholz, 2006: 49). In such moments of meeting, the ashamed other becomes a participant in the emotional world of the other, and is, even if only momentarily, truly involved. See also Kruger (2012).

## Notes to Appendix
1. Jackson, 2011: 190.
2. See *Prologue.*
3. Posel and Ross, 2014.
4. Geertz, 1973.
5. Bromley, 1986: 8; Willig, 2013.

6. Geertz, 1973: 60.
7. Biehl, 2013: 574.
8. Biehl, 2013: 574.
9. Biehl, 2013: 574–5.
10. Biehl, 2013: 575. Biehl relates a conversation he had with Clifford Geertz in 2003: 'I am sore tired of hearing the question "What is your contribution to theory?" I told Geertz. "How would you respond?"' Geertz replied without a missing a beat: 'Subtraction' (Biehl, 2013: 573).
11. See the section 'On Theory' in chapter on *Distress*.
12. Biehl, 2013: 583.
13. Important examples of medical practitioners writing about their cases include Farmer (2005); Gawande (2008, 2011, 2014); Mukherjee (2011); Sacks (1995, 2013a, 2013b, 2015) and Sweet (2012). Similarly, there are many powerful examples of psychoanalysts and psychologists writing about their cases. As in the field of medicine, some of these books are written for a more popular audience, while others are aimed at a more professional audience. See, for instance, McWilliams (1999); Orbach (2016); Wallin (2007); Yalom (2013).
14. Gabbay and Le May, 2011; Margison et al., 2000: 123.
15. Gabbard, 2000; Kantrowitz, 2006; Swartz, 1998.
16. Swartz, 2006: 428.
17. Charmaz, 1991.
18. The statistics for mothers who registered at the clinic during the four years of the study were quite similar. The average age of the 276 registered mothers was 26, the average number of children was 1.74 and average birth weight of babies was 2.975 kilograms. Forty-one were under the age of twenty.
19. See Kruger and Schoombee (2010) and Schoombee, Van der Merwe and Kruger (2005).
20. Willig, 2001.
21. See De Villiers, 2011.
22. De Villiers, 2011.
23. See Lazarus, 2007.
24. Bromley, 1986: ix.
25. Nelson and Prilleltensky, 2005; Willig, 2001.
26. Willig, 2001: 70.
27. Bromley, 1986.
28. Nelson and Prilleltensky, 2005.
29. Bromley, 1986: xi.
30. Bromley, 1986: xi.
31. Westen, Novotny and Thompson-Brenner, 2004.
32. Lazarus, 2007: 133.
33. Gibson, 2002.
34. Willig, 2001.

35. Lazarus, 2007: 140. The quote in the last line of this extract is from Gibson, 2002: 83.
36. Lazarus, 2007: 166.
37. Kruger and Lourens, 2016; Kruger et al., 2014.
38. Charmaz, 2006.
39. Charmaz, 2006.
40. For academic papers based on this study, see Kruger 2014b; Kruger and Lourens, 2016; Kruger et al., 2014.
41. South African Children's Act 38 of 2005. http://www.justice.gov.za/legislation/acts/2005-038%20childrensact.pdf.
42. Way, 1998.
43. Smith, Van Wyk and Alkana, 2013.
44. Jewkes et al., 2011.
45. Yalom and Leszcz, 2005.
46. Way, 1998.
47. Westen, Novotny and Thompson-Brenner, 2004: 658.
48. Bless, Higson-Smith and Sithole, 2013.
49. Barbour, 2007.
50. See Kruger, 2016.

# Select Bibliography

Abrahams, N., S. Mathews, R. Jewkes, L. Martin and C. Lombard. 2012. 'Every Eight Hours: Intimate Femicide in South Africa 10 Years Later'. South African Medical Research Council Research Brief. http://www.mrc.ac.za/sites/default/files/attachments/2016-06-27/everyeighthours.pdf.

Abrahams, N., S. Mathews, L.J. Martin, C. Lombard and R. Jewkes. 2013. 'Intimate Partner Femicide in South Africa in 1999 and 2009'. *PLoS Medicine* 10(4): e1001412.

Abrahams, Z., C. Lund, S. Field and S. Honikman. 2018. 'Factors Associated with Household Food Insecurity and Depression in Pregnant South African Women from a Low Socio-economic Setting: A Cross-sectional Study'. *Social Psychiatry and Psychiatric Epidemiology* 53(4): 363–72.

Adams, A.E. 1994. *Reproducing the Womb: Images of Childbirth in Science, Feminist Theory, and Literature*. Ithaca: Cornell University Press.

Adhikari, M. 2004. '"Not Black Enough": Changing Expressions of Coloured Identity in Post-apartheid South Africa'. *South African Historical Journal* 51(1): 167–78.

———. 2006. 'Hope, Fear, Shame, Frustration: Continuity and Change in the Expression of Coloured Identity in White Supremacist South Africa, 1910–1994'. *Journal of Southern African Studies* 32(3): 467–87.

Adhikari, M., ed. 2008. *Burdened by Race: Coloured Identities in Southern Africa*. Cape Town: University of Cape Town Press.

Adler, N.E., T. Boyce, M.A, Chesney, S. Cohen, S. Folkman, R.L. Khan and S.L. Syme. 1994. 'Socioeconomic Status and Health: The Challenge of the Gradient'. *American Psychologist* 49(1): 15–24.

Alcock, P. 1997. *Understanding Poverty*. London: Macmillan.

Ally, S. 2011. 'Domestics, "Dirty Work" and the Affects of Domination'. *South African Review of Sociology* 42(2): 1–7.

Als, H. 2017. 'Richard Avedon and James Baldwin's Joint Examination of American Identity'. *The New Yorker*, 13 November. https://www.newyorker.com/magazine/2017/11/13/richard-avedon-and-james-baldwins-joint-examination-of-american-identity.

Altman, N. 2004. 'History Repeats Itself in Transference-Countertransference'. *Psychoanalytic Dialogues* 14(6): 807–15.

———. 2005. 'Relational Perspectives on the Therapeutic Action of Psychoanalysis'. In *How Does Psychotherapy Work?*, edited by J. Ryan, 15–50. London: Karnac.

American Psychiatric Association. 2013. *Diagnostic and Statistical Manual of Mental Disorders: DSM-5*. Washington, DC: American Psychiatric Association.

Anderson, E. 1999. *Code of the Street: Decency, Violence, and the Moral Life of the Inner City*. New York: Norton.

Anderson, N.B. and C.A. Armstead. 1995. 'Toward Understanding the Association of Socioeconomic Status and Health: A New Challenge for the Biopsychosocial Approach'. *Psychosomatic Medicine* 57(3): 213–25.

Anker, W. 2014. *Buys: 'n grensroman*. Cape Town: Kwela Books.

———. 2018. *Red Dog*. Translated by Michiel Heyns. Cape Town: Kwela Books.

Arai, L. 2003. 'Low Expectations, Sexual Attitudes and Knowledge: Explaining Teenage Pregnancy and Fertility in English Communities; Insights from Qualitative Research'. *The Sociological Review* 51(2): 199–217.

———. 2009. *Teenage Pregnancy: The Making and Unmaking of a Problem*. Bristol: Policy Press.

Archer, S. 2011. '"Buying the Maid Ricoffy": Domestic Workers, Employers and Food'. *South African Review of Sociology* 42(2): 66–82.

Arizmendi, T.G. and D.D. Affonso. 1987. 'Stressful Events Related to Pregnancy and the Postpartum'. *Journal of Psychosomatic Research* 31(6): 743–59.

Attwell, D. 1993. *J.M. Coetzee: South Africa and the Politics of Writing*. Berkeley: University of California Press.

———. 2015. *J.M. Coetzee & the Life of Writing: Face to Face with Time*. Oxford: Oxford University Press.

Atwood, M. 2001. 'Giving Birth'. In *Mother Reader: Essential Literature on Motherhood*, edited by M. Davey, 311–24. Toronto: Seven Stories Press.

Bacal, H. 2017. 'Credo: My Psychoanalytic Adventure; A Quest to Conceptualize Therapeutic Efficacy'. *Psychoanalytic Dialogues* 27(1): 1–19.

Bakhtin, M. 1981. *The Dialogic Imagination: Four Essays by M.M. Bakhtin*. Edited by M. Holquist and translated by C. Emerson. Austin: University of Texas Press.

Bantjes, J. and L. Swartz. 2017. 'The Cultural Turn in Critical Suicidology: What Can we Claim and What do we Know?' *Death Studies* 41(8): 512–20.

Baraitser, L. 2009. *Maternal Encounters: The Ethics of Interruption*. London: Routledge.

Barbour, R. 2007. *Doing Focus Groups*. London: Sage.

Bardwick, J.M. 1971. *Psychology of Women*. New York: Harper & Row.

Barnard, R. 2012. 'Ugly Feelings, Negative Dialectics: Reflections on Postapartheid Shame'. *Safundi* 13(1–2): 151–70.

Barnes, J. 2014. *Levels of Life*. New York: Vintage.

Barr, J. and C. Beck. 2008. 'Infanticide Secrets: Qualitative Study on Postpartum Depression'. *Canadian Family Physician* 54(12): 1716–17.

Barth, R.P., B.R. Lee, M.A. Lindsey, K.S. Collins, F. Strieder, B.F. Chorpita, K.D. Becker and J.A. Sparks. 2012. 'Evidence-based Practice at a Crossroads'. *Research on Social Work Practice* 22(1): 108–19.

Bass, J.K., P.A. Bolton and L.K. Murray. 2007. 'Do Not Forget Culture When Studying Mental Health'. *Lancet* 370(9591): 918–19.

Bassin, D., M. Honey and M.M. Kaplan. 1994. *Representations of Motherhood*. New Haven: Yale University Press.

Beckett, S. 1958. *Endgame*. New York: Grove Press.

Beebe, B., S. Knoblauch, J. Rustin, D. Sorter, T.J. Jacobs and R. Pally. 2005. *Forms of Intersubjectivity in Infant Research and Adult Treatment*. New York: Other Press.

Beebe, B. and F.M. Lachmann. 2002. *Infant Research and Adult Treatment: Co-constructing Interactions*. New York: The Analytic Press/Taylor & Francis Group.

Behar, R. and D.A. Gordon, eds. 1995. *Women Writing Culture*. Berkeley: University of California Press.

Bell, K.M. and A.E. Naugle. 2008. 'Intimate Partner Violence Theoretical Considerations: Moving towards a Contextual Framework'. *Clinical Psychology Review* 28(7): 1096–107.

Belle, D. 1990. 'Poverty and Women's Mental Health'. *American Psychologist* 45(3): 385–9.

Belle, D. and J. Doucet. 2003. 'Poverty, Inequality, and Discrimination as Sources of Depression among U.S. Women'. *Psychology of Women Quarterly* 27: 101–13.

Belle, D., J. Doucet, J. Harris, J. Miller and E. Tan. 2000. 'Who is Rich? Who is Happy?' *American Psychologist* 55(10): 1160–1.

Benedek, T. 1970. *The Psychology of Pregnancy*. Edited by A. Benedek and T. Anthony. Boston: Little, Brown and Company.

Benjamin, J. 1988. *The Bonds of Love: Psychoanalysis, Feminism, and the Problem of Domination*. New York: Pantheon.

———. 2004. 'Beyond Doer and Done to: An Intersubjective View of Thirdness'. *The Psychoanalytic Quarterly* LXXIII(1): 5–46.

Bester, L. and L-M. Kruger. 2018. 'Beyond the DSM Diagnosis of Depression: One Woman's Experience of Her Psychological Distress'. Unpublished paper, Department of Psychology, Stellenbosch University.

Bhabha, H.K. 1998. 'The White Stuff'. *Artforum International Magazine* 36(9): 21–3.

Bibring, G.L. 1959. 'Some Considerations of the Psychological Processes in Pregnancy'. *Psychoanalytical Study of the Child* 14(1): 113–21.

Bibring, G.L., T.F. Dwyer, D.S. Huntington and A.F. Valenstein. 1961. 'A Study of the Psychological Processes in Pregnancy and the Earliest Mother-Child Relationship: Some Propositions and Comments'. *Psychoanalytical Study of the Child* 16: 9–27. https://archive.org/stream/in.ernet.dli.2015.138796/2015.138796.The-Psychoanalytic-Study-Of-The-Child-Vol-Xvi_djvu.txt.

Biehl, J. 2013. 'Ethnography in the Way of Theory'. *Cultural Anthropology* 28(4): 573–97.

Bion, W.R. 1962a. *Learning from Experience*. London: Karnac.

———. 1962b. 'A Theory of Thinking'. In *Melanie Klein Today: Developments in Theory and Practice, Volume I: Mainly Theory*, edited by E. Spillius, 178–86. London: Routledge.

———. 1967. *Second Thoughts*. London: Heinemann.

Biran, H. 2003. 'The Difficulty of Transforming Terror into Dialogue'. *Group Analysis* 36(4): 490–502.

Black, M.C. 2011. 'Intimate Partner Violence and Adverse Health Consequences'. *American Journal of Lifestyle Medicine* 5(5): 428–39.

Blake, P. 2013. 'Diagnosis and the Obscuring of Anger'. Unpublished paper. Department of Psychology, Stellenbosch University.

Blatt, S.J., G. Shafar and D.C. Zuroff. 2001. 'Anaclitic (Sociotropic) and Introjective (Autonomous) Dimensions'. *Psychotherapy* 38(4): 449–54.

Blatt, S.J. and D.C. Zuroff. 1992. 'Interpersonal Relatedness and Self-definition: Two Prototypes for Depression'. *Clinical Psychology Review* 12(5): 527–62.

Bless, C., C. Higson-Smith and S. Levy Sithole. 2013. *Fundamentals of Social Research Methods: An African Perspective*. 5th edition. Cape Town: Juta.

Blomquist, J.L., L.H. Quiroz, D. MacMillan, A. Mccullough and V.L. Handa. 2011. 'Mothers' Satisfaction with Planned Vaginal and Planned Cesarean Birth'. *Obstetrical & Gynecological Survey* 66(9): 531–2.

Blum, L. 2007. 'Psychodynamics of Postpartum Depression'. *Psychoanalytic Psychology* 24(1): 45–62.

Bollas, C. 1987. *The Shadow of the Object: Psychoanalysis and the Unthought Known*. London: Free Association Books.

Boonzaier, F. 2003. 'Women Abuse: A Critical Review'. In *Social Psychology: Identities and Relationships*, edited by K. Ratele and N. Duncan, 177–97. Cape Town: University of Cape Town Press.

———. 2008. '"If the Man Says You Must Sit, Then You Must Sit": The Relational Construction of Woman Abuse; Gender, Subjectivity and Violence'. *Feminism & Psychology* 18(2): 183–206.

Borges, J.L. 1998. *Jorge Luis Borges: Conversations*. Edited by R. Burgin. Jackson: University Press of Mississippi.

Borgogno, F., S.A. Merciai and P.B. Talamo. 1998. *Bion's Legacy to Groups*. New York: Routledge.

Branson, N., C. Ardington and M. Leibbrandt. 2013. 'Trends in Teenage Childbearing and Schooling Outcomes for Children Born to Teens in South Africa'. Southern Africa Labour and Development Research Unit, Cape Town, Working Paper No. 98. http://www.opensaldru.uct.ac.za/bitstream/handle/11090/614/2013_98.pdf?sequence=1.

Brault, P-A. and M. Naas. 2003. *The Work of Mourning*. Chicago: University of Chicago Press.

Brezinka, C., O. Huter, W. Biebl and J. Kinzl. 1994. 'Denial of Pregnancy: Obstetrical Aspects'. *Journal of Psychosomatic Obstetrics and Gynaecology* 15(1): 1–8.

Brock, K. 2002. 'Introduction: Knowing poverty; Critical Reflections on Participatory Research and Policy'. In *Knowing Poverty: Critical Reflections on Participatory Research and Policy*, edited by K. Brock and R. McGee, 1–11. London: Earthscan Publications.

Brockington, I. 1996. *Motherhood and Mental Health*. New York: Oxford University Press.

Bromley, D.B. 1986. *The Case-Study Method in Psychology and Related Disciplines*. New Jersey: John Wiley & Sons.

Bronfenbrenner, U. 1979. *The Ecology of Human Development: Experiments by Nature and Design*. Cambridge: Harvard University Press.

Brown, B.A. 2005. 'The Incorporation of Poverty into Adult Identity over Time: Implications for Adult Education'. *International Journal of Lifelong Education* 24(5): 393–404.

Bryanton, J., A. Gagnon, C. Johnston and M. Hatem. 2008. 'Predictors of Women's Perceptions of the Childbirth Experience'. *Journal of Obstetric, Gynecologic and Neonatal Nursing* 37(1): 24–34.

Burdette, A.M., T.D. Hill and L. Hale. 2011. 'Household Disrepair and the Mental Health of Low-income Urban Women'. *Journal of Urban Health* 88(1): 142–53.

Burgess, R. 2016. 'Dangerous discourses? Silencing Women within "Global Mental Health" Practice?' In *Handbook on Gender and Health*, edited by J. Gideon, 79–97. Cheltenham: Edward Elgar Publishing.

Burgess, R. and C. Campbell. 2014. 'Contextualising Women's Mental Distress and Coping Strategies in the Time of AIDS: A Rural South African Case Study'. *Transcultural Psychiatry* 51(6): 875–903.

Burman, E. 2011. 'Desiring Development? Psychoanalytic Contributions to Antidevelopmental Psychology'. *Journal of Qualitative Studies in Education* 26(1): 56–74.

Burmeister-Nel, H. 2005. 'A Review of the Literature on the Psychological Experience of Pregnancy: Possible Implications for Low-income Women in South Africa'. Master's thesis, University of Stellenbosch, Stellenbosch.

Burnett, C., D. Schminkey, J. Milburn, J. Kastello, L. Bullock, J.C. Campbell and P.W. Sharps. 2016. 'Negotiating Peril: The Lived Experience of Rural, Low-income Women Exposed to IPV during Pregnancy and Postpartum'. *Violence Against Women* 22(8): 943–65.

Butler, J. 2004. *Precarious Life: The Powers of Mourning and Violence*. London: Verso.

Byatt, A.S. 1995. *The Matisse Stories*. New York: Random House.

———. 2001. *The Biographer's Tale*. London: Vintage.

Callister, L.C., I. Khalaf, S. Semenic, R. Kartchner and K. Vehvilainen-Julkunen. 2003. 'The Pain of Childbirth: Perceptions of Culturally Diverse Women'. *Pain Management Nursing* 4(4): 145–54.

Calvino, I. 1972. *Invisible Cities*. Turin: Giulio Einaudi Editore.

Campbell, S., A. Morgan-Lopez, M. Cox and V. McLoyd. 2009. 'A Latent Class Analysis of Maternal Depressive Symptoms over 12 Years and Offspring Adjustment in Adolescence'. *Journal of Abnormal Psychology* 118(3): 479–93.

Caplan, P. 1997. *Food, Health and Identity*. London: Routledge.

Capogrosso, P., M. Colicchia, E. Ventimiglia, G. Castagna, M.C. Clementi, N. Suardi, F. Castiglione, A. Briganti, F. Cantiello, R. Damiano, F. Montorsi and A. Salonia.

2013. 'One Patient out of Four with Newly Diagnosed Erectile Dysfunction is a Young Man: Worrisome Picture from the Everyday Clinical Practice'. *The Journal of Sexual Medicine* 10(7): 1833–41.

Carty, E. and D. Tier. 1989. 'Birth Planning: A Reality-based Script for Building Confidence'. *Journal of Nurse-Midwifery* 34(3): 111–14.

Ceci, C. 2004. 'Nursing, Knowledge and Power: A Case Analysis'. *Social Science and Medicine* 59(9): 1879–89.

Chadwick, R. 2017. 'Ambiguous Subjects: Obstetric Violence, Assemblage and South African Birth Narratives'. *Feminism & Psychology* 27(4): 489–509. https://doi.org/10.1177/0959353517692607.

———. 2018. *Bodies that Birth: Vitalizing Birth Politics*. New York: Routledge.

Chadwick, R.J., D. Cooper and J. Harries. 2014. 'Narratives of Distress about Birth in South African Public Maternity Settings: A Qualitative Study'. *Midwifery* 30(7): 862–8.

Charles, N. and M. Kerr. 1986. 'Food for Feminist Thought'. *Sociological Review* 34(3): 537–72.

Charmaz, K. 1991. 'Methodological Appendix'. In *Good Days, Bad Days: The Self in Chronic Illness in Time*, edited by K. Charmaz, 271–7. New Brunswick: Rutgers.

———. 2006. *Constructing Grounded Theory: A Practical Guide through Qualitative Analysis*. London: Sage.

Charos, C. 2009. 'States of Shame: South African Writing after Apartheid'. *Safundi* 10(3): 273–304.

Chase, E. and R. Walker. 2013. 'The Co-construction of Shame in the Context of Poverty: Beyond a Threat to the Social Bond'. *Sociology* 47(4): 739–54.

Chesler, P. 1972. *Women and Madness*. Orlando: Harcourt Brace Jovanovich.

Christiaens, W. and P. Bracke. 2007. 'Assessment of Social Psychological Determinants of Satisfaction with Childbirth in a Cross-national Perspective'. *BMC Pregnancy and Childbirth* 7: 26–38.

Chodorow, N. 1995. 'Gender as a Personal and Cultural Construction'. *Signs* 20(3): 516–44.

———. 1999. *The Power of Feelings: Personal Meaning in Psychoanalysis, Gender, and Culture*. New Haven: Yale University Press.

Chomsky, N. and R.W. McChesney. 2011. *Profit over People: Neoliberalism and Global Order*. New York: Seven Stories Press.

Coast, E., T. Leone, A. Hirose and E. Jones. 2012. 'Poverty and Postnatal Depression: A Systematic Mapping of the Evidence from Low and Lower Middle Income Countries'. *Health Place* 18(5): 1188–97.

Cock, J. 2011. 'Challenging the Invisibility of Domestic Workers'. *South African Review of Sociology* 42(2): 132–3.

Coetzee, J.M. 1998. *White Writing: On the Culture of Letters in South Africa*. London: Yale University Press.

———. 1999. *Disgrace*. London: Secker & Warburg.

————. 2007. *Diary of a Bad Year*. London: Random Secker.

Cole, S.M. and G. Tembo. 2011. 'The Effect of Food Insecurity on Mental Health: Panel Evidence from Rural Zimbabwe'. *Social Science and Medicine* 73: 1071–9.

Coleman, L. and S. Cater. 2006. 'Planned Teenage Pregnancy: Perspectives of Young Women from Disadvantaged Backgrounds in England'. *Journal of Youth Studies* 9(5): 593–614.

Collins, B. 2007. 'Representations of Landscape and Gender in Lady Anne Barnard's *Journal of a Month's Tour into the Interior of Africa*'. MPhil thesis, University of Stellenbosch, Stellenbosch.

Collins, P.H. 1994a. 'Shifting the Centre: Race, Class, and Feminist Theorizing about Motherhood'. In *Mothering: Ideology, Experience, and Agency*, edited by E.N. Glenn, G. Chang and L.R. Forcey, 45–65. New York: Routledge.

————. 1994b. 'The Social Construction of Black Feminist Thought'. In *The Woman Question*, edited by M. Evans, 82–103. London: Sage.

Connolly, D. 2000. 'Mythical Mothers and Dichotomies of Good and Evil: Homeless Mothers in the United States'. In *Ideologies and Technologies of Motherhood: Race, Class, Sexuality, Nationalism*, edited by H. Ragone and F.W. Twine, 263–94. New York: Routledge.

Conroy, C.C. and B.H. Cottrell. 2015. 'The Influence of Skin-to-Skin Contact after Cesarean on Breastfeeding Rates, Infant Feeding Responses, and Maternal Satisfaction'. *Journal of Obstetric, Gynecologic & Neonatal Nursing* 44: S61–S62.

Cook, K. and C. Loomis. 2012. 'The Impact of Choice and Control on Women's Childbirth Experiences'. *Journal of Perinatal Education* 21(3): 158–68.

Cooper, D.G. 1971. *The Death of the Family*. Harmondsworth: Penguin.

Cordes, K., C. Baldwin and S. Mthathi. 2011. *Ripe with Abuse: Human Rights Conditions in South Africa's Fruit and Wine Industries*. New York: Human Rights Watch.

Cosslett, T. 1994. *Women Writing Childbirth: Modern Discourses of Motherhood*. Manchester: Manchester University Press.

Crofford, J. 2007. 'Violence, Stress, and Somatic Syndromes'. *Trauma, Violence and Abuse* 8(3): 299–313.

Crossley, M.C. 2007. 'Childbirth, Complications and the Illusion of "Choice": A Case Study'. *Feminism & Psychology* 17(4): 543–63.

Crowe, M. 2000. 'The Nurse-Patient Relationship: A Consideration of Its Discursive Context'. *Journal of Advanced Nursing* 31(4): 962–7.

Cuomo, C.J. and K.Q. Hall. 1999. *Whiteness: Feminist Philosophical Reflections*. Lanham, MA: Rowman & Littlefield.

Currier, D. 2004. 'Review: The Psychology of Female Violence; Crimes against the Body'. *Feminism & Psychology* 14(4): 601–3.

Cuthbert, B. and T. Insel. 2013. 'Toward the Future of Psychiatric Diagnosis: The Seven Pillars RDoC'. *BMC Medicine* 14(11): 126.

Danforth, D.N. 1982. *Obstetrics and Gynecology*. Philadelphia: Harper & Row.

Dannenbring, D., M.J. Stevens and A.E. House. 1997. 'Predictors of Childbirth Pain and Maternal Satisfaction'. *Journal of Behavioral Medicine* 20: 127–42.

Davis, K. 1997. *Embodied Practices: Feminist Perspectives on the Body*. London: Sage.

Davis-Floyd, R.E. 1994. 'The Technocratic Body: American Childbirth as Cultural Expression'. *Social Science and Medicine* 38(8): 1125–40.

———. 2000. 'Anthropological Perspectives on Global Issues in Midwifery'. *Midwifery Today* 53: 12–16, 68–69.

Dawes, A., Z. de Sas Kropiwnicki, Z. Kafaar and L. Richter. 2005. 'Survey Examines South Africa's Attitude towards Corporal Punishment'. *Article 19* 1(2): 1–3.

Dawjee, H.M. 2018. *Sorry, Not Sorry: Experiences of a Brown Woman in a White South Africa*. Cape Town: Random House Struik.

Deaton, A. 2004. 'Health in an Age of Globalization'. NBER Working Paper No. 10669. Cambridge, MA: National Bureau of Economic Research. https://www.nber.org/papers/w10669.pdf.

Dekel, B. and M. Andipatin. 2016. 'Abused Women's Understandings of Intimate Partner Violence and the Link to Intimate Femicide'. *Forum: Qualitative Social Research* 17(1). Art. 9. http://www.qualitative-research.net/index.php/fqs/article/view/2394/3939.

De Marneffe, D. 2009. *Maternal Desire: On Children, Love, and the Inner Life*. New York: Little, Brown & Co.

Dermott, E. 2012. 'Poverty, Parenting and Outcomes'. Poverty and Social Exclusion Conceptual Note No. 1. http://www.poverty.ac.uk/working-papers-parenting-poverty-child-poverty-families-government-policy-conceptual-notes/poverty.

Devereux, S. and K. Roelen. 2016. 'Hunger, Social Protection and Shame in South Africa'. Workshop report, Cape Town.

De Villiers, S. 2011. 'Mothering as a Three-Generational Process: The Psychological Experiences of Low-income Mothers Sharing Childcare with Their Mothers'. PhD dissertation, University of Stellenbosch, Stellenbosch.

Dewing, S., M. Tomlinson, I.M. le Roux, M. Chopra and A.C. Tsai. 2013. 'Food Insecurity and Its Association with Co-occuring Postnatal Depression, Hazardous Drinking, and Suicidality among Women in Peri-urban South Africa'. *Journal of Affective Disorders* 150(2): 460–5.

Dimen, M. 1992. 'Power, Sexuality, and Intimacy'. In *Gender/Body/Knowledge: Feminist Reconstructions of Being and Knowing*, edited by A. Jaggar and S. Bordo, 34–51. New Brunswick: Rutgers University Press.

———. 2011. *With Culture in Mind: Psychoanalytic Stories*. London: Routledge.

D'Oliveira, A.F.L., S. Grilo Diniz and L. Blima Schraiber. 2002. 'Violence against Women in Health-Care Institutions: An Emerging Problem'. *Lancet* 359(9336): 1681–5.

Douglas, M. 1966. *Purity and Danger: An Analysis of Concepts of Pollution and Taboo*. London: Routledge & Kegan Paul.

Dukas, C. and L-M. Kruger. 2016. 'A Feminist Phenomenological Description of Depression in Low-income South African Women'. *International Journal of Women's Health and Wellness* 1(1). https://pdfs.semanticscholar.org/763a/4c942f5c2c8704858fca410843101a86392b.pdf.

Duncan, S., R. Edwards and C. Alexander. 2010. *Teenage Parenthood: What's The Problem?* London: Tufnell Press.

Dunn, E.A. and C. O'Herlihy. 2005. 'Comparison of Maternal Satisfaction Following Vaginal Delivery after Caesarean Section and Caesarean Section after Previous Vaginal Delivery'. *European Journal of Obstetrics & Gynecology and Reproductive Biology* 121(1): 56–60.

Dunne, C.L., J. Fraser and G.E. Gardner. 2014. 'Women's Perceptions of Social Support during Labour: Development, Reliability and Validity of the Birth Companion Support Questionnaire'. *Midwifery* 30(7): 847–52.

Du Plessis, J. 2016. 'Essential Paradigm Shifts in Land and Housing'. Unpublished presentation.

Duras, M. 1985. *The Lover*. New York: Pantheon Books.

Du Toit, A. 2002. 'On Poverty, the Suffering in Poverty, and Researching it'. Unpublished paper, University of the Western Cape.

———. 2004. '"Social Exclusion" Discourse and Chronic Poverty: A South African Case Study'. *Development and Change* 35(5): 987–1010.

———. 2005. 'Chronic and Structural Poverty in South Africa: Challenges for Action and Research'. CPRC Working Paper 56, PLAAS.

———. 2006. 'Poverty Measurement Blues: Some Reflections on the Space for Understanding "Chronic" and "Structural" Poverty in South Africa'. Chronic Poverty Research Centre Working Paper No. 55. https://ssrn.com/abstract=1753682.

Edwards, R. 2018. 'An Exploration of Maternal Satisfaction with Breastfeeding as a Clinically Relevant Measure of Breastfeeding Success'. *Journal of Human Lactation* 34(1): 93–6.

Eliot, G. 1873. *Middlemarch: A Study of Provincial Life*. London: William Blackwood and Sons.

El-Nemer, A., S. Downe and N. Small. 2006. '"She Would Help me from the Heart": An Ethnography of Egyptian Women in Labour'. *Social Science and Medicine* 62(1): 81–92.

Enander, V. 2010. 'Jekyll and Hyde or "Who is This Guy?" Battered Women's Interpretations of Their Abusers as a Mirror of Opposite Discourses'. *Women's Studies International Forum* 33(2): 81–90.

———. 2011. 'Leaving Jekyll and Hyde: Emotion Work in the Context of Intimate Partner Violence'. *Feminism & Psychology* 21(1): 29–48.

Erasmus, Z. 2001. *Coloured by History, Shaped by Place: New Perspectives on Coloured Identities in Cape Town*. Cape Town: Kwela Books.

———. 2017. *Race Otherwise: Forging a New Humanism for South Africa*. Johannesburg: Wits University Press.

Erenoglu, R. and M. Baser. 2019. 'Effect of Expressive Touching on Labour Pain and Maternal Satisfaction: A Randomised Controlled Trial'. *Complementary Therapies in Clinical Practice* 34(1): 268–74.

Erickson, M.T. 1976. 'The Influence of Health Factors on Psychological Variables Predicting Complications of Pregnancy'. *Journal of Psychosomatic Research* 20(1): 21–4.

Esprey, Y. 2013. 'Raising the Colour Bar: Exploring Issues of Race, Racism and Racialised Identities in the South African Therapeutic Context'. In *Psychodynamic psychotherapy in South Africa*, edited by C. Smith, G. Lobban and M. O'Loughlin, 35–53. Johannesburg: Wits University Press.

Euripides. 2002. *Euripides: Medea*. Edited by Donald. J. Mastronard. Cambridge: Cambridge University Press.

Evens, E., E. Tolley, J. Headley, D.R. McCarraher, M. Hartmann, V.T. Mtimkulu, K.N. Manenzhe, G. Hamela and F. Zulu. 2015. 'Identifying Factors That Influence Pregnancy Intentions: Evidence from South Africa and Malawi'. *Culture, Health & Sexuality* 17(3): 374–89.

Fairbridge, D. 1924. *Lady Anne Barnard at the Cape of Good Hope 1797–1802*. Oxford: Clarendon Press.

Farmer, P. 2000. 'Foreword'. In *Dying for Growth: Global Inequality and the Health of the Poor*, edited by J.Y. Kim, J.V. Millen, A. Irwin and J. Gershman, xii–xv. Monroe, ME: Common Courage Press.

———. 2004. 'An Anthropology of Structural Violence'. *Current Anthropology* 45(3): 305–25.

———. 2005. *Pathologies of Power: Health, Human Rights and the New War on the Poor*. Berkeley: University of California Press.

Feachem, R.G.A. 2001. 'Globalisation is Good for Your Health, Mostly'. *BMJ* 323(7311): 504–6.

Felski, R. 2000. 'Commentary on Sylvia Walby's *Beyond the Politics of Location: The Power of Argument in a Global Era*', *Feminist Theory* 1(2): 225–9.

Fernando, S. 2012. 'The Roads Less Travelled: Mapping Some Pathways on the Global Mental Health Roadmap'. *Transcultural Psychiatry* 49(3–4): 396–417.

Flax, J. 1990. *Thinking Fragments: Psychoanalysis, Feminism and Post-modernism in the Contemporary West*. Berkeley: University of California Press.

———. 1993. *Disputed Subjects: Essays on Psychoanalysis, Politics and Philosophy*. New York: Routledge.

Fleming, K. and Kruger, L-M. 2013. '"She Keeps His Secrets": A Gendered Analysis of the Impact of Shame on the Non-disclosure of Sexual Violence in One Low-income South African Community: Original Contributions'. *African Safety Promotion* 11(2): 107–24.

Flyvbjerg, B. 2006. 'Five Misunderstandings about Case-Study Research'. *Qualitative Inquiry* 12(2): 219–45.

Fonagy, P. 1999. 'Psychoanalysis and Attachment Theory'. In *Handbook of Attachment: Theory, Research, and Clinical Applications*, edited by J. Cassidy and P. Shaver, 595–624. New York: Guilford Press.

Fonn, S., M. Xaba, K. Tint, D. Conco and S. Varkey. 1998. 'Maternal Health Services in South Africa: During the 10th Anniversary of the WHO "Safe Motherhood" Initiative'. *South African Medical Journal* 88(6): 687–702.

Fosshage, J. 2005. 'The Explicit and Implicit Domains in Psychoanalytic Change'. *Psychoanalytic Inquiry* 25(4): 516–39.

Foucault, M. 1961. *Madness and Civilization: A History of Insanity in the Age of Reason.* New York: Vintage Books.

———. 1977. *Discipline and Punish: The Birth of the Prison.* London: Penguin.

———. 1980. *Power/Knowledge: Selected Interviews and Other Writings 1972–1977.* Brighton: Harvester Press.

———. 1988. *The History of Sexuality.* New York: Vintage Books.

———. 1989. *The Birth of the Clinic.* London: Routledge.

———. 1995. *Discipline and Punish: The Birth of the Prison.* 2nd edition. New York: Vintage Books.

———. 2002. *The Order of Things: An Archaeology of the Human Sciences.* London: Routledge.

Frank, J.D. and J.B Frank. 1993. *Persuasion and Healing: Comparative Study of Psychotherapy.* 3rd edition. Baltimore: Johns Hopkins University Press.

Frankenberg, R. 1997. *Displacing Whiteness: Essays in Social and Cultural Criticism.* Durham: Duke University Press.

Frenkel, L. 2002. '"You Get Used to it". Working with Trauma in a Burns Unit of a South African Children's Hospital'. *Psychodynamic Practice* 8(4): 483–502.

Freud, S. 1912. 'Recommendations to Physicians on Practicing Psycho-analysis'. In *Standard Edition,* 12, 111–20. London: Hogarth Press.

———. 1989. *The Freud Reader.* Edited by P. Gay. New York: W.W. Norton.

Frosh, S. 1989. *Psychoanalysis and Psychology: Minding the Gap.* New York: New York University Press.

———. 1999. *The Politics of Psychoanalysis.* London: Palgrave.

———. 2006. *For and against Psychoanalysis.* London: Routledge.

Frosh, S., A. Phoenix and R. Pattman. 2000. '"But it's Racism I Really Hate": Young Masculinities, Racism and Psychoanalysis'. *Psychoanalytic Psychology* 17(2): 225–42.

Frosh, S. and L. Saville Young. 2017. 'Psychoanalytic Approaches to Qualitative Psychology'. In *The Sage Handbook of Qualitative Research in Psychology,* edited by W. Stainton Rogers and C. Willig, 109–26. London: Sage.

Frost, J., C. Pope, R. Liebling and D. Murphy. 2006. 'Utopian Birth and the Discourse of Natural Birth'. *Social Theory and Health* 4(4): 299–318.

Gabbard, G.O. 2000. 'A Neurobiologically Informed Perspective on Psychotherapy'. *British Journal of Psychiatry* 177(2): 117–22.

———. 2014. *Psychodynamic Psychiatry in Clinical Practice.* Washington, DC: American Psychiatric Publishing.

Gabbay, J. and A. le May. 2011. *Practice-based Evidence for Healthcare: Clinical Mindlines.* New York: Routledge.

Galeano, E. 1992. *The Book of Embraces.* Translated by C. Belfrage. New York: W.W. Norton.

Gama, N. and L. Willemse. 2015. 'A Descriptive Overview of the Education and Income of Domestic Workers in Post-apartheid South Africa'. *GeoJournal* 80(5): 721–41.

Garisch, D. 2012. *Eloquent Body*. Cape Town: Modjaji Books.

Gass, J.D., D.J. Stein, D.R. Williams and S. Seedat. 2011. 'Gender Differences in Risk for Intimate Partner Violence among South African Adults'. *Journal of Interpersonal Violence* 26(14): 2764–89.

Gawande, A. 2008. *Better: A Surgeon's Notes on Performance*. London: Picador.

———. 2011. *The Checklist Manifesto: How to Get Things Right*. London: Picador.

———. 2014. *Being Mortal: Medicine and What Matters in the End*. New York: Henry Holt.

Gay, P. 1988. *Freud: A Life for Our Time*. New York: Anchor Books.

Geerds, K. 1992. *Woeste grond: Gedichten*. Amsterdam: Arbeiderspers.

Geertz, C. 1973. *The Interpretation of Cultures*. New York: Basic Books.

———. 1995. *After the Fact: Two Countries, Four Decades, One Anthropologist*. Cambridge: Harvard University Press.

Gibbs, A., R. Jewkes, S. Willan and L. Washington. 2018. 'Associations between Poverty, Mental Health and Substance Use, Gender Power, and Intimate Partner Violence amongst Young (18–30) Women and Men in Urban Informal Settlements in South Africa: A Cross-Sectional Study and Structural Equation Model'. *PLOS One* 13(10): e0204956. https://journals.plos.org/plosone/article?id=10.1371/journal.pone.0204956.

Gibson, D. 2004. 'The Gaps in the Gaze in South African Hospitals'. *Social Science and Medicine* 59(10): 2013–24.

Gibson, K. 2002. 'Politics and Emotion in Work with Disadvantaged Children: Case Studies in Consultation from a South African Clinic'. PhD dissertation, University of Cape Town, Cape Town.

Gilbert, P. 1998. 'What is Shame? Some Core Issues and Controversies'. In *Shame: Interpersonal Behavior, Psychopathology, and Culture*, edited by P. Gilbert and B. Andrews, 3–38. New York: Oxford University Press.

Gillies, V. 2007. *Marginalised Mothers: Exploring Working-class Experiences of Parenting*. London: Routledge.

Gilligan, J. 2003. 'Shame, Guilt, and Violence'. *Social Research* 70(4): 1149–80.

Gizzo, S., M. Noventa, S. Fagherazzi, L. Lamparelli, E. Ancona, S. di Gangi, C. Saccardi, D. D'Antona and G.B. Nardelli. 2014. 'Update on Best Available Options in Obstetrics Anaesthesia: Perinatal Outcomes, Side Effects and Maternal Satisfaction; Fifteen Years Systematic Literature Review'. *Archives of Gynecology and Obstetrics* 290(1): 21–34.

Graham, L.V. 2014. '"A Strange Antipathy": Elsa Joubert and "Poppie Nongena"'. *Bulletin of the National Library of South Africa* 68(2): 174–86.

Graves, R. 1927. 'The Cool Web'. *Poetry* 30(1): 16–17.

Greenberg, J.R. and S.A. Mitchell. 1983. *Object Relations in Psychoanalytic Theory*. Cambridge: Harvard University Press.

Grisaru, N., R. Kaufman, J. Mirsky and E. Witztum. 2011. 'Food Insecurity and Mental Health: A Pilot Study of Patients in a Psychiatric Emergency Unit in Israel'. *Community Mental Health Journal* 47(5): 513–19.

Gross, E. 1990. 'The Body of Signification'. In *Abjection, Melancholia, and Love: The Work of Julia Kristeva*, edited by J. Fletcher and A. Benjamin, 80–103. London: Routledge.

Grosz, E. 1990. *Jacques Lacan: A Feminist Introduction*. London: Routledge.

Gungor, I. and N.K. Beji. 2012. 'Development and Psychometric Testing of the Scales for Measuring Maternal Satisfaction in Normal and Caesarean Births'. *Midwifery* 28(3): 348–57.

Hadley, C. and C.C. Patil. 2006. 'Food Insecurity in Rural Tanzania is Associated with Maternal Anxiety and Depression'. *American Journal of Human Biology* 18(3): 359–68.

Hall, P.J., J.W. Foster, K.M. Yount and B.M. Jennings. 2018. 'Keeping it Together and Falling Apart: Women's Dynamic Experience of Birth'. *Midwifery* 58: 130–6.

Hamman, C. and L-M. Kruger. 2017. 'Gossip Girls: The Power of Girls' Gossip in a Low-income South African Community'. *Critical Arts* 31(1): 1–17.

Hanandita, W. and G. Tampubolon. 2014. 'Does Poverty Reduce Mental Health? An Instrumental Variable Analysis'. *Social Science and Medicine* 113(7): 59–67.

Handsel, V.A. 2007. 'Psychological Variables in Battered Women's Stay/Leave Decisions: Risk-taking, Perceived Control, and Optimistic Bias'. Master's thesis, University of North Carolina Wilmington, Wilmington.

Harding, S. 2001. 'Comments on Walby's "Against Epistemological Chasms: The Science Question in Feminism Revisited: Can Democratic Values and Interests Ever Play a Rationally Justifiable Role in the Evaluation of Scientific Work?"'. *Signs* 26(2): 511–36.

Hartley, M. and L-M. Kruger. 2017. 'On Being Human: The Power of Specificity in Psychotherapy in the South African Context'. *Psycho-analytic Psychotherapy in South Africa* 25(2): 75–115.

Hastings-Tolsma, M., A.G.W. Nolte and A. Temane. 2018. 'Birth Stories from South Africa: Voices Unheard'. *Women and Birth* 31(1): 45–50.

Haugen, M.S. and M. Villa. 2006. 'Big Brother in Rural Societies: Youths' Discourses on Gossip'. *Norwegian Journal of Geography* 60(3): 209–16.

Hayes, S. 2015. 'The Big Question: Why Women Stay in Abusive Relationships'. Paper presented to the RPI Conference, Hobart, 23–25 March. https://www.rpiassn.org/wp-content/uploads/2015/04/Hayes_Sharon_The-Big-Question_2.pdf.

Hayes, S. and S. Jeffries. 2013. 'Why do They Keep Going Back? Exploring Women's Discursive Experiences of Intimate Partner Violence'. *International Journal of Criminology and Sociology* 2: 57–71.

Heim, E., I. Ajzen, P. Schmidt and D. Seddig. 2018. 'Women's Decisions to Stay in or Leave an Abusive Relationship: Results from a Longitudinal Study in Bolivia'. *Violence against Women* 24(14): 1639–57.

Helman, C.G. 2001. *Culture, Health and Illness*. 4th edition. London: Arnold.

Henderson, A. 1994. 'Power and Knowledge in Nursing Practice: The Contribution of Foucault'. *Journal of Advanced Nursing* 20(5): 935–9.

Hendricks, L., S. Swartz and A. Bhana. 2010. 'Why Young Men in South Africa Plan to Become Teenage Fathers: Implications for the Development of Masculinities within Contexts of Poverty'. *Journal of Psychology in Africa* 20(4): 527–36.

Hill, M. 1997. *Whiteness: A Critical Reader*. New York: New York University Press.

Hill, T. and B. Needham. 2013. 'Rethinking Gender and Mental Health: A Critical Analysis of Three Propositions'. *Social Science and Medicine* 92(1): 83–91.

Hirsch, M. 1989. *The Mother/Daughter Plot: Narrative, Psychoanalysis, Feminism*. Bloomington: Indiana University Press.

Hoagland, T. 2010. *Unincorporated Persons in the Late Honda Dynasty: Poems*. Minneapolis: Graywolf Press.

———. 2015. *Application for Release from the Dream*. Minneapolis: Graywolf Press.

Hodnett, E.D. 2002. 'Pain and Women's Satisfaction with the Experience of Childbirth: A Systematic Review'. *American Journal of Obstetrics and Gynecology* 186(5): 160–72.

Hollway, W. 2006. *The Capacity to Care: Gender and Ethical Subjectivity*. London: Routledge.

———. 2015. *Knowing Mothers: Researching Maternal Identity Change*. London: Palgrave Macmillan.

Hornstein, G.A. 2005. *To Redeem One Person is to Redeem the World: The Life of Frieda Fromm-Reichmann*. New York: Other Press.

Hotelling, B.A. 2004. 'Is Your Perinatal Practice Mother-Friendly? A Strategy for Improving Maternity Care'. *Birth* 31(2): 143–7.

Howell-White, S. 1997. 'Choosing a Birth Attendant: The Influence of a Woman's Childbirth Definition'. *Social Science and Medicine* 45(6): 925–36.

Hrdy, S.B. 1999. *Mother Nature: A History of Mothers, Infants, and Natural Selection*. New York: Pantheon Books.

Hudson, P.A. 1986. 'Causality and the Subject in a "Discourse-Theoretical" Approach to Marxism'. *Studies in Marxism* (7).

Huffer, L. 2009. *Mad for Foucault: Rethinking the Foundations of Queer Theory*. New York: Columbia University Press.

Hughes, J.M. 1989. 'Melanie Klein: The World of Internal Objects'. In *Reshaping the Psychoanalytic Domain: The Work of Melanie Klein, W.R.D. Fairbairn & D.W. Winnicott*, edited by J.M. Hughes, 44–88. Berkeley: Universtity of California Press.

Hwa-Froelich, D.A., C.A. Loveland Cook and L.H. Flick. 2008. 'Maternal Sensitivity and Communication Styles: Mothers with Depression'. *Journal of Early Intervention* 31(1): 44–66.

Hyde, A., M.M. Treacy, A.P. Scott, P. Mac Neela, M. Butler, J. Drennan, I. Kate and A. Byrne. 2006. 'Social Regulation, Medicalisation and the Nurse's Role: Insights from an Analysis of Nursing Documentation'. *International Journal of Nursing Studies* 43(6): 735–44.

Hydén, M. 1999. 'The World of the Fearful: Battered Women's Narratives of Leaving Abusive Husbands'. *Feminism & Psychology* 9(4): 449–69.

Illich, I. 1995. 'Death Undefeated'. *British Medical Journal* 311: 1652–3.

Ingleby, D. 1981. *Critical Psychiatry: The Politics of Mental Health*. London: Penguin.

Insel, T. 2013. 'Post by Former NIMH Director Thomas Insel: Transforming Diagnosis'. National Institute of Mental Health. https://www.nimh.nih.gov/about/directors/thomas-insel/blog/2013/transforming-diagnosis.shtml.

Insel, T., B. Cuthbert, M. Garvey, R. Heinssen, D.S. Pine, K. Quinn, C. Sanislow and P. Wang. 2010. 'Research Domain Criteria (RDoC): Toward a New Classification Framework for Research on Mental Disorders'. *American Journal of Psychiatry* 167(7): 748–51.

Ivers, L.C. and K.A. Cullen. 2011. 'Food Insecurity: Special Considerations for Women'. *American Journal of Clinical Nutrition* 94(6): 1740S–4S.

Ivey, G. 2006. 'A Method of Teaching Psychodynamic Case Formulation'. *Psychotherapy* 43(3): 322–36.

Jack, D. 1991. *Silencing the Self: Women and Depression*. Cambridge: Harvard University Press.

———. 1999. *Behind the Mask: Destruction and Creativity in Women's Aggression*. Cambridge: Harvard University Press.

Jack, K.M. 2014. 'Lived Experiences of Women Staying in Physically Abusive Relationships'. Master's thesis, University of South Africa, Pretoria.

Jackson, M. 2011. *Life within Limits: Well-Being in a World of Want*. Durham: Duke University Press.

Jacobs, L. 1996. 'Shame in the Therapeutic Dialogue'. In *The Voice of Shame: Silence and Connection in Psychotherapy*, edited by R. Lee and G. Wheeler, 294–314. Hillsdale, NJ: The Analytic Press.

Jansen, E. 2015. *Soos familie: Stedelike huiswerkers in Suid-Afrikaanse tekste*. Johannesburg: Proteaboekhuis.

Javier, R.A. and W.G. Herron. 2002. 'Psychoanalysis and the Disenfranchised: Countertransference Issues'. *Psychoanalytic Psychology* 19(1): 149–66.

Jensen, T. 2010. 'Warmth and Wealth: Re-imagining Social Class in Taxonomies of Good Parenting'. *Studies in the Maternal* 2(1): 1–13.

Jewkes, R., N. Abrahams and Z. Mvo. 1998. 'Why do Nurses Abuse Patients? Reflections from South African Obstetric Services'. *Social Science and Medicine* 47(11): 1781–95.

———. 2001. 'Health Care-Seeking Practices of Pregnant Women and the Role of the Midwife in Cape Town, South Africa'. *Journal of Midwifery & Women's Health* 46(4): 240–7.

Jewkes, R., A. Gevers, P. Cupp, C. Mathews, M. Russell, C. LeFleur-Bellerose and A. Flisher. 2011. *Respect4U*. South Africa: Medical Research Council.

Jo, Y.N. 2013. 'Psycho-Social Dimensions of Poverty: When Poverty Becomes Shameful'. *Critical Social Policy* 33(3): 514–31.

Johnson, M.P. and K.J. Ferraro. 2000. 'Research on Domestic Violence in the 1990s: Making Distinctions'. *Journal of Marriage and Family* 62(4): 948–63.

Johnson, R. 2010. 'Athol Fugard Finds Truth and Reconciliation in "The Train Driver"'. *Los Angeles Times*, 15 October. http://www.latimes.com/archives/la-xpm-2010-oct-15-la-athol-fugard-20101015-story.html.

Johnson, S., A. Burrows and I. Williamson. 2004. '"Does my Bump Look Big in This?" The Meaning of Bodily Changes for First-Time Mothers-to-be'. *Journal of Health Psychology* 9(3): 361–74.

Johnstone, L. and M. Boyle. 2018. *The Power Threat Meaning Framework: Overview.* Leicester: British Psychological Society.

Jolly, M. 1998. 'Introduction: Colonial and Postcolonial Plots in Histories of Maternities and Modernities'. In *Maternities and Modernities: Colonial and Postcolonial Experiences in Asia and the Pacific*, edited by K. Ram and M. Jolly, 1–25. Cambridge: Cambridge University Press.

Jordans, M.J.D, I.H. Komproe, W.A. Tol, J. Nsereko and J.T.V.M de Jong. 2013. 'Treatment Processes of Counseling for Children in South Sudan: A Multiple n = 1 Design'. *Community Mental Health Journal* 49(3): 354–67.

Joubert, E. 1980. *The Long Journey of Poppy Nongena.* Johannesburg: Jonathan Ball.

———. 1986. 'Agterplaas'. In *A Land Apart: A South African Reader*, edited by A.P. Brink and J.M. Coetzee, 219–30. London: Faber & Faber.

Kabakian-Khasholian, T., O. Campbell, M. Shediac-Rizkallah and F. Ghorayeb. 2000. 'Women's Experiences of Maternity Care: Satisfaction or Passivity'. *Social Science and Medicine* 51(1): 103–13.

Kabura, P., L.M. Fleming and D.J. Tobin. 2005. 'Microcounseling Skills Training for Informal Helpers in Uganda'. *International Journal of Social Psychiatry* 51(1): 63–70.

Kadish, Y.A. 2012. 'Investigating Defensive Organisations and Psychic Retreats in Anorexia'. PhD dissertation, University of Witwatersrand, Johannesburg.

———. 2016. 'Reaching across the Divide: Considering the Challenges for Intercultural Therapeutic Dyads Embedded in Previously Oppressive Social Contexts'. *Psycho-analytic Psychotherapy in South Africa* 24(1): 109–38.

Kafka, F. 1970. *The Great Wall of China: Stories and Reflections.* New York: Schocken Books.

Kagee, A. 2006a. 'The Complexity of Evidence Notwithstanding: A Reply to Swartz'. *South African Journal of Psychology* 36(2): 255–8.

———. 2006b. 'Where is the Evidence in South African Clinical Psychology?' *South African Journal of Psychology* 36(2): 233–48.

Kagee, A. and E. Breet. 2015. 'Psychologists' Endorsements of Empirically Unsupported Statements in Psychology: Noch Einmal'. *South African Journal of Psychology* 45(3): 397–409.

Käll, L.F., ed. 2013. *Dimensions of Pain: Humanities and Social Science Perspectives*. London: Routledge.

Kalmanofsky, A. 2008. 'Israel's Baby: The Horror of Childbirth in the Biblical Prophets'. *Biblical Interpretation* 16(1): 60–82.

Kamfer, R.S. 2011. *grond/Santekraam*. Cape Town: Kwela Books.

———. 2016. *Hammie*. Cape Town: Kwela Books.

Kaminer, D., A. Grimsrud, L. Myer, D.J. Stein and D.R. Williams. 2008. 'Risk for Post-traumatic Stress Disorder Associated with Different Forms of Interpersonal Violence in South Africa'. *Social Science and Medicine* 67(10): 1589–95.

Kantrowitz, J.L. 2006. *Writing about Patients: Responsibilities, Risks and Ramifications*. New York: Other Press.

Kapp, T. 2015. 'Buite blaf die honde swart'. Afrikaans translation of Bernard-Marie Koltés's play *Combat de nègre et de chiens*. First performed at the Klein Karoo National Arts Festival in 2015.

Kazdin, A.E. 2016. 'Evidence-based Psychosocial Treatment: Advances, Surprises, and Needed Shifts in Foci'. *Cognitive and Behavioural Practice* 23(4): 426–30.

Keys, A., A. Henschel and J. Brožek. 1950. *The Biology of Human Starvation*. Minneapolis: University of Minnesota Press.

Kiernan, K.E. and M.C. Huerta. 2008. 'Economic Deprivation, Maternal Depression, Parenting and Children's Cognitive and Emotional Development in Early Childhood'. *British Journal of Sociology* 59(4): 783–806.

Kirmayer, L.J. and D. Crafa. 2014. 'What Kind of Science for Psychiatry?' *Frontiers in Human Neuroscience* 8(435): 1–12.

Kiss, L., L.B. Schraiber, L. Heise, C. Zimmerman, N. Gouveia and C. Watts. 2012. 'Gender-Based Violence and Socioeconomic Inequalities: Does Living in More Deprived Neighbourhoods Increase Women's Risk of Intimate Partner Violence?' *Social Science and Medicine* 74(8): 1172–9.

Klein, M. 1975. 'Envy and Gratitude: A Study of Unconscious Sources'. In *Melanie Klein: Envy and Gratitude and Other Works, 1946–1963*, edited by R. Money-Kyrle, 176–235. New York: Delacorte Press.

———. 2011. *Love, Guilt and Reparation And Other Works, 1921–1945*. New York: Free Press.

Klein, N. 2007. *The Shock Doctrine: The Rise of Disaster Capitalism*. New York: Henry Holt.

Kleinman, A. 1986. *Social Origins of Distress and Disease: Depression, Neurasthenia, and Pain in Modern China*. New Haven: Yale University Press.

———. 1988. *Rethinking Psychiatry: From Cultural Category to Personal Experience*. New York: Free Press.

Koblinsky, M., Z. Matthews, J. Hussein, D. Mavalankar, M.K. Mribha, I. Anwar, E. Achadi, S. Adjei, P. Padmanabhan and W. van Lerberghe. 2006. 'Going to Scale with Professional Skilled Care'. *Lancet* 368(9554): 1377–86.

Kohrt, B.A., M.J. Jordans, S. Rai, P. Shrestha, N.P. Luitel, M.K. Ramaiya, D.R. Singla and V. Patel. 2015. 'Therapist Competence in Global Mental Health: Development of the ENhancing Assessment of Common Therapeutic Factors (ENACT) Rating Scale'. *Behaviour Research and Therapy* 69: 11–21.

Kohut, H. 1971. *The Analysis of the Self: A Systematic Approach to the Psychoanalytic Treatment of Narcissistic Personality Disorders*. London: Hogarth Press.

———. 1984. *How Does Analysis Cure?* Chicago: University of Chicago Press.

———. 2009. *The Restoration of the Self*. Chicago: University of Chicago Press.

Kolb, P. 1967. *The Present State of the Cape of Good Hope*. New York: Johnson Reprint Corporation.

Kornelsen, J. 2005. 'Essences and Imperatives: An Investigation of Technology in Childbirth'. *Social Science and Medicine* 61(7): 1495–504.

Kottler, A. and K. Togashi. 2015. *Kohut's Twinship across Cultures: The Psychology of Being Human*. London: Routledge.

Krauss, N. 2005. *The History of Love*. New York: W.W. Norton.

Kristeva, J. 1980. *Desire in Language: A Semiotic Approach to Literature and Art*. Edited by L. Roudiez. New York: Columbia University Press.

———. 1982. *Powers of Horror: An Essay on Abjection*. New York: Columbia University Press.

Krog, A. 1981. *Otters in Bronslaai*. Cape Town: Human & Rousseau.

———. 1989. *Lady Anne: A Chronicle in Verse*. Lanham, Maryland: Bucknell University Press.

———. 1996. 'Overwhelming Trauma of the Truth'. *Mail & Guardian*, 24 December. https://mg.co.za/article/1996-12-24-overwhelming-trauma-of-the-truth.

———. 2014. *Mede-wete*. Cape Town: Human & Rousseau.

Kruger, L.-M. 2003a. '"My Mother Pooped out a Baby": The Theoretical and Clinical Relevance of Psychoanalysis to Poor Black Mothers Living in South Africa'. Paper presented at Psychoanalysis, Gender and Race Conference, London.

———. 2003b. 'Narrating Motherhood: The Transformative Potential of Individual Stories'. *South African Journal of Psychology* 33(4): 198–204.

———. 2005. 'Childbirth and the Breakdown of the Narrative Order: Implications for Mental Health'. *Psycho-analytic Psychotherapy in South Africa* 13(2): 1–23.

———. 2006a. 'Motherhood'. In *The Gender of Psychology*, edited by T. Shefer, F. Bezuidenhoudt and P. Kiguwa, 182–97. Cape Town: Juta.

———. 2006b. 'A Tribute to 150 Years of Sigmund Freud: Not Mastering the Mind: Freud and the "Forgotten Material" of Psychology'. *Psycho-analytic Psychotherapy in South Africa* 14(2): 1–12.

———. 2007. '"Elke Vroumens Moet Daardeur" (Every Woman Has to Do it): Childbirth and Agency in One Low-Income South African Community.' Invited lecture, Department of Obstetrics and Gynaecology, Stellenbosch University.

———. 2012. '"Vrot Kolletjies": Shame, Silence and Enactment in Psychotherapy with Impoverished Clients'. *Psycho-analytic Psychotherapy in South Africa* 20(2): 1–32.

———. 2014a. 'The Slow Violence of Poverty: Notebook of a Psycho-ethnographer'. In *Winelands, Wealth and Work: Transformations in the Dwars River Valley, Stellenbosch*, edited by K. van der Waal, 125–9. Pietermaritzburg: University of KwaZulu-Natal Press.

———. 2014b. 'The Whales beneath the Surface: The Muddled Story of Doing Research with Poor Mothers in a Developing Country'. *Health Care for Women International* 35(7–9): 1010–21.

———. 2016. 'When Virtuous ("Deugsame") Women Flee: A Reflection on Dread and Flight in Group Therapy in One South African Setting'. *Psycho-analytic Psychotherapy in South Africa* 24(2): 35–78.

Kruger, L-M. and M. Lourens. 2013. 'Die subjektiewe ervaring van depressie onder Suid-Afrikaanse vroue in n lae-inkomste gemeenskap'. *Social Work/Maatskaplike Werk* 49(2): 248–70.

———. 2016. 'Motherhood and the "Madness of Hunger": ". . . Want Almal Vra vir my vir 'n Stukkie Brood" (Because Everyone Asks me for a Little Piece of Bread)'. *Culture, Medicine and Psychiatry* 40(1): 124–43.

Kruger, L-M. and K. Marquard. 2018. 'Of Suffering, Shame and Hope: Intimate Partner Violence and the Women Who Stay'. Unpublished paper, Department of Psychology, Stellenbosch University.

Kruger, L-M. and C. Schoombee. 2010. 'The Other Side of Caring: Violence in the Maternity Ward'. *Journal of Reproductive and Infant Psychology* 28(1): 84–101.

Kruger, L-M., T. Shefer and A. Oakes. 2015. '"I Could Have Done Everything and Why Not?" Young Women's Complex Constructions of Sexual Agency in the Context of Sexualities Education in Life Orientation in South African Schools'. *Perspectives in Education* 33(2): 30–48.

Kruger, L-M. and T.M. van der Spuy. 2007. '"Om Langs die Pad te Kraam": A Feminist Psychoanalytic Perspective on Undisclosed Pregnancy'. *South African Journal of Psychology* 37(1): 1–24.

Kruger, L-M., K. van Straaten, L. Taylor, M. Lourens and C. Dukas. 2014. 'The Melancholy of Murderous Mothers: Depression and the Medicalization of Women's Anger'. *Feminism & Psychology* 24(4): 461–78.

Kumar, R. and K.M. Robson. 1984. 'A Prospective Study of Emotional Disorders in Childbearing Women'. *British Journal of Psychiatry* 144(1): 35–47.

Kunitz, S. 2000. *The Collected Poems*. New York: W.W. Norton.

Lafrance, M.N. and S. McKenzie-Mohr. 2013. 'The DSM and Its Lure of Legitimacy'. *Feminism & Psychology* 23(1): 119–40.

Laing, R.D. 1967. *The Politics of Experience*. New York: Pantheon.

Lambert, M.J. and A.E. Bergin. 1994. 'The Effectiveness of Psychotherapy'. In *Handbook of Psychotherapy and Behaviour Change*, edited by A.E. Bergin and S.L. Garfield, 143–89. Oxford: John Wiley & Sons.

Lane, K. and J. Garrod. 2016. 'The Return of the Traditional Birth Attendant'. *Journal of Global Health* 6(2): e020302.

Langellier, K.M. 1989. 'Personal Narratives: Perspectives on Theory and Research'. *Text and Performance Quarterly* 9(4): 243–75.

Langenhoven, C. n.d. 'Siembaba'. http://tortel.net/~lochner/blerkas/woorde/190.txt.

Langer, A., L. Campero, C. Garcia and S. Reynoso. 1998. 'Effects of Psychosocial Support during Labour and Childbirth on Breastfeeding, Medical Interventions, and Mothers' Wellbeing in a Mexican Public Hospital: A Randomised Clinical Trial'. *British Journal of Obstetrics and Gynaecology* 105(10): 1056–63.

La Vita, M. 2014. 'En ôs stuck innie mirrel'. *Netwerk24*, 7 November. http://www. netwerk24.com/stemme/2014-11-07-en-s-stuck-innie-mirrel.

La Vita, M. and H.M. Dawjee. 2018. 'Waarom wit mense my bang maak'. *Netwerk24*, 18 May. https://www.netwerk24.com/Stemme/Profiele/waarom-wit-mense-my-bang-maak-20180517.

Lazarus, J. 2007. 'First Contact: An Exploratory Study of the Role of Psychoanalytic Infant Observation in South African Community Psychology Interventions'. DPhil dissertation, University of Stellenbosch, Stellenbosch.

Lederman, R.P. 1984. *Psychosocial Adaption in Pregnancy: Assessment of Seven Dimensions of Maternal Development*. New York: Springer.

———. 1996. *Psychosocial Adaption in Pregnancy: Assessment of Seven Dimensions of Maternal Development*. 2nd edition. New York: Springer.

Leifer, M. 1977. 'Psychological Changes Accompanying Pregnancy and Motherhood'. *Genetic Psychology Monographs* 95(1): 55–96.

———. 1980. 'Childbirth'. In *Psychological Effects of Motherhood: A Study of First Pregnancy*, edited by M. Leifer, 117–54. Westport: Praeger.

Lenta, M. 1989. 'Intimate Knowledge and Wilful Ignorance: White Employers and Black Employees in South African Fiction'. In *Women and Writing in South Africa: A Critical Anthology*, edited by C. Clayton, 241–2. Johannesburg: Heinemann.

Leonhardt-Lupa, M. 1995. *A Mother is Born: Preparing for Motherhood during Pregnancy*. Westport: Praeger.

Levenson, E.A. 1988. *The Purloined Self: Interpersonal Perspectives in Psychoanalysis*. New York: Routledge.

Levin, G. 2001. *The Complete Watercolors of Edward Hopper*. New York: Whitney Museum of Modern Art.

Light, A. 2007. *Mrs Woolf and the Servants: The Hidden Heart of Domestic Service*. London: Penguin.

Loewald, H. 1980. 'The Waning of the Oedipus Complex'. In *Papers on Psychoanalysis*, 384–404. New Haven: Yale University Press.

Loewenstein, E.A. 1991. 'Psychoanalytic Life History: Is Coherence, Continuity, and Aesthetic Appeal Necessary?' *Psychoanalysis and Contemporary Thought* 14(1): 3–28.

Long, W. 2017. 'Alienation: A New Orientating Principle for Psychotherapists in South Africa'. *Psycho-analytic Psychotherapy in South Africa* 25(1): 68–90.

———. 2019. 'Shame, Envy, Impasse and Hope: The Psychopolitics of Violence in South Africa'. Seminar presented at the Wits Institute for Economic and Social Research, University of the Witwatersrand, 11 March. https://wiser.wits.ac.za/content/shame-envy-impasse-and-hope-psychopolitics-violence-sa-13219.

Lorde, A. 1973. *From a Land Where Other People Live*. Detroit: Broadside Press.

————. 1984. *Sister Outsider: Essays and Speeches*. New York: Crossing Press.

Lorenz, H.S. and M. Watkins. 2001. 'Silenced Knowings, Forgotten Springs: Paths to Healing in the Wake of Colonialism'. *Radical Psychology* 2(2): 1–19.

Lott, B. and H.E. Bullock. 2001. 'Who Are the poor?' *Journal of Social Issues* 57(2): 189–206.

Lubbe, T. 2014. 'Some Considerations of the Role of Food in Community Work: Forum'. *Psycho-analytic Psychotherapy in South Africa* 22(1): 70–91.

Lund, C. 2014. 'Poverty and Mental Health: Towards a Research Agenda for Low- and Middle-Income Countries; Commentary on Tampubolon and Hanandita (2014)'. *Social Science and Medicine* 111: 134–6.

Lund, C., A. Breen, A.J. Flisher, R. Kakuma, J. Corriqall, J.A. Joska, L. Swartz and V. Patel. 2010. 'Poverty and Common Mental Disorders in Low- and Middle-Income Countries: A Systematic Review'. *Social Science and Medicine* 71(3): 517–28.

Lund, C. and A. Cois. 2018. 'Simultaneous Social Causation and Social Drift: Longitudinal Analysis of Depression and Poverty in South Africa'. *Journal of Affective Disorders* 229: 396–402.

Lupton, D. 1994. *Medicine as Culture: Illness, Disease and the Body in Western Societies*. London: Sage.

————. 1996. *Food, the Body and the Self*. London: Sage.

Lyman, B. 1989. *A Psychology of Food: More than a Matter of Taste*. New York: Van Nostrand Reinhold.

Lyons-Ruth, K. 1998. 'Implicit Relational Knowing: Its Role in Development and Psychoanalytic Treatment'. *Mental Health Journal* 19(3): 282–9.

Maboyana, Y. and L. Sekaja. 2015. 'Exploring the Bullying Behaviours Experienced by South African Domestic Workers'. *Journal of Psychology in Africa* 25(2): 114–20.

Macleod, C. 2001. 'Teenage Motherhood and the Regulation of Mothering in the Scientific Literature: The South African Example'. *Feminism & Psychology* 11(4): 493–510.

————. 2002. 'Economic Security and the Social Science Literature on Teenage Pregnancy in South Africa'. *Gender and Society* 16(5): 647–64.

————. 2010. *Adolescence, Pregnancy and Abortion: Constructing a Threat of Degeneration*. New York: Routledge.

————. 2011. *'Adolescence', Pregnancy and Abortion: Constructing a Threat of Degeneration*. 2nd edition. New York: Routedge.

Macleod, C.I. and T. Tracey. 2010. 'A Decade Later: Follow-up Review of South African Research on the Consequences of and Contributory Factors in Teen-Aged Pregnancy'. *South African Journal of Psychology* 40(1): 18–31.

Madhok, S. 2013. *Rethinking Agency: Developmentalism, Gender and Rights*. New Delhi: Routledge.

Maes, K.C., C. Hadley, F. Tesfaye and S. Shifferaw. 2010. 'Food Insecurity and Mental Health: Surprising Trends among Community Health Volunteers in Addis Ababa, Ethiopia during the 2008 Food Crisis'. *Social Science and Medicine* 70(9): 1450–7.

Mahopo, Z. 2018. '"Nurses Beat me up while I Was Giving Birth at Hospital"'. *Sowetan Live*, 8 November. https://www.sowetanlive.co.za/news/south-africa/2018-11-08-nurses-beat-me-up-while--i-was-giving-birth-at-hospital/.

Mannell, J. 2014. 'Adopting, Manipulating, Transforming: Tactics Used by Gender Practitioners in South African NGOs to Translate International Gender Policies into Local Practice'. *Health and Place* 30: 4–12.

Manuel, J.I., M.L. Martinson, S.E. Bledsoe-Mansori and J.L. Bellamy. 2012. 'The Influence of Stress and Social Support on Depressive Symptoms in Mothers'. *Social Science and Medicine* 75(11): 2013–20.

Marais, A. 2009. 'A Narrative Analysis of Young People's Talk of Intimate Partner Violence'. PhD dissertation, University of Cape Town, Cape Town.

Margison, F.R., M. Barkham, C. Evans, G. McGrath, J.M. Clark, K. Audin and J. Connell. 2000. 'Measurement and Psychotherapy: Evidence-based Practice and Practice-based Evidence'. *British Journal of Psychiatry*, 177(2): 123–30.

Marias, J. 2006. *Your Face of Tomorrow 1: Fever and Spear*. London: Vintage.

Marks, S. 1994. *Divided Sisterhood: Race, Class and Gender in the South African Nursing Profession*. London: St Martin's Press.

Marshall, H. and M. Wetherall. 1989. 'Talking about Career and Gender Identities: A Discourse Analysis Perspective'. In *The Social Identity of Women*, edited by S. Skevington and D. Baker, 67–98. London: Sage.

Marshall, H. and A. Woollett. 2000. 'Fit to Reproduce? The Regulative Role of Pregnancy Texts'. *Feminism & Psychology* 10(3): 351–66.

Martin, E. 1987. *The Woman in the Body: A Cultural Analysis of Reproduction*. Milton Keynes: Open University Press.

Marx, H. 2008. 'South African Soap Opera as the Other: The Deconstruction of Hegemonic Gender Idenitities in Four South African Soap Operas'. *South African Journal for Communication Theory and Research* 34(1): 80–94.

Matthee, D. 2001. 'Acts of Eating: The Everyday Eating Rituals of Female Farm Workers of Color in the Western Cape'. Master's thesis, University of Stellenbosch, Stellenbosch.

Mathews, S., N. Abrahams L.J. Martin, L. van der Merwe and R. Jewkes. 2004. 'Every Six Hours a Woman is Killed by Her Intimate Partner: A National Study Of Female Homicide in South Africa'. Cape Town: Medical Research Council.

McCue, M.L. 2008. *Domestic Violence: A Reference Handbook*. Santa Barbara: ABC-CLIO.

McIntyre, L., N.T. Glanville, S. Officer, B. Anderson, K.D. Raine and J.B. Dayle. 2002. 'Food Insecurity of Low-Income Lone Mothers and Their Children in Atlantic Canada'. *Canadian Journal of Public Health* 93(6): 411–15.

McKay, S. and T.L. Barrows. 1992. 'Reliving Birth: Maternal Responses to Viewing Videotapes of Their Second Stage Labors'. *Image: Journal of Nursing Scholarship* 24(1): 27–31.

McLaughlin, K.A., J.G. Green, M. Alegría, E.J. Costello, M.J. Gruber, N.A. Sampson and R.C. Kessler. 2012. 'Food Insecurity and Mental Disorders in a National Sample of U.S. Adolescents'. *Journal of the American Academy of Child & Adolescent Psychiatry* 51(12): 1293–303.

McWilliams, N. 1999. *Psychoanalytic Case Formulation*. New York: Guilford Press.

———. 2011. *Psychoanalytic Diagnosis: Understanding Personality Structure in the Clinical Process*. 2nd edition. New York: Guilford Press.

Mechanic, M.B., T.L. Weaver and P.A. Resick. 2008. 'Mental Health Consequences of Intimate Partner Abuse'. *Violence against Women* 14(6): 634–54.

Melender, H.L. 2002. 'Experiences of Fears Associated with Pregnancy and Childbirth: A Study of 329 Pregnant Women'. *Birth* 29(2): 101–11.

Melender, H.L. and S. Lauri. 1999. 'Fears Associated with Pregnancy and Childbirth: Experiences of Women Who Have Recently Given Birth'. *Midwifery* 15(3): 177–82.

Meyer, H.M. 2008. '"Erger as 'n vuishou": Adolescents' Experience of Pain in Chilbirth'. Master's thesis, Department of Psychology, Stellenbosch University.

Millar, K.M. 2014. 'The Precarious Present: Wageless Labor and Disrupted Life in Rio de Janeiro, Brazil'. *Cultural Anthropology* 29(1): 32–53.

Millen, J.V., A. Irwin and J.Y. Kim. 2000. 'Introduction: What is Growing? Who is Dying?' In *Dying for Growth: Global Inequality and the Health of the Poor*, edited by J.Y. Kim, J.V. Mullen, A. Irwin and J. Gershman, 3–10. Monroe, ME: Common Courage Press.

Miller, L.J. and A. Shah. 1999. 'Major Mental Illness during Pregnancy'. *Primary Care Update for OB/GYNS* 6(5): 163–8.

Mills, M. 1996. 'Shanti: An Intercultural Psychotherapy Centre for Women in the Community'. In *Planning Community Mental Health Services for Women: A Multiprofessional Handbook*, edited by K. Abel, M. Buszewicz, S. Davison, S. Johnson and E. Staples, 219–30. London: Routledge.

Miłosz, C. 2017. *Selected and Last Poems, 1931–2004*. London: Penguin.

Milton, V.C. 2008. '"Local is Lekker": Nation, Narration and the SABC's Afrikaans Programmes'. *South African Journal for Communication Theory and Research*, 34(2): 255–77.

Minh-Ha, T. 1989. *Woman, Native, Other: Writing Postcoloniality and Feminism*. Bloomington: Indiana University Press.

Mischler, E.G. 1984. *The Discourse of Medicine: Dialectics of Medical Interviews*. Norwood, NJ: Ablex.

Mitchell, S.A. and M.J. Black. 1995. *Freud and Beyond: A History of Modern Psychoanalytic Thought*. New York: BasicBooks.

Mkhize, N., J. Bennett, V. Reddy and R. Moletsane. 2010. *The Country we Want to Live in: Hate Crimes and Homophobia in the Lives of Black Lesbian South Africans*. Cape Town: HSRC Press.

Mkhwanazi, N. 2010. 'Understanding Teenage Pregnancy in a Post-apartheid South African Township'. *Culture, Health & Sexuality* 12(4): 347–58.

Moffett, H. 2006. '"These Women, They Force us to Rape Them": Rape as Narrative of Social Control in Post-apartheid South Africa', *Journal of Southern African Studies* 32(1): 129–44.

Morrison, A.P. 1994. 'The Breadth and Boundaries of a Self-psychological Immersion in Shame: A One-and-a-Half-Person Perspective.' *Psychoanalytic Dialogues* 4(1): 19–35

———. 2008. 'Shame: Considerations and Revisions; Discussion of Papers by Sandra Buechler and Donna Orange'. *Contemporary Psychoanalysis* 44(1): 105–9.

Motz, A. 2001. *The Psychology of Female Violence: Crimes against the Body*. New York: Routledge.

———. 2014. *Toxic Couples: The Psychology of Domestic Violence*. New York: Routledge.

Mrdjenović, S., S. Anton and N. Topuzović. 1999. 'Evaluation and Meaning of Emotional Reactions of Fear during the Pregnancy'. *European Psychiatry* 11(4): 323s.

Mukherjee, S. 2011. *The Emperor of All Maladies: A Biography of Cancer*. London: Fourth Estate.

Murray, L. and M. Finn. 2012. 'Good Mothers, Bad Thoughts: New Mothers' Thoughts of Intentionally Harming Their Newborns'. *Feminism & Psychology* 22(1): 41–59.

Myburgh, N. 2006. 'Violence in Nursing: Competing Discourses of Power, Care and Responsibility'. Master's thesis, University of Stellenbosch, Stellenbosch.

Myerhoff, B. 1992. *Remembered Lives: The Work of Ritual, Storytelling and Growing Older*. Edited by M. Kaminsky. Ann Arbor: University of Michigan Press.

Myers, J.E. and C.S. Gill. 2004. 'Poor, Rural and Female: Under-studied, Under-counseled, More-at-Risk'. *Journal of Mental Health Counseling* 26(3): 225–42.

Nahum, J. 2002. 'Explicating the Implicit: The Local Level and the Microprocess of Change in the Analytic Situation; The Boston Change Process Study Group (CPSG)'. *International Journal of Psychoanalysis* 83(1): 1051–62.

Nakayama, T.K. and J.N. Martin. 1998. *Whiteness: The Communication of Social Identity*. Thousand Oaks: Sage.

Naong, M.N. 2011. 'Learner Pregnancy: Perceptions on Its Prevalence and the Child Support Grant (CSG) Being the Possible Cause in South African Secondary Schools'. *Journal of Youth Studies* 14(8): 901–20.

Narayan, D. 2000. *Voices of the Poor: Can Anyone Hear us?* Oxford: Oxford University Press.

Narayan, D. and P. Petesch. 2002. *Voices of the Poor: From Many Lands*. New York: Oxford University Press.

Naylor, B. 2001. 'The "Bad Mother" in Media and Legal Texts'. *Journal of Social Semantics* 11(2): 155–76.

Nelson, G. and I. Prilleltensky. 2005. *Community Psychology : In Pursuit Of Liberation And Well-Being*. New York: Palgrave Macmillan.

Neruda, P. 1974. *The Book of Questions*. Port Townsend: Copper Canyon Press.

Newman, J.L., D.R. Fuqua, E.A. Gray and D.B. Simpson. 2006. 'Gender Differences in the Relationship of Anger and Depression in a Clinical Sample'. *Journal of Counseling and Development* 84(2): 157–62.

Nichols, M.R. 1993. 'Paternal Perspectives of the Childbirth Experience'. *Maternal-Child Nursing Journal* 21(3): 99–108.

Nixon, R. 2011. *Slow Violence and the Environmentalism of the Poor*. Cambridge: Harvard University Press.

Noah, T. 2016. *Born a Crime*. New York: Spiegel & Grau.

Nolte, A. 1998. 'Traditional Birth Attendants in South Africa: Professional Midwives' Beliefs and Myths'. *Curationis* 21(3): 59–66.

Norbeck, J.S. and V. Peterson Tilden. 1983. 'Life Stress, Social Support, and Emotional Disequilibrium in Complications of Pregnancy: A Prospective, Multivariate Study'. *Journal of Health and Social Behaviour* 24(1): 30–46.

Nouvet, E. 2014. 'Some Carry on, Some Stay in Bed: (In)convenient Affects and Agency in Neo-liberal Nicaragua'. *Cultural Anthropology* 29(1): 80–102.

Nussbaum, M. 2005. 'Women's Bodies: Violence, Security, Capabilities'. *Journal of Human Development* 6(2): 167–83.

Nuttall, S. 2009. *Entanglement: Literary and Cultural Reflections on Post-apartheid*. Johannesburg: Wits University Press.

Odent, M. 1984. *Birth Reborn*. New York: Pantheon Books.

Ogden, T.H. 1994. 'The Analytic Third: Working with Intersubjective Clinical Facts'. *International Journal of Psychoanalysis* 75: 3–20.

———. 1997. 'Reverie and Interpretation'. *Psychoanalytic Quarterly* 66(4): 567–95.

———. 1999. *Reverie and Interpretation: Sensing Something Human*. London: Karnac Books.

———. 2004. 'The Analytic Third: Implications for Psychoanalytic Theory and Technique'. *Psychoanalytic Quarterly* 73(1): 167–95.

———. 2005. *The Art of Psychoanalysis: Dreaming Undreamt Dreams and Interrupted Cries*. London: Routledge.

O'Grady, H. 2005. *Woman's Relationship with Herself: Gender, Foucault and Therapy*. London: Routledge.

Orange, D. 2005. 'Foreword'. In *Practicing Intersubjectively* by P. Buirski, xi–xii. Maryland: Jason Aronson.

———. 2006. 'For Whom the Bell Tolls: Context, Complexity, and Compassion in Psychoanalysis'. *International Journal of Psychoanalytic Self Psychology* 1(1): 5–21.

———. 2008. 'Whose Shame is it Anyway? Lifeworlds of Humiliation and Systems of Restoration (or "The Analyst's Shame")'. *Contemporary Psychoanalysis* 44(1): 83–100.

———. 2009. 'Kohut Memorial Lecture: Attitudes, Values and Intersubjective Vulnerability'. *International Journal of Psychoanalytic Self Psychology* 4(2): 235–53.

————. 2011. 'Speaking the Unspeakable: "The Implicit," Traumatic Living Memory, and the Dialogue of Metaphors'. *International Journal of Psychoanalytic Self Psychology* 6(2): 187–206.

Orange, D., G. Atwood and R. Stolorow. 1997. *Working Intersubjectively: Contextualism in Psychoanalytic Practice*. Hillsdale, NJ: The Analytic Press.

Orbach, S. 2016. *In Therapy: How Conversations with Psychotherapists Really Work*. London: Profile Books.

Orr, D.M.R. 2013. '"Now he Walks and Walks, as if he Didn't Have a Home Where he Could Eat": Food, Healing, and Hunger in Quechua Narratives of Madness'. *Culture, Medicine and Psychiatry* 37(4): 694–710.

Parker, I. 1989. 'Discourse and Power'. In *Texts of Identity*, edited by J. Shotter and K.J. Gergen, 56–69. London: Sage.

————. 1997. 'Culture and Nature after Enlightenment'. In *Psychoanalytic Culture: Psychoanalytic Discourse in Western Society*, edited by I. Parker, 161–85. London: Sage.

Parker, R. 1995. *Torn in Two: The Experience of Maternal Ambivalence*. London: Virago.

————. 1997. 'The Production and Purposes of Maternal Ambivalence'. In *Mothering and Ambivalence*, edited by W. Hollway and B. Featherstone, 17–36. London: Routledge.

Patel, V. 2014a. 'Global Mental Health: An Interview with Vikram Patel'. *BMC Medicine* 12(1). http://bmcmedicine.biomedcentral.com/articles/10.1186/1741-7015-12-44.

————. 2014b. 'Rethinking Mental Health Care: Bridging the Credibility Gap'. *Intervention* 12(1): 15–20.

————. 2017. 'Talking Sensibly about Depression'. *PLoS Medicine* 14(4): e1002257.

Peacock, M., P. Bissell and J. Owen. 2014. 'Dependency Denied: Health Inequalities in the Neo-liberal Era'. *Social Science and Medicine* 118: 173–80.

Peltzer, K., S. Pengpid, J. McFarlane and M. Banyini. 2013. 'Mental Health Consequences of Intimate Partner Violence in Vhembe District, South Africa'. *General Hospital Psychiatry* 35(5): 545–50.

Penn-Kekana, L. and D. Blaauw. 2002. *A Rapid Appraisal of Maternal Health Services in South Africa: A Health Systems Approach*. Johannesburg: Centre for Health Policy, Health Systems Development Programme, University of the Witwatersrand.

Peterman, A., J. Bleck and T. Palermo. 2015. 'Age and Intimate Partner Violence: An Analysis of Global Trends among Women Experiencing Victimization in 30 Developing Countries'. *Journal of Adolescent Health* 57(6): 624–30.

Petrus, T. and W. Isaacs-Martin. 2012. 'The Multiple Meanings of Coloured Identity in South Africa'. *Africa Insight* 42(1): 87–102.

Pfigu, T., C. Gabriel and K. van der Waal. 2014. 'Patrolling Respectability: Neighbourhood Watches as a Form of Community Policing'. In *Winelands, Wealth and Work: Transformations in the Dwars River Valley, Stellenbosch*, edited by K. van der Waal, 174–96. Pietermaritzburg: University of KwaZulu-Natal Press.

Phillips, L. 2011. '"I am Alone. I am a Woman. What Are my Children Going to Eat?" Domestic Workers and Family Networks'. *South African Review of Sociology* 42(2): 29–44.

Pike, I.L. and C.L. Patil. 2006. 'Understanding Women's Burdens: Preliminary Findings on Psychosocial Health among Datoga and Iraqw Women of Northern Tanzania'. *Culture, Medicine and Psychiatry* 30(3): 299–330.

Pillay, A.L. and A.J. Kriel. 2006. 'Mental Health Problems in Women Attending District-Level Services in South Africa'. *Social Science and Medicine* 63(3): 587–92.

Pinto, R. J., P. Correia-Santos, A. Levendosky and I. Jonenelen. 2016. 'Psychological Distress and Posttraumatic Stress Symptoms: The Role of Maternal Satisfaction, Parenting Stress, and Social Support among Mothers and Children Exposed to Intimate Partner Violence'. *Journal of Interpersonal Violence* 34(19): 1–23.

Posel, D. 2001. 'What's in a Name? Racial Categorisations under Apartheid and Their Afterlife'. *Transformation* 106(47): 50–74.

Posel, D. and F.C. Ross. 2014. *Ethical Quandaries in Social Research*. Cape Town: HSRC Press.

Quandt, S.A., J.I. Shoaf, J. Tapia, M. Hernández-Pelletier, H.M. Clark and T.A. Arcury. 2006. 'Experiences of Latino Immigrant Families in North Carolina Help Explain Elevated Levels of Food Insecurity and Hunger'. *Journal of Nutrition* 136(10): 2638–44.

Randle, T. 2014. 'The Inheritance of Loss'. In *Winelands, Wealth and Work: Transformations in the Dwars River Valley, Stellenbosch*, edited by K. van der Waal, 27–54. Pietermaritzburg: University of KwaZulu-Natal Press.

Raphael-Leff, J. 1982. 'Psychotherapeutic Needs of Mothers-to-be'. *Journal of Child Psychotherapy* 8(1): 3–13.

———. 1991. *Psychological Processes of Childbearing*. London: Chapman & Hall.

———. 1993. *Pregnancy: The Inside Story*. London: Jason Arsonson.

———. 2010. 'Healthy Maternal Ambivalence'. *Studies in the Maternal* 2(1): 1–15.

Reading, A.E. 1983. 'The Influence of Maternal Anxiety on the Course and Outcome of Pregnancy: A Review'. *Journal of Health Psychology* 2(2): 187–202.

Reid, C. and A. Tom. 2006. 'Poor Women's Discourses of Legitimacy, Poverty, and Health'. *Gender and Society* 20(3): 402–21.

Rich, A. 1986. *Of Woman Born: Motherhood as Experience and Institution*. New York: W.W. Norton.

Richter, I., S. Mathews, J. Kagura and E. Nonterah. 2018. 'A Longitudinal Perspective on Violence in the Lives of South African Children from the Birth to Twenty Plus Cohort Study in Johannesburg-Soweto'. *South African Medical Journal* 108(3): 181–6.

Robins, S. 2014. 'Development and Dystopia: An Afterword'. In *Winelands, Wealth and Work: Transformations in the Dwars River Valley, Stellenbosch*, edited by K. van der Waal, 219–29. Pietermaritzburg: University of KwaZulu-Natal Press.

Rodrigues, M., V. Patel, S. Jaswal and N. de Souza. 2003. 'Listening to Mothers: Qualitative Studies on Motherhood and Depression from Goa, India'. *Social Science and Medicine* 57(10): 1797–806.

Rogers, W. 1997. 'Sources of Abjection in Western Responses to Menopause'. In *Reinterpreting Menopause: Cultural and Philosophical Issues*, edited by P.A. Komesaroff, P. Rothfield and J. Daly, 225–38. New York: Routledge.

Roodt, V. 2012. 'Arendt, Stiegler en die lewe van die gees'. *Tydskrif vir Geesteswetenskappe* (March): 5–18.

Rose, E. 2015. 'A Feminist Reconceptualisation of Intimate Partner Violence against Women: A Crime against Humanity and a State Crime'. *Women's Studies International Forum* 53(Nov–Dec): 31–42.

Rose, N. 1985. *The Psychological Complex: Psychology, Politics, and Society in England, 1869–1939*. London: Routledge and Kegan Paul.

Rosenzweig, S. 1936. 'Some Implicit Common Factors in Diverse Methods of Psychotherapy'. *American Journal of Orthopsychiatry* 6(3): 412–15.

Ross, F. 2002. *Bearing Witness: Women and the Truth and Reconciliation Commission*. London: Pluto Press.

———. 2005. 'Codes and Dignity: Thinking about Ethics in Relation to Research on Violence'. *Anthropology Southern Africa* 28(3–4): 991–1107.

———. 2010. *Raw Life, New Hope: Decency, Housing and Everyday Life in a Post-apartheid Community*. Cape Town: University of Cape Town Press.

———. 2015. 'Raw Life and Respectability: Poverty and Everyday Life in a Postapartheid Community'. *Current Anthropology* 56(S11): S97–S107.

Roth, S. 2000. *Psychotherapy: The Art of Wooing Nature*. London: Jason Aronson.

Rowley, H. and E. Grosz. 1990. 'Psychoanalysis and Feminism'. In *Feminist Knowledge: Critique and Construct*, edited by S. Gunew, 175–204. London: Routledge.

Ruddick, S. 1994. 'Thinking Mothers/Conceiving Birth'. In *Representations of Motherhood*, edited by D. Bassin, M. Honey and M.M. Kaplan, 29–45. New Haven: Yale University Press.

———. 1996. 'Reason's "Femininity": A Case for Connected Knowing'. In *Knowledge, Difference, and Power: Essays Inspired by 'Women's Ways of Knowing'*, edited by N.R. Goldberger, J.M. Tarule, B. Clinchy McVicker and M.F. Belenky, 248–70. New York: Basic Books.

Russell, P. 1998. 'The Role of Paradox in the Repetition Compulsion'. In *Trauma, Repetition, and Affect Regulation: The Work of Paul Russell*, edited by J.G. Teicholz and D. Kriegman, 1–22. New York: Other Press.

Sacks, O. 1995. *An Anthropologist on Mars: Seven Paradoxical Tales*. New York: Vintage.

———. 2013a. *Awakenings*. New York: Knopf Doubleday.

———. 2013b. *Hallucinations*. New York: Vintage.

———. 2015. *Gratitude*. New York: Knopf Doubleday.

Salinger, J.D. 1951. *The Catcher in the Rye*. New York: Little, Brown and Company.

Salmon, P., R. Miller and N.C. Drew. 1990. 'Women's Anticipation and Experience of Childbirth: The Independence of Fulfilment, Unpleasantness and Pain'. *British Journal of Medical Psychology* 63: 255–9.

Salo, E. 2009. 'Coconuts do Not Live in Townships: Cosmopolitanism and Its Failures in the Urban Peripheries of Cape Town'. *Feminist Africa* 13: 11–21.

Sayer, R.A. 2016. *Why we Can't Afford the Rich*. Bristol: Policy Press.

Scarry, E. 1985. *The Body in Pain: The Making and Unmaking of the World*. New York: Oxford University Press.

Schafer, R. 1992. 'Narratives of the Self'. In *Retelling a Life: Narration and Dialogue in Psychoanalysis*, 21–35. New York: Basic Books.

Scheff, T. 1966. *Being Mentally Ill: A Sociological Theory*. Chicago: Aldine.

Scheffer Lindgren, M. and B. Renck. 2008. 'Intimate Partner Violence and the Leaving Process: Interviews with Abused Women'. *International Journal of Qualitative Studies on Health and Well-Being* 3(2): 113–24.

Schein, V.E. 1995. *Working from the Margins: Voices of Mothers in Poverty*. Ithaca, NY: ILR.

Scheper-Hughes, N. 1992. *Death without Weeping: The Violence of Everyday Life in Brazil*. Berkeley: University of California Press.

Scheper-Hughes, N. and P.I. Bourgois, eds. 2004. *Violence in War and Peace: An Anthology*. Malden, MA: Blackwell.

Schneider, Z. 2002. 'An Australian Study of Women's Experiences of their First Pregnancy'. *Midwifery* 18(3); 238–9.

Schoombee, C., M. van der Merwe and L-M Kruger. 2005. 'The Stress of Caring: The Manifestation of Stress in the Nurse-Patient Relationship'. *Social Work* 41(4): 388–408.

Schwartz, A. 2018. '"I Don't Think Character Exists Anymore": A Conversation with Rachel Cusk'. *The New Yorker*, 18 November. https://www.newyorker.com/culture/the-new-yorker-interview/i-dont-think-character-exists-anymore-a-conversation-with-rachel-cusk.

Scott-Palmer, J. and S.M. Skevington. 1981. 'Pain during Childbirth and Menstruation: A Study of Locus of Control'. *Journal of Psychosomatic Research* 25(3): 151–5.

Seeley, J. and C. Plunkett. 2002. *Women and Domestic Violence: Standards for Counselling Practice*. St Kilda: The Salvation Army Crisis Service.

Semrad, E.V., S. Rako and H. Mazer. 2003. *Semrad: The Heart of a Therapist*. Lincoln: iUniverse.

Sen, A. 2005. 'Foreword'. In *Pathologies of Power: Health, Human Rights and the New War on the Poor* by P. Farmer, xi–xvii. Berkeley: University of California Press.

Sen, B. and D. Hulme, eds. 2006. *Chronic Poverty in Bangladesh: Tales of Ascent, Descent, Marginality and Persistence*. Dhaka, Bangladesh: Bangladesh Institute of Development Studies.

Sen, G., B. Reddy and A. Iyer. 2018. 'Beyond Measurement: The Drivers of Disrespect and Abuse in Obstetric Care'. *Reproductive Health Matters* 26(53): 6–18.

Sénuin, L., L. Potvin, M. St Denis and L. Loiselle. 1995. 'Chronic Stressors, Social Support, and Depression during Pregnancy'. *Obstetrics & Gynecology* 85(4): 583–9.

Seu, B.I. 2006. 'Shameful Selves: Women's Feelings of Inadequacy and Constructed Facades'. *European Journal of Psychotherapy and Counselling* 8(3): 285–303.

Seuss, Dr. 1990. *Oh, the Places You'll go!* New York: Random House.

Shefer, T. 2012. 'Fraught Tenderness: Narratives on Domestic Workers in Memories of Apartheid'. *Peace and Conflict: Journal of Peace Psychology* 18(3): 307–17.

Shefer, T., D. Bhana and R. Morrell. 2013. 'Teenage Pregnancy and Parenting at School in Contemporary South African Contexts: Deconstructing School Narratives and Understanding Policy Implementation'. *Perspectives in Education* 31(1): 1–10.

Shefer, T., L-M. Kruger, C. Macleod, J. Baxen and L. Vincent. 2015. '". . . A Huge Monster That Should be Feared and Not Done": Lessons Learned in Sexuality Education Classes in South Africa'. *African Safety Promotion Journal* 13(1): 71–87.

Sideris, T. 2013. 'Intimate Partner Violence in Post-apartheid South Africa: Psychoanalytic Insights and Dilemmas'. In *Psychodynamic Psychotherapy in South Africa: Contexts, Theories and Applications*, edited by C. Smith, G. Lobban and M. O'Laughlin, 169–93. Johannesburg: Wits University Press.

Siefert, K., T.L. Finlayson, D.R. Williams, J. Delva and A.I. Ismail. 2007. 'Modifiable Risk and Protective Factors for Depressive Symptoms in Low-Income African American Mothers'. *American Journal of Orthopsychiatry* 77(1): 113–23.

Silverstein, M., S. Reid, K. DePeau, J. Lamberto and W. Beardslee. 2010. 'Functional Interpretations of Sadness, Stress and Demoralization among an Urban Population of Low-Income Mothers'. *Journal of Maternal and Child Health* 14(2): 245–53.

Simkin, P. 1991. 'Just Another Day in a Woman's Life? Women's Long-Term Perceptions of Their First Birth Experience: Part I'. *Birth* 18(4): 203–10.

———. 1992. 'Just Another Day in a Woman's Life? Part II: Nature and Consistency of Women's Long-Term Memories of Their First Birth Experiences'. *Birth* 19(2): 64–81.

Simmons, L.A., C. Huddleston-Casas and A.A. Berry. 2007. 'Low-Income Rural Women and Depression: Factors Associated with Self-Reporting'. *American Journal of Health Behavior* 31(6): 657–66.

Smith, M., S. van Wyk and L. Alkana. 2013. 'Adolescent Girls' Experience of Termination in a Community-Based Intervention'. *Social Work Practitioner-Researcher* 25(2): 120–35.

Smith, Z. 2003. *The Autograph Man: A Novel*. London: Hamish Hamilton.

Sontag, S. 1979. *Illness as Metaphor*. New York: Vintage.

Sperberg, E.D. and S.D. Stabb. 1998. 'Depression in Women as Related to Anger and Mutuality in Relationships'. *Psychology of Women Quarterly* 22(2): 223–38.

Sperry, E. 2013. 'Dupes of Patriarchy: Feminist Strong Substantive Autonomy's Epistemological Weaknesses'. *Hypatia* 28(4): 887–904.

Spillius, E. 1992. 'Clinical Experiences of Projective Identification'. In *Clinical Lectures on Klein and Bion*, edited by R. Anderson, 59–73. London: Routledge.

Spillius, E. and E. O'Shaughnessy. 2013. *Projective Identification: The Fate of a Concept*. New York: Routledge.

Spivak, G.C. 1998. 'Cultural Talks in the Hot Peace: Revisiting the "Global Village"'. In *Cosmopolitics: Thinking and Feeling beyond the Nation*, edited by P. Cheah and B. Robbins, 329–48. Minneapolis: University of Minnesota Press.

Squire, C. 1998. 'Women and Men Talk about Aggression: An Analysis of Narrative Genre'. In *Standpoints and Differences: Essays in the Practice of Feminist Psychology*, edited by K. Henwood, C. Griffin and A. Phoenix, 65–90. London: Sage.

Stainton, M. 1994. 'Commentary by Stainton'. *Western Journal of Nursing Research* 16: 618–20.

Standing, G. 2011. *The Precariat: The New Dangerous Class*. London: Bloomsbury.

Stange, K.C. and R.L. Ferrer. 2009. 'The Paradox of Primary Care'. *Annals of Family Medicine* 7(4): 293–9.

Stark, E. and A. Flitcraft. 1995. 'Killing the Beast within: Woman Battering and Female Suicidality'. *International Journal of Health Services* 25(1): 43–64.

Stein, D.J., S. Seedat, A. Herman, H. Moomal, S.G. Heeringa, R.C. Kessler and D.R. Williams. 2008. 'Lifetime Prevalence of Psychiatric Disorders in South Africa'. *British Journal of Psychiatry* 192(2): 112–17.

Steinberg, J. 2005. *The Number: One Man's Search for Identity in the Cape Underworld and Prison Gangs*. Cape Town: Jonathan Ball.

———. 2008. *Thin Blue: The Unwritten Rules of Policing South Africa*. Cape Town: Jonathan Ball.

———. 2015a. *A Man of Good Hope*. Cape Town: Jonathan Ball.

———. 2015b. 'Why I'm Moving back to South Africa'. https://www.sagoodnews. co.za/why-im-moving-back-to-south-africa/.

Stewart, R.C., J. Bunn, M. Vokhiwa, E. Umar, F. Kauye and M. Fitzgerald. 2010. 'Common Mental Disorder and Associated Factors amongst Women with Young Infants in Rural Malawi'. *Social Psychiatry and Psychiatric Epidemiology* 45(5): 551–9.

Stiglitz, J. 2013. 'The Price of Inequality'. *New Perspectives Quarterly* 30(1): 52–3.

Stiver, I.P. 1991. 'Beyond the Oedipus Complex: Mothers and Daughters'. In *Women's Growth in Connection: Writings from the Stone Center* by J.V. Jordan, A.G. Kaplan, J.B. Miller, I.P. Stiver and J.L. Surrey, 97–121. New York: Guilford Press.

Stoppard, J.M. 2000. 'Understanding Women's Depression: Limitations of Mainstream Approaches and a Material-Discursive Alternative'. In *Women's Health: Contemporary International Perspectives*, edited by J.M. Ussher, 405–14. Leicester: BPS Books.

———. 2010. 'Moving towards an Understanding of Women's Depression'. *Feminism & Psychology* 20(2): 267–71.

Strube, M.J. and L.S. Barbour. 1983. 'The Decision to Leave an Abusive Relationship: Economic Dependence and Psychological Commitment'. *Journal of Marriage and the Family* 45(4): 785–93.

Strydom, D-M. 2007. 'Ma vang self baba in hospitaalgang'. *Die Burger*, 15 June, p. 2.

Summerfield, D. 2008. 'How Scientifically Valid is the Knowledge Base of Global Mental Health?' *BMJ* 336(7651): 992–4.

Swartz, L. 1991. 'The Reproduction of Racism in South African Mental Health Care'. *South African Journal of Psychology* 21(4): 240–6.

———. 1998. 'Ways of Seeing'. In *Culture and Mental Health: A Southern African View*, edited by L. Swartz, 3–22. Cape Town: Oxford University Press.

Swartz, S. 1999. 'Using Psychodynamic Formulations in South African Clinical Settings'. *South African Journal of Psychology* 29(1): 42–8.

———. 2006. 'The Third Voice: Writing Case-Notes'. *Feminism & Psychology* 16(4): 427–44.

Swartz, S. 2012. 'The Broken Mirror: Difference and Shame in South African Psychotherapy'. *International Journal of Psychoanalytic Self Psychology* 7(2): 196–212.

———. 2013. 'Feminism and Psychiatric Diagnosis: Reflections of a Feminist Practitioner'. *Feminism & Psychology* 23(1): 41–8.

———. 2015. *Homeless Wanderers: Movement and Mental Illness in the Cape Colony in the Nineteeth Century*. Cape Town: University of Cape Town Press.

Sweet, V. 2012. *God's Hotel: A Doctor, a Hospital, and a Pilgrimage to the Heart of Medicine*. New York: Riverhead Books.

Swinburne, M. 2000. '"Home is Where the Hate is"'. *Psychoanalytic Psychotherapy* 14(3): 223–38.

Szasz, T. 1974. *The Myth of Mental Illness: Foundations of a Theory of Personal Conduct*. New York: Harper & Row.

Szymborska, W. 1988. *Poems: New and Collected, 1957–1997*. London: Faber & Faber.

Tasseau, A., E. Walter-Nicolet and F. Autret. 2018. 'Management of Healthy Newborns in the Delivery Room and Maternal Satisfaction'. *Archives de pédiatrie* 25(5): 309–14.

Taylor, L. 2011. '"Mad, Bad and Sad" – but Still Coping: An Intersubjective Psychoanalytic Case Study of Depression in One Low-Income South African Woman'. Master's thesis, University of Stellenbosch, Stellenbosch.

Teicholz, J.G. 2006. 'Qualities of Engagement and the Analyst's Theory'. *International Journal of Psychoanalytic Self Psychology* 1(1): 47–77.

Terreblanche, C. 2007. 'Nurses Play God at E Cape Hospital'. *The Sunday Independent*, 15 July. https://www.iol.co.za/news/south-africa/nurses-play-god-at-e-cape-hospital-362031.

Thomson, R., M.J. Kehily, L. Hadfield and S. Sharpe. 2011. *Making Modern Mothers*. Bristol: Policy Press.

Tolstoy, L. 1877. *Anna Karenina*. Moscow: The Russian Messenger.

Tomkins, S. 1963. *Affect, Imagery, Consciousness: Volume II; The Negative Affects*. New York: Springer.

Tomlinson, M., M.J. O'Connor, I.M. le Roux, J. Stewart, N. Mbewu, J. Harwood and M.J. Rotheram-Borus. 2013. 'Multiple Risk Factors during Pregnancy in

South Africa: The Need for a Horizontal Approach to Perinatal Care'. *Society for Prevention Research* 15(3): 277–82.

Tong, H.Q. 2010. 'Larry Beutler on Science and Psychotherapy'. *Psychotherapy.net*. https://www.psychotherapy.net/interview/larry-beutler.

Toska, E., L.D. Cluver, M. Boyles, M. Pantelic and C. Kuo. 2015. 'From "Sugar Daddies" to "Sugar Babies": Exploring a Pathway among Age-Disparate Sexual Relationships, Condom Use and Adolescent Pregnancy in South Africa'. *Sexual Health* 12(1): 59–66.

Towns, A.J. and P.J. Adams. 2009. 'Staying Quiet or Getting out: Some Ideological Dilemmas Faced by Women Who Experience Violence from Male Partners'. *British Journal of Social Psychology* 48(4): 735–54.

Trad, P.V. 1990. 'On Becoming a Mother: In the Throes of Developmental Transformation'. *Psychoanalytic Psychology* 7(3): 341–61.

———. 1991. 'Adaptation to Developmental Transformations during the Various Phases of Motherhood'. *Journal of the American Academy of Psychoanalysis* 19(3): 403–21.

Trantraal, A., C. Trantraal and N. Trantraal. 2010. *Coloureds*. Cape Town: Jincom Publishing.

Trantraal, N. 2018. *Wit issie 'n colour nie: Angedrade stories*. Edited by R.S. Kamfer and M. Steenkamp. Cape Town: Kwela Books.

Treichler, P.A. 1990. 'Feminism, Medicine, and the Meaning of Chilbirth'. In *Body/Politics: Women and the Discourses of Science*, edited by M. Jacobus, E. Fox Keller and S. Shuttleworth, 113–38. New York: Routledge.

Tronick, E.Z. 2003. 'Of Course All Relationships Are Unique: How Co-creative Processes Generate Unique Mother-Infant and Patient-Therapist Relationships and Change Other Relationships'. *Psychoanalytic Inquiry* 23: 473–91.

Truyts, C. 2016. 'One Meal at a Time: Nourishment in the Cape Winelands'. Master's thesis, University of Cape Town, Cape Town.

Tshifhumulo, R. and P. Mudhovozi. 2013. 'Behind Closed Doors: Listening to the Voices of Women Enduring Battering'. *Gender and Behaviour* 11(1): 5080–8.

Turgo, N. 2013. '"Here, we Don't Just Trade Goods, we Also 'Sell' People's Lives": Sari-Sari Stores as Nodes of Partial Surveillance in a Philippine Fishing Community'. *Singapore Journal of Tropical Geography* 34(3): 373–89.

Udjo, E.O. 2014. 'The Relationship between the Child Support Grant and Teenage Fertility in Post-apartheid South Africa'. *Social Policy and Society* 13(4): 505–19.

Ussher, J.M. 2010. 'Are we Medicalizing Women's Misery? A Critical Review of Women's Higher Rates of Reported Depression'. *Feminism & Psychology* 20(1): 9–35.

Van Coller, H. and A. van Jaarsveld. 2009. 'Identiteitskepping en die strooisage: Die geval van *7de Laan*'. *Stilet: Tydskrif van die Afrikaanse Letterkundevereniging* 21 (1): 19–38.

Van der Gucht, N. and K. Lewis. 2015. 'Women's Experiences of Coping with Pain during Childbirth: A Critical Review of Qualitative Research'. *Midwifery* 31(3): 349–58.

Van der Kolk, B. 2014. *The Body Keeps the Score: Brain, Mind, and Body in the Healing of Trauma*. New York: Penguin.

Van der Waal, C.S. 2005. 'Spatial and Organisational Complexity in the Dwars River Valley, Western Cape'. *Anthropology Southern Africa* 28(1–2): 8–21.

Van der Westhuizen, C. 2018. *Sitting Pretty: White Afrikaans Women in Postapartheid South Africa*. Pietermaritzburg: University of KwaZulu-Natal Press.

Van Niekerk, M. 2004. 'Labour'. In *The New Century of South African Short Stories*, edited by M. Chapman, 301–18. Johannesburg: Ad Donker.

Van Niekerk, M. and A. van Zyl. 2006. *Memorandum : A Story with Paintings*. Cape Town: Human & Rousseau.

Van Robbroeck, L. 2006. 'Writing White on Black: Modernism as Discursive Paradigm in South African Writing on Modern Black Art'. PhD dissertation, University of Stellenbosch, Stellenbosch.

Van Schalkwyk, S., F. Boonzaier and P. Gobodo-Madikizela. 2014. '"Selves" in Contradiction: Power and Powerlessness in South African Shelter Residents' Narratives of Leaving Abusive Heterosexual Relationships'. *Feminism & Psychology* 24(3): 314–31.

Vetten, L. 2014. 'Rape and Other Forms of Sexual Violence in South Africa'. Institute for Security Studies. https://issafrica.org/research/policy-brief/rape-and-other-forms-of-sexual-violence-in-south-africa.

Vice, S. 2010. '"How do I Live in This Strange Place?"'. *Journal of Social Philosophy* 41(3): 323–42.

Vladislavić, I. 2006. *Portrait with Keys: Joburg & What-What*. Cape Town: Umuzi.

Vollenhoven, S. 2016. *The Keeper of the Kumm: Ancestral Longing and Belonging of a Boesmankind*. Cape Town: Tafelberg.

Vyas, S., J. Mbwambo and L. Heise. 2015. 'Women's Paid Work and Intimate Partner Violence: Insights from Tanzania'. *Feminist Economics* 21(1): 35–58.

Walby, S. 2001. 'Against Epistemological Chasms: The Science Question in Feminism Revisited'. *Signs* 26(2): 485–540.

Waldenstrom, U. 1999. 'Experience of Labor and Birth in 1 111 Women'. *Journal of Psychosomatic Research* 47(5): 471–82.

Walker, L. and L. Gilson. 2004. '"We Are Bitter but we Are Satisfied": Nurses as Street-Level Bureaucrats in South Africa'. *Social Science and Medicine* 59(6): 1251–61.

Walker, M.B. 1998. *Philosophy and the Maternal Body: Reading Silence*. New York: Routledge.

Wall, G. 2001. 'Moral Constructions of Motherhood in Breastfeeding Discourse'. *Gender and Society* 15(4): 592–610.

Wallin, D.J. 2007. *Attachment and Psychotherapy*. New York: Guilford Press.

Walsh, M.B. 2015. 'Feminism, Adaptive Preferences, and Social Contract Theory'. *Hypatia* 30(4): 829–45.

Wampold, B.E. 2011. 'The Research Evidence for the Common Factors Models: A Historically Situated Perspective'. In *The Heart and Soul of Change: Delivering*

*What Works in Therapy*, edited by B.L. Duncan, S.D. Miller, B.E. Wampold and M.A. Hubble, 49–81. Washington, DC: American Psychological Association.

Way, N. 1998. *Everyday Courage: The Lives and Stories of Urban Teenagers*. New York: New York University Press.

Weaver, J.J. 2000. 'Childbirth'. In *Women's Health: Contemporary International Perspectives*, edited by J.M. Ussher, 307–12. Leicester: BPS Books.

Weissmann, M.M., E.S. Paykel and G.L. Klerman. 1972. 'The Depressed Woman as a Mother'. *Social Psychiatry* 7(2): 98–108.

Wertz, R.W. and D.C. Wertz. 1977. *Lying-in: A History of Childbirth in America*. New York: Free Press.

West, M. 2005. 'Speaking with a Forked Tongue: Marlene van Niekerk's "Labour" as an Examination of Black Labour and White Dis-ease in Suburban South Africa'. *Current Writing* 17(1): 149–65.

———. 2009. *White Women Writing White: Identity and Representation in (Post-) Apartheid Literatures of South Africa*. Cape Town: David Philip.

Westen, D., C.M. Novotny and H. Thompson-Brenner. 2004. 'The Empirical Status of Empirically Supported Psychotherapies: Assumptions, Findings, and Reporting in Controlled Clinical Trials. *Psychological Bulletin* 130(4): 631–63.

Whitaker, R.C., S.M. Phillips and S.M. Orzol. 2006. 'Food Insecurity and the Risks of Depression and Anxiety in Mothers and Behaviour Problems in their Preschool-Aged Children'. *Pediatrics* 118(3): e859–68.

White, E. 2000. 'Me and my Shrinks.' *The Guardian*, 8 October. https://www.theguardian.com/books/2000/oct/08/biography.features.

Whitford, M. 1991. 'Maternal Genealogy and the Symbolic'. In *Luce Irigaray: Philosophy in the Feminine*, edited by M. Whitford, 75–97. London: Routledge.

Wicomb, Z. 1998. 'Shame and Identity: The Case of the Coloured in South Africa'. In *Writing South Africa: Literature, Apartheid, and Democracy, 1970–1995*, edited by D. Attridge and R. Jolly, 91–107. Cambridge: Cambridge University Press.

Wiesel, E. 1986. 'Insight: Perspectives on the World'. *The Arizona Republic*, 26 October.

Willemse, H. 2011. 'A Coloured Expert's Coloured'. In *Reshaping Remembrance: Critical Essays on Afrikaans Places of Memory*, edited by S. Huigen and A. Grundlingh, 23–32. Amsterdam: SAVUSA.

Williams, P.J. 1988. 'On Being the Object of Property'. *Signs* 14(1): 5–24.

Willig, C. 2001. *Introducing Qualitative Research in Psychology: Adventures in Theory and Method*. Buckingham: Open University Press.

———. 2013. *Introducing Qualitative Research in Psychology*. Buckingham: Open University Press.

Wilshire, D. 1989. 'The Uses of Myth, Image, and the Female Body in Re-visioning Knowledge'. In *Gender/Body/Knowledge: Feminist Reconstructions of Being and Knowing*, edited by A.M. Jaggar and S. Bordo, 92–114. New Brunswick: Rutgers University Press.

Wilson, K.L. and F.M. Sirois. 2010. 'Birth Attendant Choice and Satisfaction with Antenatal Care: The Role of Birth Philosophy, Relational Style, and Health Self-Efficacy'. *Journal of Reproductive and Infant Psychology* 28(1): 69–83.

Winnicott, D.W. 1949. 'Hate in the Counter-Transference'. *International Journal of Psychoanalysis* 30: 69–74.

———. 1960. 'The Theory of the Parent-Infant Relationship'. *International Journal of Psychoanalysis* 41: 585–95.

———. 1984. *Deprivation and Delinquency*. London: Tavistock.

———. 1992. *Psycho-analytic Explorations*. Edited by C. Winnicott, R. Shepherd and M. Davis. Cambridge: Harvard University Press.

Winterbach, Ingrid. 2015. *Vlakwater*. Cape Town: Human & Rousseau.

———. 2017. *The Shallows*. Translated by Michiel Heyns. Cape Town: Human & Rousseau.

Wolf, M. 1992. *A Thrice-Told Tale: Feminism, Postmodernism & Ethnographic Responsibility*. Tanford: Tanford University Press.

Wolman, W., B. Chalmers, G.J. Hofmeyr and V.C. Nikodem. 1993. 'Postpartum Depression and Companionship in the Clinical Birth Environment: A Randomized, Controlled Study'. *American Journal of Obstetrics and Gynecology* 168(5): 1388–93.

Woods, J. 2017. 'W.G. Sebald, Humorist'. *The New Yorker*, 5 June. https://www.newyorker.com/magazine/2017/06/05/w-g-sebald-humorist.

World Health Organisation. 2012. 'Femicide (1)'. http://apps.who.int/iris/bitstream/handle/10665/77421/WHO_RHR_12.38_eng.pdf?sequence=1.

Wright, G., M. Noble, P. Ntshongwana, D. Neves and H. Barnes. 2014. 'The Role of Social Security in Respecting and Protecting the Dignity of Lone Mothers in South Africa: Final Report'. Centre for the Analysis of South African Social Policy. https://core.ac.uk/download/pdf/43542923.pdf.

Yalom, I.D. 2013. *Love's Executioner and Other Tales of Psychotherapy*. Cape Town: Penguin.

Yalom, I.D. and M. Leszcz. 2005. *The Theory and Practice of Group Psychotherapy*. New York: Basic Books.

Young, G.H. and S. Gerson. 1991. 'New Psychoanalytic Perspectives on Masochism and Spouse Abuse'. *Psychotherapy* 28(1): 30–8.

Young, R. 2004. *White Mythologies: Writing History and the West*. London: Routledge.

Youngleson, A. 2007. 'The Impossibility of Ideal Motherhood: The Psychological Experiences and Discourse of Motherhood amongst South African Low-Income Coloured Mothers Specifically in the Kylemore Community'. Master's thesis, University of Stellenbosch, Stellenbosch.

# Acknowledgements

*Ek kon dit nie verduur om in die dorp aan te bly waar boom en berg onverskillig staan teenoor iedere menslike lotgeval nie . . . Soos jy, ervaar ek die dorp as 'n verraderlike plek, waar 'n mens ongesiens kan ondergaan, al is die maan hier glorieryker as elders. In die nag tydens volmaan maak ek my mond oop. Die wind waai daardeur soos deur 'n spelonk. Dit voel vir my ek eet die wind, en word daardeur gevul.*[1]

I admire my friend Ingrid Winterbach's sentences simply for their beauty. In these particular words from her book *Vlakwater*, she also very succinctly captures the difficulty of living in a deeply unequal world. However, she also reminds me that we are never alone in this compromised world. '*Soos jy* (Like you),' she says. She is not speaking to me specifically, but I hear her.

This book is about poverty. It is about the emotional impact of poverty on people – those who are poor and those who are not. It was a difficult book to write. It took years. After all these years I remain in

---

1. Ingrid Winterbach, *Vlakwater* (Cape Town: Human & Rousseau, 2015), 9 and 318. The English translation reads:

    I could not stand staying on in a town where mountains and trees alike are indifferent to every human vicissitude . . . Like you I experience the town as a treacherous place, where some could perish in obscurity, even though the moon here is more glorious than anywhere else. At night when the moon is full I open my mouth. The wind blows through it as if through a grotto. It feels as if I am eating the wind and fulfilled by it.

Ingrid Winterbach, *The Shallows*, translated by Michiel Heyns (Cape Town: Human & Rousseau, 2017), 8 and 267.

awe of the people who are the focus of this book: their resilience, their agency, their willingness to continue, their capacity for engagement and sharing, their insistence on caring – even if their means are limited.

I have patients (still a better word than clients). In my almost 25 years of practising as a therapist in my town and in my valley, I have been privileged to encounter and to develop relationships with some of the most incredible people I know. My patients, while often coming to me troubled and vulnerable, with dread and with hope, have taught me in very moving ways about resilience and strength. They also continue to remind me on a daily basis about the power of connection and human relationships. My work with them keeps me going. It has always been and will remain my most important vocation.

I have students. I teach because it is the best way of learning. My students have generously allowed me a space to think and talk and discuss and continue to learn. Their insights and questions have forced me to stay humble and alert and curious. Their energy, enthusiasm and commitment continue to give me hope. While writing this book I went through hundreds of student journals and was deeply moved by what students go through when doing clinical work and research. Their journals reveal the extent to which difficult encounters make them feel vulnerable, ashamed, guilty, afraid, alone, dispirited and overwhelmed – but they always continue. Their ability to feel gratitude, despite the ordeals we put them through, always amazes me. I have enjoyed teaching at all levels, but became most intimately acquainted with my clinical Master's students. Getting to know these students, and being part of their development for so many years, has been a privilege. I have also had two writing groups that provided important and valued contexts for collegial reflection. The first included Suzanne de Villiers, Jana Lazarus and Maxine Spedding; the second, Ronald Davies, Melinda Fouche, Diane Nell and Mariam Salie. These groups have anchored me in very important ways.

I have had dedicated research assistants, many of them now valued colleagues and close friends: Trish Blake, Josie Greenhalgh, Colette Hamman, Maxine Spedding, Dannah Sutter and Tanya van der Spuy. There is no adequate way of thanking them for what they did and what they had to put up with. Trish was involved when I started sending away book proposals. Colette, Dannah and Josie shared with me the last long furlongs of the book. It felt never-ending and exhausting. I don't know how many times I said, 'We are nearly there.' I did most of the translations myself, but consulted Michiel Heyns often when I got stuck. Just before first submission Carine Janse van Rensburg, a wonderful and experienced translator and editor, came to the rescue and swiftly and expertly translated the quotes that still had to be done.

My publisher put at my disposal a generous, patient and supportive group of people. Louis Gaigher asked me to submit a proposal to University of KwaZulu-Natal Press while he was still working for the press as commissioning editor. He also introduced me to the art of Tanya Poole, whose work *Girl with Blue Hands* I subsequently used as a cover image. After the proposal was accepted, publisher Debra Primo was remarkably engaged and consistent, never losing faith that the book would eventually emerge, even though it took me many years. Sally Hines, the project manager, moved the project along gently, but also firmly when needed. Greater patience no one has. Editor Alison Lockhart was meticulous, but also very generous in trying to understand my thinking. I feel incredibly privileged to have worked with this team.

I have colleagues and mentors. My colleagues in the Department of Psychology inspired and supported me in different ways, especially during this last year. My dear friends Ursula Hartzenberg and Sherine van Wyk played an important role in my life during the years of writing the book. I have had many mentors and role models over the years. At Stellenbosch I think of Johann Degenaar, André du Toit, Andries du Toit, Andrew Nash and Betsie Nel. In Boston I was fortunate to learn from the finest of feminist supervisors and teachers: Debbie Belle, Leslie Brody, Fran Grossman and Catherine Riessman. Academic role models whom I was fortunate to get to know personally and who became friends include Jane Flax, Carol Gilligan, James Gilligan, Anna Motz, Rob Nixon, Alessandra Piontelli, Annemiek Richters, Tammy Shefer and Kees van der Waal. Debbie Belle's early work on poverty was definitive in directing my interests as a researcher and clinician. Alessandra Piontelli felt like a soulmate in the years of conceiving the book. Her way of combining psychoanalysis and ethnography has been formative for me, as well as her insistence always to be interested in those on the margins.

Other mentors were there for me in other ways and kept me relatively sane and healthy: Ruth Eastwood, Aletta Elders, Jacques Human, Anne Levett, Margaret Orr and Solair Terblanche. Ruth Eastwood became like a second mother.

I have friends, people who take care of me in different ways and whom I regularly break bread with. Many close friends read the manuscript or drafts of chapters. Pieter Fourie was the first one to read the entire manuscript and told me on a winter afternoon in Suki Thai that he thought there was something here. Bea Roberts, my oldest friend, read and proofread the whole manuscript with great care in one weekend and gave me permission to go on. Other close friends and exceptional readers read draft chapters and did so with care and attention: Pierre de Vos, Louise Gelderblom, Sandra Kriel, Stephanus Muller, Carel van der Merwe, Sherine van Wyk, Jurie Wessels and Ingrid Winterbach. All of them found the kindest ways of saying the very good words, 'There is something here, but you are not yet there. Keep on trying.' Stephanus Muller was pivotal in saying, 'You are in trouble. Go for it, anyway.' After all the rewriting, I still think this is where the book is at. It will always remain an attempt at something, despite the incredible readers I have had. My friends who are novelists, poets and scriptwriters produced text after text. Their work and my conversations with them about work inspire me and continue to keep me convinced that novelists and poets know more about people and life than psychologists: Tom Dreyer, Pieter Fourie, Damon Galgut, Michiel Heyns, Murray la Vita, Stephanus Muller, Fanie Naudé, Louis Pretorius, Malan Steyn, Carel van der Merwe and Ingrid Winterbach. Other close and supportive people, breakers of bread, include Rita Barnard, Pierre Brugman, Jacques du Plessis, Jean du Plessis, Ockie Dupper, Amanda Gouws, Andries Gouws, Stuart Mathews, Elmi Muller, Roopa Nair, Roddy Payne, Chris Petty, Mareli Pretorius, Vasti Roodt, Lomin Saayman, Lwando Scott, John Solomon, Maxine Spedding, Nina Swart, Sandra Swart, Hugo Theart, Barbara Thompson, Lize van Robbroek, Stella Viljoen, Andries Visagie, Anthony Waddell, David Waddilove and Graham Walker. I also have my so-called study groups, the fabulous feminist reading group, the departmental symposium group (Bronwyne Coetzee, Zuhayr Kafaar, Desmond Paynter, Rizwana Roomaney and Mariam Salie) and then the Peaches. I think the never-ending book and my clumsy attempts at coping with the stress must have been frustrating and puzzling to all who know me, but my dear friends and colleagues stayed kind and supportive and interested. As Jacques du Plessis said to me recently: '*Ouma verstaan nie, maar Ouma is trots.*' Psychologists call this unconditional love.

I have a family. My mother and father taught me that reading, music and art are the best ways to understand what the world is about (and also the best ways to escape it). My mother loves me so much that she read the entire manuscript twice, and is willing to read it again. My father (*die Reus van Groenberg*), sadly, is not here to read it. My mother's brother, Michiel Heyns, has compelled me to read novels and poetry since I was fortunate enough to become his student (and one of his many fans) in my first year at university. He is also a best friend. My oldest brother, John, my academic reading partner and sounding board, introduced me to many of the texts I cite in this book and kept on reading with me throughout the writing process. Most importantly, as a developmental economist, he was pivotal in making me understand how the personal is political and vice versa. My other brothers, Tindall and Louis, have been important in the writing of this book in ways that are more indirect and hard to describe, but no less important. They were just there, bridges over troubled waters.

This book is for my daughter, Mia. The book became part of her life, as it was part of mine, for 19 years (she is only 23). She lived through its writing with grace and kindness and love (and some well-justified grumpiness). While I was so busy and slightly obsessed, she quietly became a person of whom I am in awe. *Verwonderd.*

These acknowledgements are about the simple fact that, even if writing this book at times felt like a lonely ordeal, I was never alone. I am fortunate to share my life with extraordinary people. I thank them all.

# Index